Aviation Medicine and the Airline Passenger

Edited by

Andrew RC Cummin MA DM FRCP
Consultant in Respiratory Medicine, Charing Cross Hospital, London
Honorary Senior Lecturer, National Heart and Lung Institute, Faculty of Medicine,
Imperial College of Science, Technology and Medicine, University of London
Lately, Senior Medical Officer (Research), Royal Air Force Institute of Aviation Medicine

and

Anthony N Nicholson OBE DSc MD(hc) PhD FRCP(Lond) FRCP(Ed) FRCPath FFOM FRAeS
Visiting Professor of Medicine, National Heart and Lung Institute, Faculty of Medicine,
Imperial College of Science, Technology and Medicine, University of London
Visiting Professor of Aviation Medicine, Department of Human Physiology and Aerospace Medicine,
King's College School of Medicine, University of London
Lately, Commandant and Director of Research, Royal Air Force Institute and School of Aviation Medicine

A member of the Hodder Headline Group
LONDON·NEW YORK·NEW DELHI

First published in Great Britain in 2002 by
Arnold, a member of the Hodder Headline Group,
338 Euston Road, London NW1 3BH

http://www.arnoldpublishers.com

Distributed in the United States of America by
Oxford University Press Inc.,
198 Madison Avenue, New York, NY10016
Oxford is a registered trademark of Oxford University Press

British Library Cataloguing in Publication Data
A catalogue record for this book is available from the British Library

Library of Congress Cataloging-in-Publication Data
A catalog record for this book is available from the Library of Congress

ISBN 0 340 80637 0 (hb)

1 2 3 4 5 6 7 8 9 10

Commissioning Editor: Joanna Koster
Production Editor: Anke Ueberberg
Production Controller: Iain McWilliams
Cover Designer: Terry Griffiths/Mouse Mat Design

Typeset in 10/12 Pts Minion by Integra Software Services Pvt. Ltd., Pondicherry, India
www.integra-india.com
Printed and bound in Italy by Giunti

Contents

List of contributors

MICHAEL BAGSHAW MB BCh MFOM DAvMed FRAeS
Head of Medical Services, British Airways Health
Services, Harmondsworth, United Kingdom

DEVINDER S BANSI MD MRCP
Consultant Physician, Department of
Gastroenterology, Charing Cross Hospital, London,
United Kingdom

DOUGLAS A CHAMBERLAIN CBE HonDSc MD FRCP FRCA
Honorary Professor of Resuscitation Medicine,
University of Wales College of Medicine, Cardiff,
United Kingdom

GEOFFREY VP CHAMBERLAIN RD MD FRCS FRCOG HonFACOG
Lately, Professor and Chairman, Department of
Obstetrics and Gynaecology, St George's Hospital
Medical School, London
Honorary Consultant Obstetrician and
Gynaecologist, British Airways Health Services,
United Kingdom

MARTIN P CONNOR MSc MBChB MRCPath DTM&H
Consultant Microbiologist, Department of Pathology,
Royal Hospital Haslar, Gosport, United Kingdom

ANDREW RC CUMMIN MA DM FRCP
Consultant in Respiratory Medicine, Charing Cross
Hospital, London
Honorary Senior Lecturer, National Heart and
Lung Institute, Faculty of Medicine, Imperial
College of Science, Technology and Medicine,
London, United Kingdom

BRIAN M FRIER BSc MD FRCP(Ed) FRCP(Glas)
Consultant Physician and Honorary Professor in
Diabetes, Royal Infirmary of Edinburgh, Edinburgh,
United Kingdom

PAUL LF GIANGRANDE BSc MD FRCP(Lond) FRCP(Ed) FRCPath
Director and Consultant Haematologist, Oxford
Haemophilia Centre and Thrombosis Unit,
The Churchill Hospital, Oxford
Honorary Senior Lecturer in Haematology,
University of Oxford, United Kingdom

ANDREW J GIBBONS MA MBBChir FRCS FDS
Senior Specialist in Maxillofacial Surgery, Royal Air
Force

J SIMON R GIBBS MA MD FRCP
Senior Lecturer in Cardiology, National Heart and
Lung Institute, Faculty of Medicine, Imperial College
of Science, Technology and Medicine, London
Honorary Consultant in Cardiology, Charing Cross
Hospital, London, United Kingdom

ANDREW D GREEN MBBS FRCPath MFPHM DTM&H
Armed Forces Consultant in Communicable
Disease Control, Surgeon General's Department,
United Kingdom

BOB GROVER BSc MBBS MRCP
Specialist Registrar, Department of
Gastroenterology, Charing Cross Hospital, London,
United Kingdom

ROBERT MC HUNTER MSc MBBS MFOM DAvMed
Head of Aeromedical Centre, Safety Regulation
Group, Civil Aviation Authority, Gatwick Airport,
United Kingdom

DAVID A JONATHAN MBBS FRCS
Consultant in Otolaryngology, Frimley Park
Hospital, Camberley, United Kingdom
Consultant Adviser in Otolaryngology, Civil
Aviation Authority, United Kingdom

E GRAHAM LUCAS MBChB FRCP(Ed) FRCPsych FFOM D(Obst)RCOG
Emeritus Consultant Psychiatrist, Maudsley
Hospital, London
Consultant Psychiatrist, Foreign and
Commonwealth Office and Civil Aviation
Authority, United Kingdom
Visiting Professor, Postgraduate Medical School,
University of Guildford, United Kingdom

PETER MARTIN HonCRAeS FRAeS
Honorary Solicitor, Royal Aeronautical Society,
United Kingdom

VINCENT McAULAY MBChB MRCP
Specialist Registrar in Medicine, Royal Infirmary of
Edinburgh, Edinburgh, United Kingdom

COLIN AB McCLAREN OStJ MBChB FRCA
Lately, Consultant Adviser in Anaesthetics,
Royal Air Force

FRANCIS G MISKELLY MSc MD PhD MRCP
Senior Lecturer, Faculty of Medicine, Imperial College
of Science, Technology and Medicine, London
Honorary Consultant Physician, Department of
General Medicine and Care of the Elderly, Charing
Cross Hospital, London, United Kingdom

ANTHONY N NICHOLSON OBE DSc MD(hc) PhD FRCP(Lond)
FRCP(Ed) FRCPath FFOM FRAeS
Visiting Professor of Medicine, National Heart and
Lung Institute, Faculty of Medicine, Imperial College
of Science, Technology and Medicine, London
Visiting Professor of Aviation Medicine, Department
of Human Physiology and Aerospace Medicine,
King's College School of Medicine, London,
United Kingdom

MICHAEL D O'BRIEN MD FRCP
Physician for Nervous Diseases, Department of
Neurology, Guy's Hospital, London, United Kingdom

MARTIN P SAMUELS MD FRCP FRCPCH
Consultant Paediatrician and Senior Lecturer in
Paediatrics, Keele University, Academic Department
of Paediatrics, North Staffordshire Hospital, Stoke
on Trent, United Kingdom

PAUL E STEVENS BSc MBBS FRCP
Consultant Nephrologist, Department of Renal
Medicine, Kent and Canterbury Hospital,
Canterbury, United Kingdom

JR ROLLIN STOTT MA MBBChir MRCP DAvMed DCH DIC
Principal Medical Officer, QinetiQ Centre for
Human Sciences, Farnborough
Lately, Senior Medical Officer (Research), Royal Air
Force Institute of Aviation Medicine, United Kingdom

ANDREW V THILLAINAYAGAM MD FRCP
Consultant Physician, Gastroenterology Unit,
Hammersmith Hospitals, London
Honorary Senior Lecturer in Medicine,
Faculty of Medicine, Imperial College of Science,
Technology and Medicine, London, United Kingdom

But a Samaritan who was making the journey came upon him, and when he saw him was moved to pity. He went up and bandaged his wounds, bathing them with oil and wine. Then he lifted him on to his own beast, brought him to an inn, and looked after him there. Next day he produced two silver pieces, and gave them to the innkeeper, and said, 'Look after him; and if you spend any more, I will repay you on my way back'.

Gospel According to Luke
Chapter 10 Verses 33–35
The New English Bible, 1972

Preface

Over the years the medical concerns and well-being of the airline passenger have been a rather neglected aspect of aviation medicine. Aeromedical practitioners have traditionally focused their attention on the aircrew where they have striven to ensure realistic medical standards and maintain health and well-being. Indeed, even in countries with major international carriers, neither the national regulatory authority nor the airlines has claimed to have any statutory commitment to the health of the passenger, although most airlines give advice on specific problems to the medical practitioner and provide extra assistance to the passenger.

Nevertheless, the potential hiatus in medical care has given rise to public concern and, in some countries, government institutions have now committed themselves to ensuring that adequate attention will be given to the healthy, as well as to the ill, passenger – at least in flight. It is widely accepted that air travel does not have a serious impact on the health of the vast majority of passengers and that many complaints are concerned with comfort – though the latter cannot be necessarily dismissed. But, there are problems in a minority that need attention, and these are likely to grow in importance with the increasing travel of the elderly and of those with a clinical disorder or disability.

Now that the book is at hand, we hope that it will fulfil our aim to provide an authoritative text on medicine as it applies to pre-flight assessment and to in-flight assistance. The book is directed to the medical professional in its widest sense. It will be of value to the specialists of many disciplines whose advice may be sought by their colleagues, to occupational physicians who advise the employees of their company on worldwide travel, to general practitioners who day-by-day deal with the enquiries of their patients, often elderly and perhaps disabled, and to those in the nursing and allied professions who are involved in aviation medicine.

It will be of equal value to physicians who act as 'Good Samaritans', particularly on long-haul flights, and the text gives sound advice on handling in-flight events. In this way the book will be useful for those whose skills are not directly related to the problem at hand, but, nevertheless, may be the only practitioner on board. The lone psychiatrist may have to face an in-flight delivery, the dermatologist cope with a pneumothorax and the gynaecologist handle air rage. We hope that the airlines will have the book available on their flights, and that they will find it useful in the training of their cabin staff.

We are indebted to the authors who have brought their undoubted experience and expertise in acute medicine and in aviation medicine to this book, and we have worked closely with the authors to provide overall consistency of the text. We are indebted to Mrs Janet James MBE who prepared the final manuscript for the publishers and to Dr Joanna Koster, Arnold Publishers, for her counsels and advice.

Andrew Cummin
Anthony Nicholson
April 2002

Medico-legal issues: the Good Samaritan

PETER MARTIN

Good Samaritans, whether they be physicians or others in the professions ancillary to medicine, who give emergency medical services to fellow passengers, are often concerned about their legal liability, if, as a result of medical malpractice or error in the giving of those services, the passenger treated dies or is injured. The purpose of this chapter is to describe the legal environment in which the Good Samaritan may operate, and to explain the complicated liability issues that may arise for doctors and airlines from the provision of emergency medical relief. The subject, which is highly legalistic, is not made easier to explain to lawyers, let alone laymen, by a remarkable lack of authority from the courts on the relationship between the Good Samaritan, the passenger and the airline. There is no universal system of air or medical malpractice law that governs all the possible events which may occur in the course of international carriage by air. This chapter attempts to give an overview that may need to be adapted to various international jurisdictions.

In the first place it is useful to provide a brief summary of the general recommendations. When asked to act as a Good Samaritan, the medical practitioner should ensure that any medical problems that exist before embarkation are referred to the ground medical services, if at all possible. In flight, the medical practitioner should refuse to intervene if not competent or incapacitated, and should seek an immediate landing if the emergency cannot

reasonably be treated on board with available equipment before the next scheduled landing. The practitioner should have evidence of qualifications, in addition to documents providing evidence of identity. A full record of what has been done for a patient should be made and indemnity from the aircraft commander or the station manager should be sought before leaving the destination airport. The names of the aircraft captain and station manager should be recorded, and reasons obtained if an indemnity has been refused. The insurers for the medical practitioner should be informed of any in-flight medical intervention on return home.

LEGAL ENVIRONMENT

The international carriage by air of passengers is subject largely not to common law or codified rules, but to rules established by the international legal instruments, which together make up the so-called 'Warsaw System'. Indeed, many national legislatures have subjected domestic carriage by air to rules based upon those of the system. The principal legal regimes that currently apply to international carriage by air are the Warsaw–Hague regime which is a version of the original Warsaw Convention (1929), as amended by the Hague Protocol (1955), and the original Warsaw regime itself. The system is of growing complexity, so that its systematic nature is not always or immediately apparent, though it is not necessary to explain all the complexities, for reasons which will become clearer later. For such details the reader is referred to the textbook *Shawcross and Beaumont: Air Law* edited by Martin (2001).

In the early days of international air transport there were no uniform rules of law governing the carriage of passengers. Their rights and the liabilities of carriers by air depended on the general law, which had developed to meet the needs of those concerned with carriage by land and sea. Different legal systems approached different facts in different ways. Not only was there uncertainty as to the substantive content of air law in particular countries but, in international carriage, there were difficult choice-of-law problems. Lawyers call this 'the conflict of laws'. This is the determination of which country's law applies where the facts involve persons, firms and companies from different jurisdictions all, perhaps, flying not over the national airspace of one state but over the national airspace of a series of states or over international waters.

By providing, as it did, a set of uniform rules to replace the many and varied ones of individual states, the Warsaw Convention eliminated many of the troublesome conflicts which would otherwise arise in the event of accident, given the cross-border nature of international flights. It resolved jurisdictional questions, it prescribed a limitation period and created a uniform system of documentation. By establishing a uniform law as to the air carrier's liability in the event of death, wounding or other bodily injury, the Convention managed to sidestep, in a practical way, most questions involving conflicts of laws.

In the area of the carrier's liability, the main feature of the Convention was a reversal of the burden of proof. Under the common law system, the burden of proof of negligence falls upon the plaintiff. Under the Convention, the carrier's liability remained fault based, but fault would be assumed on proof only of damage and did not have to be established by the plaintiff. The carrier could escape liability only by proving that he, and his servants and agents, had taken all necessary measures to avoid the liability and the burden of proof of this defence fell on him.

However, to balance this valuable and practical reversal of the burden of proof, the liability of the carrier, in terms of the amount of damages that could be awarded, was limited. The Convention fixed a maximum amount, worth some £1000 in 1929 when it first was signed, for death or injury. The plaintiff could only recover more if he could prove what is now, in shorthand terms, described as intentional or reckless misconduct determined, usually, but not in every jurisdiction, by reference to a subjective test.

In the years since 1929, matters have, inevitably, moved on and, now, in the year 2002 the original Warsaw system, though very much in existence as a matter of law, has been modified by agreements between airlines and their passengers. These are known as 'special contracts', which are permissible under the Warsaw system. They improve, in favour of the passenger, not only the liability regime, but also the amounts of damages that can be recovered without the need to prove aggravated negligence. The system has also been modified in the European Community by a Regulation having the force of law in some countries.

Put in the most simple terms, which inevitably produces some distortion, the position today is that if a passenger is killed or injured on an international flight of many of the world's major carriers, damages on an unlimited basis can be obtained simply on proof of loss or damage. The carrier can attempt to limit these to the local currency equivalent of Special Drawing Rights (SDR) 100 000 on proving his freedom from negligence. (An SDR is a notional currency unit derived daily by the International Monetary Fund from the value of a basket of currencies.) If that burden cannot be discharged, and it is very difficult, almost impossible, to do so, then the carrier must compensate victims of accident fully by reference to the applicable standards in the jurisdiction in which the claim is brought. To qualify for damages from the carrier, the passenger must have suffered death, wounding or other bodily injury on board the aircraft in an accident caused by the carrier. These terms will be examined further below after introducing some ideas concerning Good Samaritans.

THE GOOD SAMARITAN

Airline cabin crew are trained in first aid and in the use of aircraft medical equipment including the emergency medical kit save for those parts designated for doctors such as oxygen sets, resuscitators, aspirators and eye irrigators. Cabin crew must not act beyond their limits of training, and so there may be occasions when advice or assistance from a medical practitioner is sought, either, and usually initially on major airlines, from a ground consultancy or a medically qualified passenger. Doctors may, therefore, be asked to give assistance to fellow-passengers in distress either by the passenger himself or by the cabin or flight crew of the aircraft. Sometimes doctors volunteer when they observe the need for assistance. The general rule adopted by airlines is that on board medical assistance will be requested when the emergency is serious or life threatening and where immediate 'hands-on' help is necessary or desirable. This must be so when the ground consultancy cannot be reached or when the consultancy recommends such assistance to the aircraft commander.

Most airlines govern crew duties on board by means of a formal manual of flying crew orders, which usually prescribes the circumstances in which, with the permission of the aircraft commander, the emergency medical kit may be opened and used by the flight crew, cabin crew or a Good Samaritan. As these usually contain certain controlled drugs and prescription-only medicines, their use must be formally authorized. It must be assumed, therefore, that if drugs or instruments from the kit are used by the Good Samaritan, it is with the knowledge and consent of the airline via the aircraft commander, and it is essential that they be used only as indicated. It is evident that the provision of drugs and instruments by the airline and authorization for their use involve the airline directly in any liability issue which may arise.

As indicated above, it is possible for a Good Samaritan to receive advice on the management of a passenger from a ground-based medical consultancy which will assist in diagnosis and treatment via radio or data link. This may involve a dialogue between the Good Samaritan and the consultants via a crew member if the Good Samaritan is too occupied with the passenger to use the radio telephone or satellite communication. This indirect communication creates the possibility of a misunderstanding. These practical issues, the existence or possibility of which must always be kept in mind, complicate what might otherwise be an answer to a relatively simple question.

Doctors may be concerned by assuming, or being asked to assume, the Good Samaritan role. Bodies which provide indemnity to medical practitioners make it clear that they should not hesitate to act as Good Samaritans whenever they believe it is reasonable to do so (Schutte 1999). Furthermore, bodies that regulate the practice of medicine consider that in an emergency the medical practitioner should offer anyone at risk the treatment that they could reasonably be expected to provide. However, there are areas of concern about acting as a Good Samaritan. These are the potential legal liability, the physical safety of the medical practitioner and the obligations that exist with respect to confidentiality.

LEGAL LIABILITY

In the airline context, potential legal liability can be considered in four parts:

- the duty of care,
- the vicarious liability of the airline,
- airline indemnity for the Good Samaritan and
- exclusivity.

A duty of care to the patient is established as soon as a doctor intervenes, whether approached by the airline or whether the practitioner has volunteered spontaneously. The medical practitioner must then recognize the limits of his professional competence and, where appropriate, should step back and allow someone else to take over. If the medical practitioner acts negligently or incompetently, given all the circumstances, he may become liable in common law if the passenger suffers further harm. What is worse is that if he is reckless, and as a result the patient dies or suffers serious harm, the doctor may become criminally liable. If sued direct, and if insured, he is likely to be entitled to discretionary assistance for claims arising from Good Samaritan acts, but it must be assumed that the discretion relates to competence. Competent intervention will be supported, but an incompetent intervention may not be supported. The question to be answered is whether it is possible for a medical practitioner to be sued successfully for negligence as primarily liable if the death, wounding or other bodily injury took place on board the aircraft. We will return to this topic later.

If a doctor responds to a call which needs emergency medical services then, although the matter is not wholly free from doubt because of a lack of judicial interpretation of the Warsaw Convention, he may become an agent of the airline when performing those services. In these circumstances, if the airline is sued in respect of any malpractice, error, or mistake by the doctor, the airline's liability will, or should be, governed by the Warsaw system and the airline's own insurance. However, it is possible that in answering a call from the aircraft commander, the doctor remains wholly independent of the airline in any contractual sense. Indeed, for the airline to be liable, there must be an 'accident'. The definition of an accident will be dealt with later.

It must also be added that there may be a difference in the liability regime if the doctor volunteers to assist without the invitation of the crew, for example, by treating a passenger beside him whose distress causes him to take action without an external call to do so. Such cases are rare as the action taken by a doctor is usually approved by the aircrew who inevitably become aware of it in the course of their duties.

The Warsaw system does not in any obvious way provide the Good Samaritan with automatic indemnity against his primary liability if the doctor is sued direct and not, as is more usual, the airline. Furthermore, few airlines automatically offer or provide such indemnity against direct liability and most are reported usually to refuse if asked, after a medical emergency on board, to provide one. Although at first surprising, it is perhaps clear that this must, on the face of it, be the case as the doctor's identity, qualifications, competence and experience are likely to be unknown to the airline and incapable of immediate proof. How could an airline automatically indemnify an officious or plausible charlatan? The question is a difficult one to answer in any definitive way. But there is a better reason why airlines may not find it necessary to provide the Good Samaritan doctor with indemnity and that lies within the exclusivity of the Warsaw system.

The Warsaw system provides that any action for damages arising from death, wounding or other bodily injury during the carriage by air, however founded, can only be brought subject to the conditions and limits set out in the Convention. The idea is that the Convention is to be the only system within which claims can be made, and that its rules are not to be circumvented by the bringing of claims outside it. This provision has been the subject of extensive interpretative litigation, as a result of which it is possible to offer some views. These views serve to explain that successful direct actions against doctors may not, for a specific legal reason unconnected with the alleged negligence itself, be successful by reason of the application of the exclusivity rule.

The intention of the Warsaw system seems to be to provide a secure regime within which restriction on the carrier's freedom of contract is to operate. The passenger receives benefits in return, but only in defined circumstances to which the limits of liability are to apply. To permit exceptions, whereby a passenger could sue outside the Convention regime for losses sustained during the international carriage by air, would distort the whole system, even in cases for which the Convention did not create any liability for the carrier. The whole purpose is to ensure, in all questions relating to the carrier's liability, that it is the Convention regime that applies.

Thus it can, and should, be argued in any case in which a doctor is sued directly as a result of an accident arising during the carriage by air, that the only party to be sued is the carrier and that there is no right of direct action against the doctor that can be properly sustained. It has to be said that such a case has yet to arise in practice. However, it is also the case that many responsible carriers make special insurance provision to ensure that this kind of liability is covered up to the limits of indemnity of the policy.

WHAT IS AN ACCIDENT?

If, then, an airline is to be liable for its own negligence and the negligence of a Good Samaritan, there must be an 'accident' on board the aircraft. In the simplest of terms, an accident is any unintended and unexpected occurrence that produces hurt or loss. The word 'accident' is often used to denote any unintended hurt or loss apart from its cause. If the cause is not known, the hurt or loss would itself certainly be called an accident. There have been a large number of cases in which the argument about the word 'accident' has centred on the passenger's state of health. A heart attack on an entirely normal flight would not be classified as an accident, even, it seems, if the passenger alleges that the cabin crew failed to provide adequate attention. The same is true even if the flight aggravates a pre-existing condition such as the effect of the relative hypoxia of the cabin on a passenger with pulmonary disease, the many risk factors inherent in a flight precipitating a thrombophlebitis or discomfort to a passenger with a hiatus hernia.

It is argued that an accident must in some way be external to the passenger, and so death on board as the result of a pre-existing medical condition does not render the airline liable. However, in the instances cited above it is evident that, though the event is not external to the passenger, their condition may be aggravated by the cabin environment. Furthermore, if emergency medical treatment is negligently or incompetently given and there is a deterioration of the passenger's condition which can be evidentially linked to that negligence or incompetence, there may be an accident creating a presumption of liability under the Convention.

If the airline is to be liable for its own negligence or the negligence of a Good Samaritan, the passenger must die, be wounded or suffer bodily injury as a direct or indirect result of that treatment. Death is death and wounding is wounding, but what is 'bodily injury' in this context? Is bodily injury palpable, conspicuous physical injury? Or does it include mental and psychosomatic injury? A current view is that there can be no recovery for 'psychological' injury unaccompanied by physical injury. However, it has been argued, not conclusively, that perhaps the right approach would be to construe it as including psychological damage, especially if it were shown by expert medical evidence to have a physical basis. It is probably prudent, given the way the law tends to develop in this sort of case, to assume that 'bodily injury' will include mental injury if it can be linked to physical damage. The risk to the airlines and the Good Samaritan is apparent.

THE AVIATION MEDICAL ASSISTANCE ACT 1998 (UNITED STATES OF AMERICA)

The Act applies only to air carriers and individuals sued in the United States Federal or State courts. It does not apply elsewhere, but it could be regarded as a model for best practice. The Act provides that in the USA an air carrier shall not be liable for damages in any action arising out of the performance of the air carrier in obtaining or attempting to obtain the assistance of a passenger in an in-flight medical emergency. This includes the acts or omissions of the passenger rendering the assistance, if the passenger is not an employee or agent of the carrier and the carrier in good faith believes the passenger is a medically qualified individual. Under the same statute, an individual shall not be liable if he renders in-flight emergency medical assistance unless he is guilty of gross negligence or wilful misconduct.

The expression 'medically qualified individual' is defined in the Act as including any person who is licensed, certified or otherwise qualified to provide medical care, including a physician, nurse, paramedic and emergency medical technician. In the USA, therefore, the *bona fide* medical practitioner is held harmless by the law, even if negligent, provided he is not guilty of aggravated negligence. The question must be, of course, whether acting outside medical competence is aggravated negligence. In the simplest terms, the airline passenger turned Good Samaritan is protected in a way that his counterpart in other countries is not.

In passing, it is worth noting here that the Act mandated the Administrator of the Federal Aviation Administration to decide whether automatic external defibrillators should be installed on both passenger aircraft and at airports. In this context he decided (6 June 2000) that it was not necessary to propose a regulation requiring automatic external defibrillators at airports because the majority had already taken steps to provide for the medical capability to address cardiac events. However, all airlines registered in the USA will be required to be equipped with automatic external defibrillators and augmented medical kits. A new rule to this effect will be in force from 12 May 2002 so as to allow for acquisition of the equipment and training of the crew.

THE WAY AHEAD

With these observations it is possible to propose, at least from a legal aspect, the measures which should be adopted by the airlines and by Good Samaritans. As far as the airlines are concerned, the flight and cabin crew must be trained to deal with medical emergencies. Appropriate medical equipment must be carried and be available. This should include automatic external defibrillators. However, they are not yet mandatory for the European Community though, as far as the USA is concerned, the Federal Aviation Administration has decided that their carriage should be required, together with enhanced medical kits. At present some airlines permit their carriage and use, but most have not yet addressed the issue. A counsel of perfection will be for all airlines to follow the advice of the Federal Aviation Administration when the rule is in force.

In the event of a medical emergency requiring a call for volunteers, volunteers should, so far as possible, be identified positively as suitably qualified with the aircraft commander as the final arbiter. Doctors and those ancillary to medicine should, as a counsel of perfection, be able, whether on holiday or a business trip, to identify themselves as suitably qualified, if they volunteer. If they feel that they are not competent to handle the event or that they are fatigued, under the influence of a sedative drug, or inebriated, they should disqualify themselves from assisting with the emergency. It must be borne in mind that to practise medicine while incompetent or incapacitated will inevitably, if a medical accident occurs, impair, if not remove, any insurance protection. Refusing to act because of incompetence or incapacity is not negligence, but very much the reverse.

The Good Samaritan should seek from the aircraft commander a contractual indemnity, and, if this is refused, as it probably will be, the refusal should be recorded in writing and signed by the aircraft commander before leaving the aircraft, with reasons. The advice, if any, of any ground-based consultant should be recorded by the doctor as well as the airline. At least the doctor will be able to demonstrate that he has tried to secure the necessary protections. Some airlines may show the doctor a document carried on board the aircraft which indicates the level of insurance cover the airline carries for its own legal liability for medical malpractice, error, or mistake by any person performing emergency medical relief on behalf of that airline. This is fine so far as it goes, and it is valuable, but, examples seen by the writer do not appear to cover the primary liability of the doctor if sued direct, however unsuccessful that direct action may ultimately be. The airline concerned must be asked, if necessary on the return of the doctor to his home base, to confirm whether a full indemnity, including a costs indemnity, is on offer in the event of action against the doctor.

The doctor must make the fullest note of what he did on board as soon as possible after the conclusion of the emergency and the intervention must be reported to the malpractice insurer as such an event may give rise to a future claim – however unlikely. In

no circumstances should the doctor ask for or accept any form of remuneration in money or money's worth for acting as a Good Samaritan. To do so may subtly alter his status *vis à vis* the airline and the passenger and, thereby, his professional indemnity cover. It may be said to create a contractual professional relationship damaging or destroying Good Samaritan protections. This may be a hard counsel to follow because some airlines are generous in the way they record their gratitude for successful interventions. An upgrade for the remainder of the journey is acceptable but cash or free tickets for a subsequent journey is quite another matter. Choices need to be made here and prudence dictates refusal of money or money's worth. The medical practitioner may wish to consider forwarding a fee note for his services to the airline on return home, but only after consultation with his defence advisor.

Better safe than sorry. Despite the obviously adverse commercial aspects of a diversionary or unscheduled landing, Good Samaritans should not hesitate formally to recommend this to the aircraft commander if they perceive the need for urgent, ground-based, medical treatment as in cases of continuing unconsciousness, acute breathing difficulties, severe and uncontrolled pain, uncontrolled bleeding, major injury and shock and, possibly, impending birth. Good Samaritans should ask for the declaration of a medical emergency so as to ensure that the landing aircraft is met at the airport by medically qualified staff. Airlines can help to avoid medical emergencies occurring in flight, just as they can help avoid potentially disruptive behaviour in flight, by the careful vigilance of the ground staff prior to boarding. If a passenger is taken ill at the airport, then, following the usual airline guidelines, which may include seeking help from a Good Samaritan if no local medical help is available, consideration must be given to denial of boarding. Remember that an accident, even a medical accident, during embarkation may be the responsibility of the carrier since embarkation is part of the carriage by air for Warsaw system purposes.

CONCLUSION

This is, as forecast, a confused and confusing area of the law in which, as usual, there are no certain answers to hypothetical questions. Some comfort may, however, reasonably be drawn from the words to be found in another air law convention, the Tokyo Convention 1963 on offences and certain other acts committed on board aircraft. This convention gives important powers to aircraft commanders for securing the safety of the aircraft and the management of dangerous behaviour on board, including restraint of passengers. It is worth noting that the commander may request and authorize, but not require, the assistance of passengers to restrain a passenger, and that no such passenger shall be held responsible in any proceedings on account of the treatment undergone by the person against whom the action was taken. By analogy, it seems reasonable to argue that, if a Good Samaritan acts competently in relation to a fellow passenger at the request of the aircraft commander, he is entitled to indemnity.

REFERENCES

Martin P, ed. *Shawcross and Beaumont: Air Law*, 4th edn. London: Butterworths, 2001 (issue 86).

Schutte P. The doctor as a Good Samaritan. *J Med Defence Union* 1999; **15**: 2–6.

The cabin environment

ANDREW RC CUMMIN AND ANTHONY N NICHOLSON

A journey in an aircraft is an unusual experience as passengers are enclosed for several hours in a cabin designed to protect them against a hostile environment. The cabin is a micro-environment which attempts to balance the physiological needs of the occupants and the engineering constraints of an aircraft operating at altitude, but the differences between the cabin environment and sea level in the fresh air can be significant, even to the well-being of the healthy. For this reason, over the past few years, much has been written about the potentially adverse effects on the health of passengers, though unfortunately many commentaries have tended to be sensational and have lacked the necessary objectivity. It is essential that the nature of the cabin environment is understood, and that it is appreciated that any potentially adverse effect is more likely to impair comfort than health. This is especially true for the healthy passenger, though the cabin environment may lead to significant problems in some individuals and have some serious effects in ill passengers.

Of prime importance to respiration and so to passengers with cardiovascular and pulmonary pathology is the reduced pressure of the cabin compared with that of sea level. The reduced pressure avoids unacceptable pressure differences across the cabin structure; however, it is acknowledged that, though the cabin altitude may be acceptable for a fit youngster, it may not be so acceptable for an elderly passenger with pulmonary disease. Another characteristic is the low humidity which, though it does not lead to systemic dehydration, can cause drying of the

mucous membranes with the sensation of thirst. Further, the quality of the cabin air is much discussed with reference to particulate and volatile contaminants, and, in this context, high quality filters and 'no smoking' restrictions are relevant. Other aspects are cosmic radiation where consideration has to be given to those who travel frequently or are pregnant, restriction of movement and lack of mobility, particularly in some cabins, which are risk factors in the genesis of deep vein thrombosis, and the existence of micro-organisms and droplets generated by passengers, which could possibly lead to the spread of infection. In this chapter we cover reduced pressure, air quality and low humidity. Other aspects of the cabin environment that could affect well-being, such as lack of mobility, are covered within chapters dealing with specific conditions, and a particular chapter is devoted to cosmic radiation.

REDUCED PRESSURE

Subsonic aircraft cruise at altitudes of up to and around 40 000 feet. Flying at these altitudes avoids turbulence and reduces drag on the aircraft, benefiting fuel consumption. The ambient atmosphere is hostile with the temperature below $-50°$ C and the pressure about 140 mmHg – just one-fifth the pressure at sea level. Of course, the concentration of oxygen in the air outside the aircraft remains around

21 per cent, though the partial pressure of oxygen itself is far too low to maintain life. It is for this reason that aircraft flying at altitude are pressurized (Figure 2.1). At cruise altitude, the maximum pressure in the cabin is influenced by the allowable differential pressure across the wall of the cabin, and this varies with aircraft design. It would be technically possible to maintain cabin pressure at sea level, and this would be physiologically ideal. However, the sigmoid shape of the haemoglobin dissociation curve is such that, in a healthy person, the low pressure within the cabin (equivalent to 8000 feet) has only a small effect on the oxygen content of the arterial blood. The regulatory authorities recognize this and 8000 feet is the maximum permitted cabin altitude, but it is important to realize that the regulations generally assume that the aircraft occupants are healthy. There is also some evidence that high level cognitive performance may be marginally impaired at such cabin altitudes, suggesting that a somewhat lower cabin altitude may be desirable for the aircrew, though this is not relevant to the passengers.

As an aircraft ascends, cabin pressure falls and this will have consequences on gases within body cavities. Body cavities are moist and gas within them is saturated with water vapour. As the pressure falls and the gas expands, water evaporates, increasing the expansion within the cavity still further. Gas expansion within a healthy distensible viscus is unlikely to cause a problem and gas within healthy rigid structures such as the paranasal sinuses and the middle ear is usually readily vented. Rapid rates of ascent are usually well tolerated, but problems may occur on descent. The reason for this is that pressure on structures such as the pharyngotympanic tube may cause occlusion, a problem that escalates as descent continues. Small changes in pressure are less likely to precipitate a problem. For this reason the rate of increase in cabin pressure is important, though rates of change of pressurization are not subject to regulation by the aviation authorities. An automatic system controls rate of change of pressure during climb and descent. Typically, rates of change of pressure after take-off are limited to an equivalent of about 500 feet per minute and on descent to 300 feet per minute. Nevertheless, many passengers, especially those with colds, experience discomfort or pain in the ears or sinuses, which can be severe. In some circumstances expansion of gas may cause particular problems. Examples include pneumothorax and gas in delicate structures such as the eye or ear following surgery. These are considered in detail elsewhere.

A further problem that can result from a fall in pressure is decompression sickness. Decompression sickness arises when tissues are saturated with nitrogen. Subatmospheric decompression sickness is very unusual below an altitude of 18 000 feet, and so the airline passenger is not at risk. The exceptions are those who have, for reasons of work or leisure, been exposed previously to an atmosphere at a higher pressure than sea level. These include recreational and professional divers, caisson workers and tunnellers. Flying before such activities is safe, but flying soon afterwards is potentially hazardous. The exact interval that needs to expire between exposure and flying, whether or not in a pressurized aircraft, depends on the frequency, duration and depth of the exposure and the nature of the gases breathed. Specialist advice from the occupational physician should be sought by any such worker prior to a flight.

Cabin decompression may occur if there is a reduction of inflow of air, an increase in the discharge of air or a failure of the cabin structure. Loss of cabin pressure due to reduced cabin air

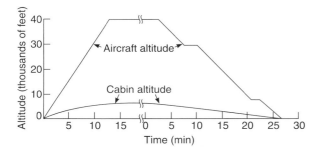

Figure 2.1 *The time course of the cabin altitude (lower curve) of a typical aircraft during a flight (aircraft altitude, upper curve) up to 40 000 feet and back to ground level (Ernsting et al. 1999).*

inflow is unlikely in multi-engined aircraft, as little inflow of air is needed for the purpose of maintaining pressure. Power from just one engine is sufficient. Failure of the pressure controller or of the discharge valves is also unlikely to cause decompression in passenger aircraft because of the duplication of the system and independent mechanisms for closing the discharge valves. Gross structural failure occurred in the early days of the jet airliner, but is not encountered nowadays as metal fatigue is better understood, though it may occur due to sabotage. Lesser defects, such as faulty seals, loss of a door or of a transparency, are rare. If the defect is small and the airliner large, the rate of fall in cabin pressure will be slow, and the fall in pressure will be moderated by continued inflow of air into the cabin. In some aircraft this can be increased in an emergency. If necessary, the pilot will initiate a descent, and, in these circumstances, the maximum cabin altitude reached will be considerably lower than the altitude at which the decompression occurred (Figure 2.2). The main risk to passengers following decompression is hypoxia. Rapid decompression at 40 000 feet while breathing air will lead to the partial pressure of oxygen in the alveoli falling to around 15 mmHg. Consciousness would be lost rapidly, but supplemental oxygen is provided by the overhead masks. These must be donned immediately. The time of useful consciousness is short so it is essential that adults with children should attend to themselves first.

AIR QUALITY

Passengers packed tightly into a metal tube need a supply of fresh air. Air is drawn from outside of the aircraft, compressed and delivered to the cabin (Figure 2.3). Cabin pressure is regulated by controlling the rate by which air is vented to the outside. This throughput provides ventilation with fresh air. However, compression of fresh air requires energy, and, with the demand for increased efficiency, fuel can be saved if some of the air is re-circulated. Re-circulation was used on earlier aircraft, but became more common in the 1980s with up to 50 per cent of the air being re-circulated. Cabin air is replenished with fresh air around 10–15 times per hour by progressive dilution. This initiative appears to have been accompanied by complaints from passengers about air quality, though it is essential to differentiate between ill health and discomfort.

One problem was that contaminants from tobacco smoke, which in older aircraft would have been vented, were being re-circulated to other parts of the aircraft. Passengers in non-smoking areas became aware of tobacco smoke and concern was exacerbated by reports on the harmful effects of passive smoking. Symptoms of eye and nose irritation related to nicotine and cotinine levels could be worse in aircraft that re-circulate air. This problem appears to have abated with the introduction of

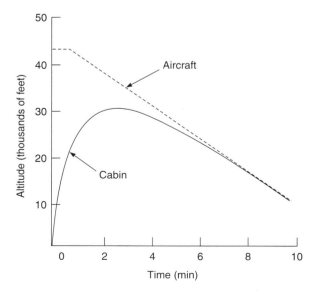

Figure 2.2 *The time course of cabin altitude when decompression occurs through a relatively small defect and descent of the aircraft is started 30 seconds after the beginning of the decompression (Ernsting et al. 1999).*

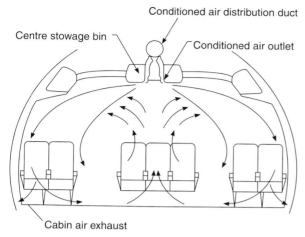

Centre stowage bin

Conditioned air distribution duct

Conditioned air outlet

Cabin air exhaust

Figure 2.3 *Typical circulation of air in a modern airliner.*

smoking bans, but the quality of cabin air still generates debate, as many do not feel comfortable when flying. Re-circulating half the cabin air creates the impression that half the air has been used already.

A continuing controversy concerns volatile organic compounds and centres around the possibility of oil leaking into the cabin air supply with the risk of exposure to the neurotoxic lubricant, tricresyl phosphate. The aviation and oil industries claim that exposure of passengers is not a hazard, but this position is not totally accepted (Winder and Balouet 2001). One of the last commercial uses of tricresyl phosphate is in aviation fuels, and there are isomers, other than tri-ortho-cresyl phosphate, which could be of greater relative toxicity, as well as N-phenyl-1-naphthylamine, which is a sensitizer. An oil leak from an engine at high temperature and pressure at altitude may not necessarily be an event of low toxicity, and such an event demands careful investigation. Even newer oils contain tricresyl phosphate.

There is also concern about the possibility of airborne transmission of infection. Re-circulated air may either be returned to the same cabin zone or mixed with fresh air and redistributed throughout the cabin. Air entering the aircraft is bled from the engine compressor at a temperature of more than 350° C and is essentially sterile. But once in the aircraft, there is the potential for contamination of the air by aerosols produced by the coughs and sneezes of passengers. Presumably disease may be transmitted from passenger to passenger in this way, as it is from person to person in close contact

in any other crowded environment. The question is whether the cabin environment might facilitate airborne transmission of disease as a result of re-circulation of the air. Microbiological studies suggest that the risks are greatest when the aircraft is on the ground and concern has been expressed about cabin conditions on the ground when aircraft ventilation systems are not operating. Transmission of influenza may have occurred in such circumstances.

On the other hand, there is no evidence of infection being spread by the air conditioning. The use of high-efficiency particulate air (HEPA) filters is not yet standard, but impressive claims based on laboratory tests are made for their effectiveness in removing both bacteria and, possibly, viral particles. Even without filters, infectious particles are likely to be reduced to below infectious levels by the addition of fresh and re-circulated air. Furthermore, the dry cabin air may reduce the time that bacteria remain viable though the opposite may be the case for viruses.

Re-circulation of cabin air has also created concern about whether there is enough fresh air. Typically aircraft cabins have 1000–2000 litres of air space per person. Aircraft without re-circulation capability tend to have higher fresh air ventilation capacities than aircraft that re-circulate cabin air, and certain parts of the aircraft may receive more fresh air per occupant than others. The flight deck is well supplied with ventilation – ten or more times higher than elsewhere. This leads to suspicions, especially from those in economy sections, that the passenger cabins are not well ventilated, but circulating air has functions other than respiration. These include cooling. The cockpit requires additional circulation because of the heat generated by the avionics and the effects of the sun. Nevertheless, on the whole, newer aircraft provide less fresh air than older types. A measure of the adequacy of the supply of fresh air is the measurement of the levels of carbon dioxide, though carbon dioxide can arise from sources such as dry ice used to chill food as well as from the occupants. The concentration of carbon dioxide in a fully laden passenger aircraft varies and tends to be highest during the ascent and descent phases. On long flights at cruising altitude typical concentrations are 500–800 p.p.m., which are well within acceptable limits.

Ozone forms in the upper atmosphere when oxygen reacts with ultra-violet light, and the ozone layer absorbs the potentially harmful ultra-violet radiation before it reaches the surface of the earth. The concentration of ozone in the atmosphere is maximal around 100 000 feet, but significant concentrations exist around 40 000 feet. These vary with respect to the seasons, being highest in the spring, and with the possibility of plumes due to weather events at high latitudes. Heating of the inlet air reduces the ozone reaching the cabin, but, nevertheless, peak concentrations in the cabin can exceed accepted levels. It is in this context that catalytic filters have been introduced, and these, together with the circulation of cabin air, lead to low levels.

Ozone could be a hazard to the well-being of the airline passenger as exposure leads to irritation of the eyes and respiratory tract with chest tightness and headache, and the pulmonary symptoms can be aggravated by exercise. Symptoms of mild exposure resolve in a few hours, but exposure to high concentrations can lead to airways damage and mental impairment. Although the possibility of any hazard to the well-being of the airline passenger due to ozone is becoming less and less an issue, certain passengers may be particularly sensitive to ozone contamination. These would include individuals with pulmonary disorders such as asthma, who could be affected in a way similar to that which can arise at sea level when the ambient ozone level is relatively high. Irritation of the eyes and of the respiratory tract similar to that known to be associated with exposure to ozone remain significant complaints even of healthy occupants, including the crew. The explanation could well relate to the low humidity of the cabin, which has similar clinical effects.

LOW HUMIDITY

Within the folklore of aviation medicine there has always resided the myth of dehydration of passengers in aircraft with low humidity cabins. So entrenched has been the belief that passengers lose excess body water during long-haul flights that many, even experienced aeromedical practitioners, have recommended the intake of extra fluid during the flight. Yet there is no physiological basis to support such advice (Nicholson 1998). Admittedly, loss of fluid from the respiratory tract and the skin may increase in an ambience of low water pressure, but even in a zero humidity environment with similar levels of cabin temperature, fluid loss over that normally experienced cannot be of clinical import. Nevertheless, although systemic dehydration is not a significant factor in healthy individuals, the low humidity can lead to dryness of the mucous membranes. Indeed, it is the dryness of the pharynx and of the skin and conjunctivae that have led to the widely held view of dehydration in flight.

The hypothalamus and posterior pituitary play the dominant part in water balance by influencing intake and urinary excretion, though intake usually exceeds the absolute requirement and the urine is rarely maximally concentrated. Impulses from the neurones of the hypothalamus lead to the rapid release of the antidiuretic hormone (ADH) stored in the secretory vesicles of the posterior pituitary gland. ADH targets the distal tubules and collecting ducts of the kidneys increasing their permeability, and so the reabsorption of water. Multiple mechanisms control sodium and water excretion by the kidneys. The two primary systems involved in regulating the concentration of sodium and the osmolality of the extracellular fluid are the osmoreceptor–ADH feedback system and the thirst mechanism (Figure 2.4). The osmoreceptor–ADH system is the sensitive mechanism which operates over the normal range of plasma osmolality whereas the osmotic thirst mechanism cuts in when the normal range is exceeded. The ADH system and thirst may also be activated in hypovolaemia, but a significant reduction in plasma volume is needed

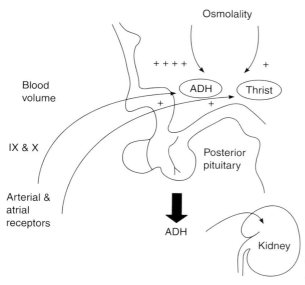

Figure 2.4 *Changes in plasma osmolality and blood volume affect the secretion of ADH and the sensation of thirst, but the secretion of ADH in response to rising plasma osmolality is the most sensitive mechanism. (Redrawn from Nicholson 1998).*

with both mechanisms involving the arterial baro-receptors and the atrial capacitance vessels.

A thirsty person experiences relief almost immediately after drinking water, even though water cannot have been absorbed from the gastrointestinal tract or yet had an effect on extracellular fluid osmolality. However, the relief of the sensation of thirst is short lived, and the desire to drink is satisfied only when the plasma osmolality or the blood volume returns to normal. A sensation of thirst due to dryness of the pharynx alone can give rise to some modulation of fluid balance even in a fully hydrated individual. The antidiuretic hormone could be released in response to a sensation of thirst, initiated peripherally, and lead to a change in plasma osmolality. This could lead to water retention followed by a compensatory diuresis due to the correcting influence of the hypothalamic osmo-receptors. The activity of such conflicting mechanisms could explain the cyclical pattern in the rate of urinary excretion observed in water loaded individuals exposed to zero humidity.

As far as current jet aircraft are concerned, the cabin air is derived from compressors, and under high altitude cruise conditions contains a negligible portion of water vapour. Without humidity control, the cabin is characterized by low humidity, and so passengers experience dryness of the upper respiratory tract and of the skin and conjunctivae. Clearly it

is possible that the low humidity environment of the cabin of modern aircraft could lead to water loss from the skin and respiratory tract above that normally experienced in the office and home environment. However, in a cabin with zero humidity for 8 hours, the maximum loss of fluid by all insensible means would only be around 100 g over that normally experienced. However, even with such a limited additional loss of fluid, the sensitive osmotic mechanisms would bring about a small change in urinary osmolality. Essentially, there is no evidence that exposure to a low humidity environment (even in the nude) can lead *per se* to dehydration. The sensation of thirst experienced by a healthy individual in the low humidity environment is due to a direct local drying of the pharyngeal membranes, and this, in itself, may generate a sensation of thirst by central mechanisms.

CONCLUSION

It is evident that the reduced pressure and reduced humidity of the aircraft cabin, as well as the quality of air, can have implications for the well-being of the healthy as well as for the ill passenger. Reduced pressure with the inevitable hypoxia of the cabin environment and the low humidity could be important issues for passengers with vascular and respiratory disorders whilst air quality could under some circumstances also influence their well-being. The low humidity of the cabin may be particularly relevant to the carriage of seriously ill patients who have a tracheotomy or are intubated, though it is more an inconvenience to the healthy passenger and, in any case, dryness of the mucous membranes can be treated locally. The clinical issues that are directly related to reduced pressure and humidity are dealt with in subsequent chapters.

REFERENCES

Ernsting J, Nicholson AN. and Rainford DJ, eds. *Aviation Medicine*. Oxford: Butterworth-Heinemann, 1999.

Nicholson AN. Dehydration and long haul flights. *Travel Med Int* 1998; **16**: 177–81.

Winder C and Balouet J. Toxic ingredients in aviation jet oils. *Proceedings of the 72nd Annual Scientific Meeting of the Aerospace Medical Association, Reno, Nevada*, May 2001, Abstract 350, page 112.

Cosmic radiation

ROBERT MC HUNTER

Cosmic radiation is from natural sources and is particularly present in the atmosphere at the operating altitudes of aircraft. It enters the aircraft cabin and poses a risk to the health of both passengers and crew. The risk is small, but as air travel is now normally such a safe activity, cosmic radiation becomes an important hazard. Moreover, the doses of radiation to passengers who fly frequently can be higher than the doses to workers employed in industries that have a more obvious association with radiation, such as radiography and nuclear power production. In this chapter the nature and the problem of cosmic radiation at altitude are discussed, as well as the uncertainty of estimates of risk.

NATURE OF COSMIC RADIATION

Cosmic radiation is the collective term for the radiation which comes from the sun (solar) and from the galaxies (galactic) (Reitz 1993). It is an ionizing radiation that can displace charged particles from atoms. This can lead to the disruption of molecules in living cells. With low doses of radiation the disruption may be repaired readily by cellular processes, but at higher doses there is an increasing chance that cell damage may occur. Cosmic radiation is not like many man-made radiations, such as

x-rays, for which a heavy material such as lead is a suitable shield. It is a complex mixture of electromagnetic and subatomic particle radiations with a wide range of energies for which light materials, such as water vapour and air, are suitable shields. In this way the atmosphere substantially protects the earth from cosmic radiation, though doses are greater with increasing altitude (Van Allen and Tatel 1948). The aluminium skin of an aircraft fuselage does not significantly shield the occupants against cosmic radiation.

Much of cosmic radiation consists of electrically charged particles; lower energy particles are deflected away from the earth or toward the polar regions by the magnetic field. Hence, doses of cosmic radiation are greater at polar latitudes (Lantos 1993). Cosmic radiation at aircraft altitudes is almost entirely galactic in origin. It comes from all directions and exposures are similar by day and by night. It is rare for the radiation from the sun to contribute directly at aircraft altitudes, but solar activity does modulate the amount of galactic cosmic radiation that reaches earth. The output of radiation from the sun varies in an approximately 11-year cycle. At times of maximum solar output associated with increasing numbers of sunspots and solar storms, the magnetic field imbedded within the sun's radiation tends to deflect the galactic cosmic component away from earth. Paradoxically, doses of cosmic radiation are usually (but not always) around 20 per cent lower during periods of solar maxima (Lantos 1993).

RADIATION EFFECTS

Cellular damage may occur when a tissue absorbs ionizing radiation. Three outcomes are possible. These are that the cell is repaired successfully by cellular processes, the cell dies or fails to reproduce, or the cell survives, though genetically altered. If within a tissue a large number of cells die, this is likely to lead to a demonstrable loss of tissue function. The probability of this effect is likely to be zero at low doses, but above a threshold dose the probability increases to 100 per cent. Above this threshold dose the severity of the harm will also increase. These effects with high doses are known as *deterministic effects*. An example of a *deterministic effect* would be a radiation burn to the skin. However, in the case of the occupants of a transport aircraft, the doses are extremely unlikely to be so high that *deterministic effects* would be seen.

When the irradiated cell survives, but is genetically altered, the cell or one of its clones, after some period of time, may become cancerous. The probability that radiation will cause cancer increases with dose, but it would seem that either there is no threshold for this effect or the threshold dose is very low. However, the severity of the cancer is not related to the dose of radiation. This effect is known as a *stochastic effect* – in plain terms, a *statistical effect*. Doses of cosmic radiation to the occupants of a transport aircraft are low, but are assumed, stochastically, to cause cancer. This assumption is made in the risk estimates of the International Commission on Radiological Protection (1990). The assumption is made because there are no human epidemiological data available from which conclusions can be drawn regarding the risks of long-term exposure to low doses of radiation at a low dose rate. Such a study would be practically impossible. The harmful effects of low levels of radiation are small increases in the rates of cancer and birth defects, which already have a relatively high prevalence in the population. It has been calculated that to assess the effect of a dose of 1 mSv

(approximately equivalent to one-third the annual dose of cosmic radiation received by aircrew) the size of population to be studied would need to be 500 000 000 (Barish 1996).

Much of our knowledge of the harmful effects of radiation has come from the study of small populations exposed to high doses at high rates and to types of radiation that are less biologically damaging, i.e. radiation incidents and medical overexposure. Linear extrapolations are made from high doses and high dose rates to low doses and low dose rates. In this way risks can be overestimated and lead to excessive protection. Indeed, some believe that low doses of radiation may be beneficial to humans. However, it is a characteristic of cosmic radiation that some of the particle energies can be enormously high, up to 10^{20} eV,[*] and there can be no doubt that a single energetic subatomic particle is capable of producing a biological effect. On this basis the linear no threshold hypothesis adopted by the International Commission on Radiation Protection (ICRP) appears prudent and conservative (Hall 1998).

UNITS OF MEASUREMENT

The unit of absorbed dose of ionizing radiation is the gray (Gy), and 1 Gy=1 joule of radiation energy absorbed per kilogram of tissue. A Gy is a large dose of radiation, and, for an acute (high dose rate) whole-body radiation exposure, approximately 3.25 Gy will prove to be fatal in 50 per cent of healthy young adults without any medical intervention (Hall 1993). The hourly absorbed dose of cosmic radiation at aircraft altitudes is approximately a million times less than this. However, equal absorbed amounts of different types of radiation may differ in the amount of biological harm they cause. To evaluate this effect, absorbed doses are multiplied by radiation weighting factors to give equivalent doses. The unit of equivalent dose is the sievert (Sv). Different tissues of the body have different sensitivities to radiation, and to allow for this, the equivalent dose to the various tissues of the body are multiplied by tissue-weighting factors, and added together to give an effective dose to the

---

[*]eV, electron volt. A unit of energy equivalent to the energy gained by an electron in passing through a potential difference of 1 volt.

whole body. The unit of effective dose is also the sievert (Sv).

To illustrate the difference between equivalent dose and effective dose, consider a chest x-ray. The equivalent dose may be about 90 μSv. However, radiosensitive organs, such as the lungs and the breasts, are exposed, but other important radiosensitive organs, such as the gonads, are not exposed. The effective dose is about 30 μSv (Barish 1996). Radiation monitors are usually calibrated in terms of the quantity of ambient dose equivalent. It is the dose equivalent at a depth of 1 cm in a theoretical sphere of tissue, and is independent of the direction of the radiation. This is particularly relevant for cosmic radiation. For one particular component of the cosmic radiation field, the proton component, the effective dose is much greater than the ambient dose equivalent, and so at aircraft altitudes the effective dose is about 20 per cent greater than the ambient dose equivalent (Bartlett 1999a).

OCCUPANTS OF TRANSPORT AIRCRAFT

Until recently, little consideration was given to protection of the occupants of transport aircraft. The reasons for this are several. Cosmic radiation is difficult to measure. Huge particle energies may be found in the cosmic radiation field (Heinrich *et al.* 1999). The genesis of such particles is not fully understood and synthetic production for reference and instrument calibration has proved to be difficult. It must also be appreciated that the study of cosmic radiation has been divided amongst a number of groups, such as geophysicists, astrophysicists, computer and power supply engineers, and there have been few opportunities for these workers to share knowledge. Further, the benefits of air transportation are clear, radiation levels at aircraft altitudes have been thought to be not readily amenable to control, and there has been a tradition of not applying radiation-protection practices to natural source radiations.

As far as those who fly frequently, this position has now changed. The International Commission on Radiation Protection (1990) has recommended that aircrew should be considered as occupationally exposed and, independent of this, that there should be an annual occupational dose limit of 20 mSv. Furthermore, attention should be given to passengers, such as couriers, who fly more frequently than most. These recommendations were adopted in a European Commission Council Directive for transposition into member states' national law on or before 13 May 2000. This Directive is commonly referred to as the Euratom Directive, and is described in greater detail later in this text.

The potentially adverse effects of cosmic radiation have come to recent prominence for a number of reasons. There has been a marked reduction in the annual occupational effective doses received by classified radiation workers (other than aircrew) over the last decade (Bartlett 1999b). In the UK, the average occupational effective dose in 1996 was 0.8 mSv, but there are some 24 000 aircrew who fly approximately 700 hours per year and whose annual occupational effective dose is between 2 and 4 mSv. Hence, aircrew can be one of the most highly exposed of working groups. Passengers who fly frequently, perhaps some 200 hours per year, may receive doses in excess of 0.8 mSv, so taking their exposure above that of most classified radiation workers. It is possible that there are some passengers flying for more hours than aircrew. They are likely to be the most highly exposed individuals.

Just as cosmic radiation may cause ionization in living cells, ionization may also arise in electronic circuits. The vulnerability of electrical equipment to cosmic radiation is increasing due to the trend toward high performance computers operating at low voltages. Moreover, there is an increasing carriage of such computers in airborne and satellite systems for global navigation, surveillance and communication. During solar maximal periods (most recently 2000–2002) radiation levels at aircraft altitudes may be expected to be generally lower. However, for brief periods during solar storms and other such solar excursions, cosmic radiation levels may be substantially elevated. Notably this occurred in 1956 when levels rose above 100 μSv h^{-1} (Armstrong *et al.* 1969) an increase above normal levels of two orders of magnitude.

Modern aircraft are optimized to fly at high altitudes, where exposures to cosmic radiation are greater. In addition to the efficiency gains at altitude, such aircraft can accept higher flight levels and so do not incur the delays associated with congested lower flight levels. The efficiency of modern aircraft has led to the development of ultra-long-haul operations where flight durations far exceeding 12 hours are possible (Bagshaw *et al.* 1996). Such flights carry a relief crew, and so the relief crew is exposed even when not operating the aircraft. The number of persons exposed to cosmic radiation in aircraft will, therefore, increase as air transportation develops. Finally, the age and sex distributions of the crew are different from those of other groups occupationally exposed to radiation. Aircrew are younger and approximately half their number are female, whereas only a few per cent of classified workers are female. The young and females are thought to be the most radiosensitive in the world of aviation.

MEASUREMENT AND CALCULATION OF DOSE

Measurement of cosmic radiation is complex. This is principally because it is a mixture of radiations to which individual detectors may or may not be sensitive, and it is difficult to produce a reference field for the calibration of instruments. Detectors typically measure only one type and energy range of radiation, and for other radiations there may be limited sensitivity. Cosmic radiation detectors may be of two types, active or passive. Active instruments are devices that measure radiation over short periods of time, such as minutes or seconds. Active instruments are useful in measuring the effects of short-term changes in dose rates as may be seen during solar flares or during rapid altitude changes. Passive instruments usually measure radiation from the time they leave the laboratory until they are returned for analysis. Active detectors are typically larger instruments whereas passive detectors are usually small and can be carried on the person.

Tissue equivalent proportional counter

The instrument generally acknowledged to be the reference for cosmic radiation dosimetry is the Tissue Equivalent Proportional Counter (TEPC). The TEPC consists of a plastic detector chamber filled with an organic gas such as propane. The wall of the chamber and the low-pressure gas within are said to be tissue equivalent as they have a similar atomic composition to tissue. When radiation interacts with the walls of the detector, charged particles are liberated. Some of these particles enter the gas cavity and cause ionization of the gas. Ionization within the gas cavity simulates the energy deposition that would take place within a small piece of tissue. To calibrate a counter, a reference field is required and a mixed high-energy particle field is used for this purpose.

Personal dose meters

Electronic personal dose meters are battery-powered devices useful for monitoring the less energetic components of the cosmic field. Passive detectors are reliable devices that are sensitive to both high- and low-energy radiations and may also be able to distinguish particle type and energy. Hence, combinations of passive detectors give information on the dose qualities required and also on the composition of the radiation field. Passive detectors usually have low sensitivity, but this disadvantage can be minimized if the detectors are flown for a prolonged period of time as on repeated flights on the same route. This gives an average route dose or, for a person flying many different routes, an accumulated dose. Film badges are radiographic film surrounded in part by various filters. They are insensitive to the neutron component of cosmic radiation and so need to be used with another monitoring device. Etch track detectors contain a plastic material and when neutrons strike the plastic they leave a track which is revealed by chemical etching and microscopy. Thermoluminescent detectors (TLDs) have also been used for in-flight dosimetry. They contain a chemical that is altered on exposure to radiation, and, when subsequently heated in the laboratory, emits light from which the radiation exposure can be derived. TLDs are sensitive to doses around 10 μGy. Superheated drop (bubble) detectors use drops of liquid which, when struck by a particle, become gaseous. These detectors can detect doses down to 1 μSv.

Computer-derived dose estimates

The Civil Aerospace Medical Institute (CAMI) of The Federal Aviation Administration (FAA) developed a computer program (CARI) that estimates the galactic radiation effective dose rate at any location in the atmosphere. The program requires the date and location of departure, the flight profile with time in ascent, cruise and descent, and the arrival location. A factor (the heliocentric potential) to allow for the modulating influence of solar activity can be applied for a given date. To understand the heliocentric potential, it is necessary to describe the interaction of galactic cosmic radiation with the space surrounding earth. The solar system is filled with an expanding ionized gas (plasma) from the sun known as the solar wind. Galactic cosmic radiation particles that enter the heliosphere (the region dominated by the solar wind which extends, at least, beyond the major planets), are scattered by the magnetic fields carried by the solar wind.

Theoretically, the effect on the galactic cosmic radiation energy spectrum (distribution of energies) of passage through this region of space is approximately the same as would be produced by a Sun-centered electric potential with a magnitude at the Earth's orbit equal to the energy lost by the galactic cosmic radiation in passing through the solar wind to that point (O'Brien et al. 1996). The activity of the sun varies during its 11-year cycle, and this alters the energy lost by the galactic cosmic radiation in penetrating the heliosphere to the earth's orbit. An increase in solar activity leads to an increase in the solar wind and an increase in heliocentric potential. This results in a reduction in the galactic cosmic radiation at earth and vice versa. For a given heliocentric potential, the amount of galactic radiation reaching ground level can be predicted and so, working back from actual ground level monitoring data, the heliocentric potential can be calculated.

The limitation of the CARI program is that it calculates the galactic component of cosmic radiation only. During exceptional solar storms the galactic component of cosmic radiation may be reduced, but the solar component may be greatly increased. In this case the program underestimates the dose for the flight. In the event of an elevated solar component, advice is posted on the FAA website. A number of other computer programs are under development, including the European Program Package for the Calculation of Aviation Route Doses (EPCARD) (Schraube et al. 1999). Table 3.1 shows the mean calculated effective route doses (μSv) on various long-haul flights during the spring and summer of 2000. The lower doses on eastbound flights on the same route but in different directions are related mainly to shorter flight times due to tail winds.

Biological dosimetry

In the world of aviation, biological dosimetry is usually taken to imply estimates of exposure based on the frequency of chromosome aberrations in T-lymphocytes. The aberration usually taken as a marker of exposure is the dicentric chromosome, i.e. a chromosome with two centromeres. A dicentric chromosome involves damage to both strands of DNA (deoxyribonucleic acid) in two chromosomes and then, if the

Table 3.1 *Mean calculated (CARI-6) route doses (effective dose μSv) for various long-haul routes*

Route	No. flights	Flight duration(h)	Mean calculated (CARI-6) route dose (effective dose μSv)
London–Tokyo	4	12.22	51.7
Tokyo–London	3	12.63	59.2
London–Los Angeles	3	10.25	51.8
Los Angeles–London	2	10.25	56.1
London–Shanghai	2	10.90	42.0
Shanghai–London	1	12.45	57.0
London–Hong Kong	1	12.02	55.9
London–New York	3	7.58	32.1
New York–London	2	5.58	27.9
London–Johannesburg	6	10.73	26.5
Johannesburg–London	5	11.20	27.9
London–Athens	4	3.30	12.0
Athens–London	4	3.37	13.6

damaged chromosomes lie physically close to one another, the two centromeric portions may join. The frequency of aberrations is taken to be a radiation response and the dose may be determined against the dose–response relationship.

Typically, the technique is used for retrospective dose estimation in cases of medical overexposure, reactor disasters and industrial incidents (Bender and Gooch 1962). In principle, the technique may be applied to air personnel when overexposure is suspected, though, to date, it has not been used to reconstruct doses following solar storms. Controversially, the technique has been used in routine assessments providing estimated annual effective dose equivalents of up to 37 mSv in some aircrew (Scheid *et al.* 1993, Heimers *et al.* 1995, Wolf *et al.* 1999, Heimers, 2000). These are substantially higher than the highest published physically derived annual dose estimate of 9 mSv (Schalch and Scharmann 1993).

There are a number of factors which may explain why biological dosimetry can produce doses much higher than those derived from physical estimates. The naturally occurring background rate of aberrations in an individual is a variable parameter, exposures to agents other than ionizing radiation may produce chromosome aberrations and ultraviolet light and radiomimetic chemicals may also induce aberrations. Given these limitations, some consider that 100 mGy is the lowest detectable exposure with this technique, and so the technique is not appropriate for low-dose cosmic radiation exposure studies. A further difficulty is that a dose–response curve for cosmic radiation does not exist.

DETRIMENT OF COSMIC RADIATION

The average annual background radiation dose in the United Kingdom is 2.2 mSv. Aircrew receive an additional average annual occupational exposure of 2–4 mSv (Bartlett 1996). The risk of radiation exposure is estimated by the International Commission on Radiological Protection (ICRP). ICRP risk estimates are derived from epidemiological studies, medical exposures and occupationally exposed persons, such as uranium miners and radium dial painters, and radiobiological research. These estimates have wide confidence limits and are probably conservative. The risk of death from a radiation-induced cancer depends on the age of the person at the time of exposure. This is in part because cancers take some time to develop and during this time an elderly person is more likely to die from other causes. For an adult working population, the risk of developing a fatal cancer is estimated at 4×10^{-2} Sv^{-1} (4 per cent per Sv). A return flight between London to New York would result in an effective dose of approximately 60 μSv or 60×10^{-6} Sv, and the risk of fatal cancer would be $60 \times 10^{-6} \times 4 \times 10^{-2} \times 100$ per cent = 0.00024 per cent. The risk of acquiring a fatal cancer in the general population is approximately 23 per cent, and so the risk after the flight has increased from 23 per cent to approximately 23.00024 per cent. In the case of a passenger making the return trip to New York every week, the annual accumulated effective dose would be 3.120 mSv. The added risk of developing a fatal cancer would be 0.0125 per cent.

The development of a fatal cancer results in a reduction in life expectancy. Calculations regarding the reduction in life expectancy rely on a number of assumptions and depend on the model chosen. There are likely to be substantial uncertainties associated with these calculations. The ICRP estimates that the risk of an attributable death in an 18-year-old professional pilot receiving an annual effective dose of 3 mSv for the maximum possible length of his career (until age 65) is 0.35–0.55 per cent. Should such an attributable death occur, the loss of life expectancy would be between 12.6 and 19.8 years, resulting in death most probably between 68 and 78 years. The added risk is very small, but it is greater than other fatal risks which air personnel face in connection with normal flying in a large commercial aircraft. The lifetime risk of a pilot being killed in a large commercial aircraft due to an accident is less than half the risk of death due to cosmic radiation exposure.

Concerns have been expressed regarding the occupants of executive jets which are capable of flying at altitudes around 50 000 ft. In accordance with the regulations of the International Civil Aviation Organization, such aircraft are not permitted to fly above 15 000 m (49 000 ft) unless active radiation monitors are carried. In practice it is only the commercial supersonic transport, Concorde, which operates routinely above this altitude and for this reason active monitoring has been installed. The smaller executive jets rarely operate up to such altitudes, as these altitudes are usually only possible when the aircraft are lightly loaded. The crew tends to fly for fewer hours than their heavy jet counterparts and on many occasions the aircraft are flown without cabin staff. The approach to passengers is, therefore, the same as that of passengers travelling by the main air carriers.

Genetic risks

A further hazard is the possibility of damage to a germ cell such that when a child is subsequently conceived there is a defect. This may be manifest in the child or in the subsequent offspring of that child. There are no direct data from human studies, but the effect is recognized from animal studies. The ICRP estimates that the risk of passing on severe hereditary effects to first generation offspring is $0.15-0.4 \times 10^{-2}$ Sv^{-1} (approximately 0.3×10^{-2} Sv^{-1}). In the case of a person of either sex flying between London and New York every week for a year and then conceiving a child, that child's risk of inheriting a radiation-induced severe defect is $0.3 \times 10^{-2} \times 0.003120 \times 100$ per cent = 0.00094 per cent. This figure may be compared with the background incidence of genetic abnormalities in the general population which has been estimated to be 4.23 per cent (Barish 1996).

Risks during pregnancy

Radiation may harm a pregnancy. Daniell *et al.* (1990) reported that air stewardesses had a relative risk of miscarriage of 1.9 compared with un-employed women and 1.3 compared with employed women. The risk to the pregnancy and the choices facing a frequent flyer who is pregnant change throughout the gestation. These risks may be best considered using practical scenarios.

RECENT CONCEPTION

A businesswoman reports that her last menstrual period was 6 weeks ago. She has a positive pregnancy test today and the likely time of conception was 4 weeks ago. In the past 4 weeks she has flown from London to New York and back every week. What have been the risks to the fetus so far? There are few data available to answer this question, and much of

the data are derived from animal studies. In the day after fertilization, should an adverse effect occur, the most likely adverse effect will be death of the embryo. If the embryo survives, then the radiation exposure on the first day is unlikely to lead to subsequent developmental defects (Friedberg *et al.* 1973). After the first day, the principal risks are miscarriage, developmental abnormalities such as physical and mental defects, and the subsequent development of cancer. However, based on mouse embryo experiments, it has been suggested that, after the first day post-conception, the embryo is much less radiosensitive, and that doses up to 20 mSv would not affect the survival of the pregnancy (Friedberg *et al.* 1987). There may be a threshold dose of 20 mSv, below which these adverse effects are not seen. It is exceptionally unlikely that the embryo would be exposed to 20 mSv during an entire pregnancy.

It is very unlikely that the mother would be aware of the death of the fetus in the first day after conception. The period is unlikely to be noticeably delayed and she would be unlikely to have had a pregnancy test. It is not possible to give an accurate estimation of the risk to the fetus on day 1, because the spontaneous miscarriage rate for early pregnancies is remarkably high. Regardless of exposure to radiation, about half of all embryos are lost before the next period is due and around 30 per cent are lost after or around the time of a missed period (Wilcox *et al.* 1988). For the duration of the entire pregnancy, exposure carries a risk of fatal cancer in later life and the risk coefficient for this is estimated to be 0.1 Sv^{-1}. In this example, the dose since conception was 240 μSv (0.000240 Sv) and the risk to the fetus developing a fatal cancer due to cosmic radiation exposure, *in utero*, is therefore $0.000240 \times 0.1 \times 100 = 0.00240$ per cent.

FLYING WHILE PREGNANT

A businesswoman who is pregnant decides to carry on travelling for the company until the scan at 12 weeks, 10 weeks post-conception, confirms the pregnancy. She flies from London to New York and back twice weekly for each of these weeks. What are the additional risks? The dose for this period is 1200 μSv, the risk of cancer is therefore $0.001200 \times 0.1 \times 100 = 0.01200$ per cent. Finally, a businesswoman informs her employers that she is pregnant. She is advised that she may continue to fly until she has been exposed to a further 1 mSv, though, with the principle of keeping doses as low as is reasonably achievable, she may if she wishes cease to travel on behalf of the company. How much more flying can she do and what are the additional risks of flying up to the 1 mSv limit? Flying London to New York twice weekly exposes her to 0.120 mSv per week. She may, therefore, continue for a further $1/0.120 = 8.3$ weeks. She travels for a further 8 weeks. The dose for this period is 0.000960 Sv, and the risk of cancer is therefore $0.000960 \times 0.1 \times 100 = 0.0096$ per cent. The risk of the child developing a fatal cancer due to the total dose of radiation from the time of conception is the sum of these risks, i.e. 0.0216 per cent.

Epidemiology

There have been several studies concerning patterns of mortality and the incidence of cancers in those who fly. Early work on mortality data for flight deck crew using the Proportional Mortality Ratio (PMR) approach (Sailsbury et al. 1991, Irvine and Davies 1992) generated hypothesis related to excesses for melanoma, colon cancer and brain cancer. Cohort studies (Band et al. 1990, Band et al. 1996, Irvine and Davies 1999) have demonstrated different patterns of excesses and deficits, however, the latter does support the excess of melanoma. The common finding from more recent cancer incidence data (Gundestrup and Storm 1999, Rafnsson et al. 2000, Haldorsen et al. 2000) is that of an excess for melanoma. Cancer incidence data for female cabin crew have shown an excess of breast cancer in two small cohorts (Pukkala et al. 1995, Rafnsson et al. 2000), but no difference from expectation in a third (Haldorsen et al. 2000). Melanoma excesses were seen in each of the studies for both sexes.

Many of the above studies lack the statistical power to draw firm conclusions and, even in the larger studies, exposure to radiation is not separated from other confounders. Aircrew and passengers are exposed to other potential carcinogens, such as, ozone, fuels, other radiations, and also to circadian rhythm disruption and different lifestyle factors. The statistical relationship between the incidence of these malignancies and radiation exposures is at best an association and no causal link has been established.

SOLAR STORMS

Solar storms are said to occur when large amounts of solar material, typically protons, are projected from the sun toward the earth. When the amount of material is considerable, it is described as a coronal mass ejection. Smaller amounts of material arise from solar flares. In either case, the scale of the event is described most accurately by the associated power per unit area arriving at the earth's surface. Where solar storms cause an increase in cosmic radiation at ground level, a ground level event is said to have occurred.

The highest recorded dose rate on board a commercial aircraft is 75.9 μSv h^{-1} (Reitz 1993). This was with Concorde in 1989. An equivalent dose of 1.1 mSv h^{-1} was estimated at an altitude of 65 000 ft (19.8 km) over the North Pole for a flare which took place in September 1989 (Barish 1990). One of the largest solar flares took place on 23rd February 1956. Dose rates were calculated as a function of altitude on the basis of ground level measurements as there were no direct measurements in the atmosphere. The upper limit of the equivalent dose rate was 30 mSv h^{-1} at 65 600 ft (20 km) altitude and 10 mSv h^{-1} at 32 800 ft (10 km) (Reitz 1993). These are high dose rates, indeed, but they are rare, and to date have only occurred for relatively short periods of time. In the 1956 event, 20 minutes after the onset of a visible flash of light on the sun, cosmic radiation at ground level increased abruptly to a very high intensity, and returned to normal within about 18 hours. The greatest risk would have been to aircraft at high altitude and high geomagnetic latitudes.

In comparison with today, there were, at that time, relatively few aircraft exposed. However, such is the concern regarding the potential harm of such an event that studies are under way to predict (Forcast) elevated levels of cosmic radiation at aircraft altitudes or provide actual information (Nowcast) on current levels. Forecasting techniques include the search for surface signatures on the sun, which may be associated with coronal mass ejections, and the observation of sound waves within the sun (helioseismology), which may predict eruptions of material. Once the radiation has left the sun, some of the radiation will be travelling at or near the speed of light. However, much of the proton radiation will be travelling more slowly than this, perhaps taking some hours to reach the earth. A number of satellites are now in position at relatively fixed points between the sun and earth which may give some 45 minutes warning of an event. The options would be to delay flights or to operate flights at lower geomagnetic latitudes and lower altitudes.

LEGISLATION

Aircraft intended to operate above 15 000 m (49 000 ft) are required to carry continuous active radiation monitoring equipment, and the pilots of such aircraft follow certain procedures in the event of a potential exposure to cosmic radiation. There are relatively few civil aircraft which have the capability of flying above 15 000 m. Concorde has an operating altitude of approximately 18 000 m (59 000 ft) and so active radiation-monitoring equipment has been carried on these aircraft. In some 100 000 flights an emergency descent has never been initiated due to radiation from a solar flare (Bagshaw 1999).

A number of small business jets is also capable of operating at altitudes above 15 000 m. At the time of writing, active radiation monitors suitable for an aircraft instrument panel are not available. Hence, most, if not all such jets that are flying commercially are certificated to fly at altitudes not above 15 000 m. In the case of the requirement to carry active monitors above 15 000 m, an alternative may be to carry out a regular monitoring programme of the flights.

The ICRP recommended limit for air personnel is that the 5-year average should not exceed 20 mSv and not exceed 50 mSv in any one year. In addition, the dose to a fetus should not exceed 1 mSv, and the FAA and the National Council on Radiation Protection and Measurements (NCRP) recommend that the equivalent dose not exceed 0.5 mSv in any one month.

European legislation can be traced to the treaty that established the European Atomic Energy Community (EURATOM) to oversee the safe development of the nuclear industry. The treaty requires the European Community to lay down basic standards for the protection of workers and the general public against ionizing radiation. These standards are laid down as Council Directives. Until 1984, the Basic Safety Standards Directive was the only legislation based on the EURATOM treaty. This Directive had incorporated recommendations of the ICRP. Since 1984 a number of other Directives have been made, but it was not until the ICRP publication

in 1990 that the recommendation was made that aircrew and frequent fliers should be considered as occupationally exposed.

The Revised Basic Safety Standards for the Protection of Workers and the General Public Against Ionising Radiation were laid down in the European Commission Council Directive of 1996. This Directive required commercial airline operators to assess the exposure of aircrew likely to receive an annual exposure of greater than 1 mSv, to organize work schedules with the aim of reducing the exposures of highly exposed aircrew, and to inform aircrew of the health risks involved. Following a declaration of pregnancy, it is necessary to ensure that the equivalent dose to the fetus will be as low as reasonably achievable, and that it is unlikely that any circumstance could lead to the dose exceeding 1 mSv during the remainder of the pregnancy. Air couriers and other frequent fliers are not mentioned in the Directive. However, it does recommend that employers of such individuals should make arrangements for determining exposure doses. In this context 'highly exposed' is taken to mean an annual exposure of greater than 6 mSv.

Flight doses have been evaluated in many research programmes. Aircrew who fly short-haul routes at lower geomagnetic latitudes are very unlikely to approach an annual exposure of 6 mSv, and for these it is suggested that, where their maximum annual doses can be shown to be less than 4 mSv, individual monitoring may be unnecessary. In cases where the assessment suggests that the maximum annual dose may be greater than 4 mSv, individual monitoring should be initiated to ensure that annual doses do not exceed 6 mSv. Records of individuals exposed to more than 6 mSv per annum must be kept for 30 years or until the individual is 75, whichever is the longer period of time. In the unlikely event of an increase in cosmic radiation exposure at aircraft altitudes due to solar particle events, calculation of aircrew and passenger doses should be undertaken using a method which includes the dose of solar cosmic radiation.

CONCLUSION

Cosmic radiation is a hazard to the health of passengers. For the most part this hazard exists in theory only as there is no experimental or medical evidence to show that low dose and low dose rates of radiation are harmful. The exception may be the fetus in the first 24 hours or so following conception when a single high-energy particle in the cosmic radiation field may prove to be fatal. However, even in the absence of occupational exposure to cosmic radiation, the spontaneous miscarriage rate at this time is very high.

Epidemiological studies do not separate the influence of confounding variables such as exposure to aviation fuels and oils. Such studies look at the effects of exposure to the totality of the aviation environment and included within this are the lifestyle factors associated with worldwide travel and frequent flying. Cosmic radiation exposure may be harmful or may, possibly, even be beneficial. However, with flights at high altitudes there is the possibility, in the event of solar flares, that cosmic radiation may be at higher doses and dose rates. In this exceptional circumstance exposure could be harmful and so consideration should be given to flight time limitations or to the operation of the aircraft at lower geomagnetic latitudes and lower altitudes.

In considering the risks of radiation in flight, thought needs to be given to the many issues which influence flight safety, and to social and economic factors. In comparison with other forms of transportation, despite whatever risks may be attributable to cosmic radiation, air travel is normally expeditious and safe. It can be concluded from the many research studies carried out that for passengers, including those pregnant and those who travel frequently, there is very little risk from cosmic radiation. As far as intense solar flares are concerned, means are being developed to monitor such events and to ensure that the operation of the aircraft is at safe altitudes and latitudes.

REFERENCES

Armstrong TW, Asmiller RG and Barrish J. Calculation of the radiation hazard at supersonic aircraft altitudes produced by an energetic solar flare. *Nucl Sci Eng* 1969; **37**: 337–42.

Bagshaw M, Irvine D and Davies DM. Exposure to cosmic radiation of British Airways flying crew on ultra long haul routes. *Occup Environ Med* 1996; **53**: 495–8.

Bagshaw M. Cosmic radiation measurements in airline service. *Radiat Prot Dosim* 1999; **86**: 333–4.

Band PR, Spinelli JJ, Ng VTY, Moody J and Gallagher RP. Mortality and cancer incidence in a cohort of commercial airline pilots. *Aviat Space Environ Med* 1990; **61**: 299–302.

Band PR *et al.* Cohort study of Air Canada pilots. Mortality, cancer incidence and leukaemia risk. *Am J Epidemiol* 1996; **143**: 137–43.

Barish RJ. Health physics concerns in commercial aviation. *Health Phys* 1990; **59**: 199–204.

Barish RJ. *The Invisible Passenger. Radiation Risks for People Who Fly.* Madison, WI: Advanced Medical Publishing, 1996.

Bartlett DT. Cosmic radiation exposure of aircraft crew. *Radiat Prot Bull* 1996; **4**: 9–16.

Bartlett DT. Radiation protection concepts and quantities for the occupational exposure to cosmic radiation. *Radiat Prot Dosim* 1999a; **86**: 263–8.

Bartlett DT. Aspects of the exposure of aircraft crew to radiation. *Radiat Prot Dosim* 1999b; **81**: 243–5.

Bender MA and Gooch PC. Persistent chromosome aberrations in irradiated human subjects. *Radiat Res* 1962; **16**: 44–53.

Daniell WE, Vaughan TL and Millies BA. Pregnancy outcomes among female flight attendants. *Aviat Space Environ Med* 1990; **61**: 840–4.

Friedberg W, Hanneman GD, Faulkner DN, Darden EB and Deal RB. Prenatal survival of mice irradiated with fission neutrons or 300 kVp X-rays during the pronuclear-zygote stage: survival curves, effect of dose fractionation. *Int J Radiat Biol* 1973; **24**: 549–60.

Friedberg W, Faulkner DN, Neas BR *et al.* Dose–incidence relationships for exencephalia, anophthalmia and prenatal mortality in mouse embryos irradiated with fission neutrons or 250kV X-rays. *Int J Radiat Biol* 1987; **52**: 223–36.

Gundestrup M and Storm HH. Radiation-induced acute myeloid leukaemia and other cancers in commercial jet cockpit crew: a population-based cohort study. *Lancet* 1999; **354**: 2029–31.

Haldorsen T, Reitan JB and Tveten U. Cancer incidence among Norwegian airline pilots. *Scand J Work Environ Health* 2000; **26**: 106–11.

Hall E. *Radiobiology for the Radiologist*, 4th edn. Philadelphia: Lippincott Williams & Wilkins, 1993.

Hall EJ. Taylor Lecture – Cancer risks in the work place. *Health Phys* 1998; **75**: 357–66.

Heimers A. Chromosome aberration analysis in Concorde pilots. *Mutat Res* 2000; **467**: 169–76.

Heimers A, Schroder H, Lengfelder E and Schmitz-feuerhake I. Chromosome aberration analysis in aircrew members. *Radiat Prot Dosim* 1995; **60**: 171–5.

Heinrich W, Roesler S and Schraube H. Physics of cosmic radiation fields. *Radiat Prot Dosim* 1999; **86**: 253–8.

International Commission on Radiological Protection. *Publication 60*. Oxford: Pergamon Press, 1990.

Irvine D and Davies DM. The mortality of British Airways pilots, 1966–1989: a proportional mortality study. *Aviat Space Environ Med* 1992; **63**: 276–9.

Irvine D and Davies DM. British Airways flightdeck mortality study, 1950–1992. *Aviat Space Environ Med* 1999; **70**: 548–55.

Lantos P. The sun and its effects on the terrestrial environment. *Radiat Prot Dosim* 1993; **48**: 27–32.

O'Brien K, Friedberg W, Sauer HH and Smart DF. Atmospheric cosmic rays and solar energetic particles at aircraft altitudes. *Environ Int* 1996; **22** (Suppl 1): S9–44.

Pukkala E, Auvinen A and Wahlberg G. Incidence of cancer amongst Finnish airline cabin attendants, 1967–1992. *Br Med J* 1995; **311**: 649–52.

Rafnsson V, Hrafnkelsson J and Tulinius H. Incidence of cancer among commercial airline pilots. *Occup Environ Med* 2000; **57**: 175–9.

Reitz G. Radiation environment in the stratosphere. *Radiat Prot Dosim* 1993; **48**: 5–20.

Sailsbury DA, Band PR, Threlfall WJ and Gallagher RP. Mortality among British Columbia Pilots. *Aviat Space Environ Med* 1991; **62**: 351–2.

Schalch D and Scharmann A. In-flight measurements at high latitudes: fast neutron doses to aircrew. *Radiat Prot Dosim* 1993; **48**: 85–91.

Scheid W, Weber J, Traut H and Gabriel HW. Chromosome aberrations induced in the lymphocytes of pilots and stewardesses. *Naturwissenschaften* 1993; **80**: 528–30.

Schraube H, Mares V, Roesler S and Heinrich W. Experimental verification and calculation of aviation route doses. *Radiat Prot Dosim* 1999; **86**: 309–15.

Vagero D, Swerdlow AJ and Beral V. Occupation and malignant melanoma. A study based on cancer registration data in England and Wales and in Sweden. *Br J Ind Med* 1990; **47**: 317–24.

Van Allen JA and Tatel HE. The cosmic ray counting rate of a single geiger counter from ground level to 161 km altitude. *Phys Rev* 1948; **73**: 245–51.

Wilcox AJ, Weinberg CR, O'Connor JF *et al*. Incidence of early loss of pregnancy. *N Engl J Med* 1988; **319**: 189–94.

Wolf G, Obe G and Bergau L. Cytogenetic investigations in flight personnel. *Radiat Prot Dosim* 1999; **86**: 275–8.

FURTHER READING

Exposure of Aircrew to Cosmic Radiation. European Commission, Luxembourg: Office for Official Publications of the European Communities, 1996.

Recommendations for the Implementation of Title VII of the European Basic Safety Standards Directive (BSS) concerning Safety. Significant Increase in Exposure due to Natural Radiation Sources. European Commission, Luxembourg: Office for Official Publications of the European Communities, 1997.

4

Pre-flight assessment and in-flight assistance

ANDREW RC CUMMIN, ANTHONY N NICHOLSON AND MICHAEL BAGSHAW

Flying as a passenger is unlikely to be a problem for the healthy and mobile individual, though as populations age increasing numbers of travellers are elderly, often with some disability. Around 5 per cent of passengers will already suffer from a chronic illness and it is in those with pre-existing illness that in-flight medical incidents are most likely to occur. Pre-existing conditions can be exacerbated by the journey and acute problems can be precipitated by the environment, and so pre-flight assessment is important to identify those at risk. In this context, most airlines will advise on fitness to travel and provide services for those needing extra help. They will tend to approach the issue of air passenger health according to their own guidelines or those of a group of airlines with which they are allied, but, in general, they are likely to be consistent with the advice of the Air Transport Medicine Committee of the Aerospace Medical Association. The deliberations of the Committee were published initially in *Aviation Space and Environmental Medicine* (1996), and later as *Medical Guidelines for Airline Travel* (1997).

PRE-FLIGHT ASSESSMENT

In the pre-flight assessment it is necessary to take into account the way in which the cabin envir-onment and other aspects of the journey may inter-act with existing pathology and possibly precipitate a potential problem. Unfortunately, it is often those passengers who need pre-flight assessment who do not consult their medical practitioner before a flight. The possibility of venous thromboembolism being associated with travel is now widely publicized, but the potentially adverse effects of a hypobaric and hypoxic environment are less well appreciated. Similarly, few patients are aware of the range of adverse effects that may arise from expansion of air in their bodies as the pressure in the cabin decreases with the operating altitude. Expansion of air may well be a problem for those who have undergone recent surgery, particularly to delicate structures such as the eye where intraocular bubbles of air could be serious. Other patients who need careful assessment are those with cardiorespiratory disease, cerebrovascular disease, coagulation disorders, anaemia, gastrointestinal bleeding, sinusitis and otitis media and infections, as well as those who are pregnant, neonates and those with fractures in plaster. This chapter outlines the general approach in handling these issues. Specific advice is given in sub-sequent chapters. A key principle for those with a problem is to ensure that treatment of the under-lying condition is optimized well before departure, and that potential problems in-flight are anticipated.

It is important to consider the journey as a whole. For many, the most difficult hurdles will be on the ground. Check-in and departure procedures may be prolonged and even healthy travellers may find them stressful. For those requiring an ambulance, wheelchair or stretcher, delays may be long and stress will be compounded. Long distances between check-in, boarding gate and the aircraft, together with the requirement for security procedures, all add to the pressures. For some, boarding coaches and climbing stairs may present a special problem. In planning the journey it is also necessary to consider whether there will be a change of aircraft and whether the transit may be difficult. Medical facilities may not be to hand if the transit is between terminals, and for some the altitude at a stopover or at the destination may be an issue.

Patients should be reminded to carry the medicines that they might possibly need during the flight on their person or in readily accessible hand luggage. Advice on the timing of ingestion of medicines, especially for diabetes and for oral contraception, is essential. The management of the diabetic is the subject of a later chapter. Some patients will need to take a summary of their medical condition and its management with them, and those on controlled drugs should ensure that these are compatible with local laws at their destination. A note from their medical practitioner giving details of any medication being carried may help to avoid difficulties at customs and immigration. Many drugs are not available in the same formulation, if at all, in other countries so patients must take a supply sufficient for their stay. However, it should be noted that it is not possible to store medications under refrigerated conditions during flight.

NEEDS OF THE PASSENGER

With the pre-flight assessment completed, the next stage is to convey the needs of the passenger to the airline. A useful document in preparing a patient for the flight is the Medical Information Form (MEDIF) published by the International Air Transport Association (IATA). It is available from the airline, completed by the medical practitioner and forwarded to the airline at the time of booking. This will ensure timely medical clearance and is essential when fitness to travel is in doubt as a result of recent illness, injury, surgery or a stay in hospital or when there is the possibility that a chronic illness may become unstable. It is also needed if special services, such as oxygen or a stretcher, are required and when equipment such as a nebulizer is to be carried. The airline must also be notified at the time of booking if a wheelchair is needed, but if passengers need personal attention during the flight, other than the normal cabin service, the airline is likely to require an adult to travel with the passenger.

When a passenger needs a stretcher, the advice of the airline must be sought in good time. All such equipment must comply with safety regulations. The stretcher must provide adequate restraint, be fixed securely and must not impede the movement of other occupants or their egress in an emergency. For this reason the airline will normally provide the stretcher. Because of the practical difficulties inherent in the operation, airlines usually require stretcher cases to be supervised by a company specializing in medical assistance. Sometimes it may be more appropriate for the patient to be carried in an air ambulance, and the carriage of the seriously ill is dealt with in a later chapter.

Arrangements for the seating of passengers with mobility problems need prior consultation with the airline. There is limited leg space in some cabins and a passenger with an above-knee plaster or with an ankylosed knee or hip may not fit into the available space. Immobility in an uncomfortable position may be painful, and may increase the risk of venous thromboembolism. These problems are not necessarily avoided in more spacious cabins. Furthermore, a passenger with a disability must not impede the free egress of other passengers in the case of an emergency. Immobile or disabled passengers cannot be seated adjacent to emergency exits, which usually have more leg room, or be permitted to stretch a leg in plaster along the aisle. The medical requirements of an individual passenger cannot be placed above the safety of all others.

Although an airline will carry oxygen supplies to cover the needs of a passenger who becomes suddenly ill, a passenger needing oxygen throughout the journey must notify the airline in advance. Not all airlines will provide this service. It is not permissible, normally, for the passenger to use their own supply as safety regulations require the use of aviation-specification oxygen. This ensures that the water content will be sufficiently low to avoid freezing of the valves and regulators at altitude. Oxygen on board an aircraft is potentially hazardous and, if a patient were to bring their own cylinder on board, the airline would not be able to ensure that it had been maintained to appropriate standards. There can be problems securing cylinders during flight and concerns related to the impossibility of inspecting the contents of a cylinder. For sick passengers needing oxygen, the airline will normally provide a cylinder or an oxygen concentrator, though on some aircraft types a supply of oxygen may be tapped from the aircraft ring main system. Airlines only provide oxygen for the flight. If supplemental oxygen is also required on the ground, additional arrangements must be made for a supply of oxygen at the airport terminal and for the collection of equipment on boarding the aircraft. However, medical oxygen is not available at all airports.

IN-FLIGHT INCIDENTS

In-flight medical incidents may be as trivial as a tension headache or as serious as a stroke, myocardial infarction, pneumothorax or a premature delivery. Cabin crew receive training in first aid and basic life support, as well as in the use of the equipment carried on board, but in difficult cases they may use a tele-medicine air-to-ground link or they may request assistance from a medically qualified passenger. In the latter case, though, the captain of the aircraft may well demand proof of qualification. National bodies regulating medical practitioners usually expect their doctors to respond to a call for help despite lack of special expertise; however, a doctor who is tired from a long journey, or perhaps unwell, or who may have had a few drinks too many may well be advised to decline to assist. As far as the airlines are concerned, they appreciate that the Good Samaritan acts in good faith whilst understanding that their training and expertise may not be in the specialist field appropriate to the event. Many airlines, but not all, provide liability coverage, and such cover may also be provided by professional insurance indemnity schemes. However, the indemnity provided by airlines may only apply provided the drugs contained within their medical kit are used

in accordance with accompanying instructions. Indeed, indemnity and the wider international position of the medical practitioner responding to an in-flight emergency are not absolutely clear, and are dealt with elsewhere.

The possibility that medical assistance may be called for during a flight inevitably raises the question of the equipment and medical supplies carried aboard. This has become an issue of increasing debate and in 1998 the Aerospace Medical Association published the deliberations of a group of physicians with an interest or expertise in aviation. The document did not constitute official policy as the Association considered that much more information on the nature of in-flight incidents was essential before general advice could be offered to airlines. Nevertheless, the deliberations of the group were useful. As a baseline they recommended that nitroglycerine, sublingual or spray, should be carried for suspected angina, diazepam for seizures, intravenous lignocaine (lidocaine) for dysrhythmias, an inhaled bronchodilator for acute asthma and intramuscular glucagon for hypoglycaemia. They also recommended the carriage of an auto-injector of adrenaline (epinephrine) and 50 per cent dextrose. Other drugs including aspirin, analgesics and antihistamines were recommended for less severe conditions, though some of these, such as aspirin, have a wide range of indications. An injectable diuretic and hydrocortisone were added as later recommendations.

IN-FLIGHT MEDICAL EQUIPMENT

It is the task of the national regulatory authority to stipulate the minimum scale and standard of medical equipment to be carried aboard aircraft which operate under their jurisdiction, but it is the airline that determines the detail of the equipment which is carried. The airline takes into consideration the route structure and length of sectors, passenger expectations, training of cabin crew, acceptability to medical practitioners from different cultures and likely emergencies, as well as the requirement to fulfil the statutory standard. The requirements for in-flight support, particularly on long-haul flights, are becoming less controversial, though equipment and medication vary between airlines. This really reflects the lack of a worldwide database on the nature of in-flight emergencies and the concern of airlines whether an appropriately qualified practitioner would be available to use more sophisticated equipment and medication. The Aerospace Medical Association has established a worldwide collection system, but it will be some years before meaningful data are available.

A basic kit does not meet the expectations of passengers and is not acceptable to medical practitioners, and so the major airlines carry a much wider range of medication and equipment. This is evident from the lists published by airlines that operate world wide. *Aviation Space and Environmental Medicine* has published the lists of medical equipment carried by several airlines (Emergency Medical Kit Ad Hoc Task Force 1998, Thibeault *et al.* 1998, Lyznicki *et al.* 2000a, 2000b). The airlines included Aeromexico, American Airlines, British Airways, Delta Airlines, El Al, Finnair, Japan Air Lines, Qantas Airways and United Airlines. It is evident that the medical advisers of many airlines are concerned to ensure adequate support to the crew and to the in-flight physician, and the in-flight medical kits cover, as far as is reasonable, in-flight medical incidents world wide. Indeed, the list of medications carried by some airlines is impressive, and many airlines carry endotracheal tubes, laryngoscopes, urinary and intravenous catheters, umbilical clamps and an array of surgical instruments. Such support cannot be anticipated from all carriers.

Cardiopulmonary resuscitation (CPR) is an essential feature of cabin crew training and has long been a statutory requirement in most countries. CPR equipment can range from a mouth-to-mouth face guard to an automated external defibrillator. The latter is becoming a more common item and cabin crews are trained in its use. Some types have a cardiac monitoring facility and such information can be useful in reaching a decision on whether to divert. An automated external defibrillator is an important item of the in-flight equipment as it affords immediate and time-critical support in the event of a cardiac arrest. However, it must be stressed that defibrillation is but part of adequate care and requires careful consideration of the range of drugs that should be carried in flight. In-flight defibrillation is the subject of a separate chapter.

IN-FLIGHT MEDICAL ADVICE

The crew of an aircraft usually defers to the advice of an assisting medical practitioner with respect to the well-being of another passenger, even when the advice implies a diversion for an unscheduled landing. It is for this reason that the medical practitioner must weigh the various issues carefully. However, the ultimate decision as to whether to divert rests with the aircraft captain who has to balance the operational and medical factors and take into consideration the availability of medical facilities at the diversion airport. It has to be accepted that in some cases the practitioner may not be sufficiently familiar with the medical problem or with the air environment to make the optimum decision. It is for this reason that air-to-ground links are useful so that the captain and the medical practitioner can discuss the situation with an experienced medical adviser. Such a facility allows the various options to be discussed. The link also provides information on the medical facilities available at the diversion airport either through the database of the airline medical department itself or through a third party. The advent of digital technology has enabled the transmission of air-to-ground clinical data including blood pressure and pulse rate, temperature, blood oxygen levels, end-tidal P_{CO_2} and respiration rate, and the electrocardiogram by means of the on-board telephone. Clinical experience is being gained using this technique.

Death in-flight is rare, but when it occurs it is a most distressing event. In view of the large number of individuals who now travel, many of them elderly, there is always the possibility that a passenger may die naturally in the course of the journey. Death can be confirmed by a medical practitioner (who is recognized as such by the captain) or by a practitioner at the airport or receiving hospital. In the absence of medical advice, the cabin crew may well continue resuscitation until the aircraft lands. If the death is confirmed in-flight, the captain records the event including the time of death and geographical coordinates. The advice of the captain and of the cabin staff should always be taken regarding the manner in which a deceased passenger is carried during the remaining part of the flight. Diversion of the aircraft is not appropriate in the event of an in-flight death. The local authorities at the destination may carry out various investigations into the circumstances of the death. These may be time consuming and could involve delay to the practitioner, the crew and the aircraft.

CONCLUSION

Careful pre-flight assessment of passengers with medical problems is the key to good in-flight support. In some cases the advice of the medical department of an airline or even of a specialized unit is necessary, and careful briefing of the passenger and of their relatives is essential. Needless to say, it is important to stress to all passengers that they should carry their medication on their person or in readily accessible hand luggage aboard the aircraft. Passengers carrying any form of medication should have to hand a letter of confirmation from their medical practitioner to ease customs and immigration formalities. In the case of some conditions and some journeys, the medication should be documented carefully in English, French and Spanish so that its nature, details of administration and purpose are clear to, and can be easily understood by, medical practitioners world wide. Advice should also be given on the need to adjust timing of administration in the event of a time-zone change. This is particularly important for diabetics and for women on oral contraceptives. Finally, it is essential that all travellers should have adequate medical insurance cover.

REFERENCES

Air Transport Medicine Committee, Aerospace Medical Association. Medical guidelines for air travel. *Aviat Space Environ Med* 1996; **67** (Suppl II): B1–16.

Emergency Medical Kit Ad Hoc Task Force, Aerospace Medical Association. Report of the inflight emergency medical kit task force. *Aviat Space Environ Med* 1998; **69**: 427–8.

Lyznicki JM, Williams MA, Deitchman SD and Howe JP III. Medical oxygen and air travel. *Aviat Space Environ Med* 2000a; **71**: 827–31.

Lyznicki JM, Williams MA, Deitchman SD and Howe JP III. Inflight medical emergencies. *Aviat Space Environ Med* 2000b; **71**: 832–8.

Medical Guidelines for Airline Travel. Alexandria, VA: Aerospace Medical Association, 1997.

Thibeault C and Air Transport Medicine Committee, Aerospace Medical Association. Special committee report: emergency medical kit for commercial airlines. *Aviat Space Environ Med* 1998; **69**: 1112–13.

5

Immunization, and infectious and tropical diseases

MARTIN P CONNOR AND ANDREW D GREEN

Modern aircraft can circumnavigate the globe in little over 24 hours, and this is well within the incubation period of almost all infectious diseases. As a result, any general practitioner can now face patients with infective conditions acquired literally anywhere in the world. Furthermore, the number of international tourists has grown exponentially for the last 40 years, reaching a total of over 500 million in 1995. It is estimated that the global trend of a 6 per cent annual increase will continue for the foreseeable future, reaching nearly 1000 million by 2010 (World Tourism Organization 1999).

Do any of these travellers actually get sick? The answer appears to be that they do. Several studies have looked at people from different nations who visited a variety of places, including both developed and developing countries. Although there is the expected variation according to geography, season and exact circumstances of travel, the overall trend is similar. On average about 30 per cent of travellers become ill during or shortly after travel, with the majority affected by gastrointestinal upset. Infective conditions also account for most of the other illness (Cossar and Reid 1989). However, these infectious diseases are not life-threatening, accounting for less than 4 per cent of total traveller deaths. Travellers generally die from trauma, if young, or cardiovascular events, if older (Hargarten *et al.* 1989).

Even if the most conservative estimates are made, there is a significant health burden related to infectious disease and travel. Over the last decade the recognition of these specific problems has led to an increased interest in travel medicine. Whilst much of the impetus has derived from physicians concerned with infectious diseases, there are many other health issues of equal merit, and these are dealt with elsewhere in this book. Importantly, most infectious diseases can be prevented by relatively simple precautions. The final point to remember about infectious diseases is their nature – they are communicable, and spread to others. This may be important, not only after return home, but also during the journey itself. In many respects, the aircraft environment is ideal for the transmission of infectious diseases (Association of Port Health Authorities 1995, Wick and Irvine 1995, Kenyon *et al.* 1996).

PREVENTION

In common with many other areas of medicine, the reduction of risk associated with infectious disease involves an integrated multi-tiered approach. It is generally unrealistic to adopt a 'no-risk' strategy, since this is both impractical and unlikely to be successful. For example, a recent study of Swiss tourists required that they be closely monitored for their choice of 'safe' foodstuffs in an African country. Despite being aware of participating in a research project, and of the close presence of an investigator complete with clipboard, more than 95 per cent made one or more dietary indiscretions within a 24-hour period (Steffen 1991). Furthermore, the infecting dose of some enteric diseases may be fewer than 10 organisms, and a single bite from an infective mosquito is sufficient to transmit some arboviral infections. Risk reduction rather than elimination should therefore be the realistic aim.

Sexually transmitted diseases

Sexual promiscuity is common in travellers. More than 40 per cent of young female holidaymakers have one or more contacts during short overseas holidays (Stricker *et al.* 1991). Travellers should be counselled about the risks associated with sexual exposure and advised of the benefits of condom use. The quality of products on sale in many countries is not ensured and they should be advised to take sufficient supplies with them. Unfortunately, many encounters follow alcohol ingestion, which in turn leads to selective amnesia. Recently reported incidents related to travel include heterosexually acquired syphilis from Russia, antibiotic-resistant gonococcal infection from South East Asia and up to 10 per cent of new HIV diagnoses.

Food poisoning

The axiomatic statement: 'If you can't wash it, boil it or peel it, forget it!' holds true. Standards of food preparation and hygiene in many parts of the globe can be variable. However, many people travel to sample local cuisine and ignore such advice, whilst others are compromised for reasons of courtesy or convention. It is difficult to decline to eat at a diplomatic banquet, or to refuse meals offered when involved in a business negotiation. In these circumstances travellers can be advised to use discretion and common sense, since dogmatic statements will inevitably be ignored. It is generally better to offer practical advice that might be followed than that which is correct, but impossible to put into practice.

The effects of alcohol

Although usually associated with traumatic injury, alcohol often plays a part in the acquisition of infectious disease. Loss of inhibition leads not only to risks from sexually transmitted and food-borne diseases, but also vector-borne disease – sleeping off a hangover on a beach is more hazardous in West Africa than in Europe. There are even specific infections related to alcohol ingestion, such as paragonimiasis associated with ingestion of 'drunken raw crabs' in China (Zhi-Biao 1991).

Sporting activities and infection

A variety of infections is associated with travellers' interest in sport. These include those associated with immersion in fresh water, such as leptospirosis and schistosomiasis. Seawater may be equally hazardous, with unusual skin and soft tissue infections found in exposure to estuarine waters. Coral injuries are notorious for producing wounds that become severely infected. Simple trauma on land may also be complicated by infection, and both cutaneous anthrax and cutaneous diphtheria have been seen in sportsmen. A recent tour of a sports team to the Pacific was severely affected by tropical ulcer infection of lower limbs caused by mixed saprophytic anaerobic organisms (Anon 1992). Education about the risks associated with water immersion should be given to those travellers planning such activities, and basic first aid measures advised for all skin trauma.

Insect bites

Travellers are usually receptive to advice on insect bite avoidance, since there is an obvious short-term benefit. Surprisingly, few are aware of the diseases spread by arthropods, and so advice is rarely wasted. Simple precautions include appropriate clothing (with or without impregnation of insecticide), use of impregnated bed nets, and proper use of insect screens in rooms. A range of personal repellent applications is now available, most either based on diethyl toluamide or natural products such as citronella. Travellers should be reminded that many disease vectors bite during daylight and not just at night.

Water quality

The quality of mains water is variable world wide, and reliable local information is essential. Where there is doubt, water purification devices should be used. A wide variety are available with a range of production capacities, although many on the market are of unproven efficacy. The most effective combine physical filtration with a residual chemical decontamination. It is important that travellers do not underestimate their water requirements in tropical environments, and most will require in excess of 20 litres each day. Reliance on bottled water is not to be encouraged, since locally produced products are often of similar quality as mains water. Taking supplies from the home country is logistically difficult, since each traveller will need two to three times their own body weight each week.

Antibiotics

The use of antibiotics during travel has been a controversial issue for several years. They can be used to prevent infection or to treat suspected or established infections. Antibiotics are not without risk, and a careful assessment of their requirement and effectiveness in a given situation should always be undertaken before they are prescribed. There is little evidence to support their use in the majority of travellers. It has been demonstrated in travellers to the tropics that a degree of protection from gastroenteritis is possible in those who have been given oral ciprofloxacin. The majority of travellers' diarrhoea is due to enterotoxigenic *Escherichia coli* and this, which occurs commonly shortly after arrival, is inclined to be mild and self-limiting (Connor and Green 1995). Antibiotic prophylaxis may be useful if it was imperative that the traveller was not troubled by diarrhoea shortly after arrival in a foreign country. This could include a businessman or politician with a vital meeting to attend, or personnel deployed rapidly to an area of political instability. One suggested regimen is ciprofloxacin 1 g as a single dose.

Antibiotic prophylaxis may be considered in the traveller with an underlying medical condition. For example, patients who are HIV positive may be exposed to higher risks from gastrointestinal pathogens that would be self-limiting in immunocompetent individuals, but may be deadly in the HIV-positive patient. It is difficult to cover all potential pathogens with a few antibiotics, and there may be interactions with concurrent antiretroviral therapy. It is safer in these situations to discuss individual cases with a microbiologist or HIV specialist before travel. Asplenic patients are required to take penicillin or erythromycin prophylaxis for life following their splenectomy. However, the sensitivity of *Streptococcus pneumoniae* to penicillin (the primary pathogen in splenectomized patients) can vary from one country to another. The prevalence of penicillin-resistant *Streptococcus pneumoniae* in the UK is only about 4 per cent, whereas the prevalence in Spain is 44 per cent. Higher levels exist in Iceland, South Africa and parts of the USA (Goldstein and Garau 1997). Asplenic travellers to these countries may be prescribed an alternative antibiotic such as co-amoxiclav.

Antibiotics may be carried in some circumstances for self-treatment. The decision to issue antibiotics in advance of travel will depend on the country being visited, the availability and quality of medical care available, the degree of isolation or terrain the traveller will cover, and the medical knowledge of the traveller or another in the party. For many travellers to the tropics this will include some antibiotic and antimotility agents for the treatment of gastroenteritis. If symptoms of diarrhoea do not improve within 24 hours or if severe abdominal cramps, fever or blood in the stool are present, then antibiotics should be started. If there is no improvement in symptoms within 24 hours, medical attention must be sought elsewhere. Antibiotics can be supplied to the isolated traveller for use in the treatment of skin or eye infections; however, not all microbes will be sensitive to routine antibiotics. It must be remembered that many antibiotics can interfere with the efficacy of oral contraceptives and an unexpected pregnancy can result if alternative contraception is not used.

HIV and antiretroviral prophylaxis

Health-care workers planning long-term service in areas with a high prevalence of HIV in the local population may be concerned about the availability of antiretroviral prophylaxis. This is recommended in some countries for those who have sustained a cutaneous injury in an HIV high-risk incident. Antiretrovirals must be started as soon as possible after the injury, and continued for 4 weeks. However, they can have severe side effects and compliance throughout the full length of the treatment period is problematical. Consideration should not only be given to prescribing such drugs, but also to the provision of an initial starter pack of therapy if it is considered that such treatment may not be easy to obtain in the country in which they will be working. In any case, arrangements for follow-up including repatriation may be necessary.

IMMUNIZATION

Immunization against infectious diseases is a mainstay of modern preventative medicine. It is of even more importance to the traveller who will be exposed to infections now regarded as rare in the home country, but remain major killers in many developing countries. Most vaccines are both effective and safe to administer with any side effects being mild and self-limiting in nature. Hypersensitivity to a vaccine component or anaphylaxis can occur rarely. For this reason, a vaccine should be administered, with resuscitation equipment at hand, by an appropriately trained worker.

A risk assessment of the whole trip is required when a traveller enquires about appropriate immunizations for a journey. This should include the geographical itinerary of the countries to be visited, locations within those countries, planned stopovers *en route* and any likely unplanned diversion or travel complications. Although useful as an *aide mémoire*, immunization wall charts should only be used as that – a guide, and not the rule for required vaccinations. Wall charts can quickly become outdated and often look at a country as a whole, without reference to the internal distribution of a particular infectious disease. A traveller may be given unnecessary injections with considerable discomfort and financial cost or miss those appropriate for a particular destination and activity. The length and nature of the journey, either business, holiday or back packing, may affect the possible hazards the traveller may encounter. Type and standard of accommodation and sources of food and water are useful indicators for an assessment of risk. The risk of acquiring infectious disease for a young back packer travelling around sub-Saharan Africa for several months is considerably greater than that of a businessman staying in a luxury hotel for a few nights in a similar area.

Costs can be quite considerable if a number of immunizations and booster doses of vaccine is required. Indeed, in the case of a student the costs may be greater than the entire travel budget. The doctor may be asked to prioritize the immunizations required for the journey, and in this situation a careful assessment is essential. Only yellow fever immunization is a legal requirement according to international health regulations, and then only for entry to some countries. A World Health Organization (WHO) certificate of immunization issued by an official centre can be presented as proof of vaccination. There is no longer a requirement by the WHO for cholera immunization before entry to any country. Advice regarding immunization and travel health can be obtained from a variety of sources. There are a number of vaccination questions which travellers frequently ask their doctor. The following cover some of the more common queries about each of the vaccines offered by travel clinics.

HEPATITIS A

A man and his 2-year-old child are going to Goa, India, for a 2-week holiday. The father was immunized 5 years ago with hepatitis A vaccine.
Hepatitis A is a hepatovirus within the family Picornaviridae, spread by the oral–faecal route. It is found throughout the Indian subcontinent. The incubation period is 15–45 days and presents as a general malaise, myalgia and fever followed by hepatitis. Hepatitis A is the commonest vaccine-preventable disease in travellers, infecting up to 20 per 1000 per month of stay (Steffen 1992). Symptomatic disease is common in adults, but rare in children, where mild or subclinical infection is usual. The formaldehyde-inactivated vaccine is effective and recommended for all non-immune travellers.

Since young children mostly suffer asymptomatic hepatitis A infections, there is an argument for not immunizing this age group. However, the vaccine is suitable for infants over the age of 12 months and as well as preventing hepatitis A in the child, it will indirectly prevent faecal–oral spread to susceptible adults and children on return to home. It is also important to remember that although most children will not suffer severe illness, a minority will. As a result, rare complications of a common disease such as hepatitis A cause a greater burden of severe disease than the common complications of rare diseases, and protection by immunization is clearly justifiable. One dose of vaccine will give protection for at least a year, but with a booster 6–12 months later, protection can last 10 years. The recommendation is for the father to have a single reinforcing booster before travel, after which his immunity should last for at least 10 years. The child should be vaccinated against hepatitis A.

YELLOW FEVER

An HIV/AIDS patient is going on holiday to Thailand for 3 weeks. He requests numerous immunizations including yellow fever.

Yellow fever is a viral haemorrhagic fever found in Africa and parts of South and Central America. It can have a mortality in excess of 50 per cent. It is caused by a flavivirus transmitted by the bite of an infective *Aedes* mosquito. Although yellow fever is not found in Thailand, there is a requirement for travellers coming directly from yellow fever regions to South East Asia to produce a valid vaccination certificate on arrival. The reason is to prevent introduction of the disease into an area that has the appropriate mosquito vectors. An International Certificate of Vaccination is valid from the 10th day after primary immunization for a 10-year period and immediately after re-immunization. These certificates are evidence of immunization and can only be issued by clinics approved by the World Health Organization.

A live attenuated vaccine has been available for nearly 50 years, and is widely recognized as being safe and effective. There have been recent deaths in tourists to sub-Saharan Africa who were not immunized with the attenuated live vaccine. An HIV/AIDS patient should not routinely be given a live vaccine. As long as he avoids yellow fever zones on route to Thailand, he will not require the immunization.

HEPATITIS B

A man is going for a 2-week holiday to Oman. Should he have hepatitis B immunization?

Hepatitis B is prevalent throughout Asia, Africa and the Middle East. The virus is a small, enveloped hepadnavirus, and generally causes an acute hepatitis.

Most adults recover from the acute infection, but up to 10 per cent develop chronic infection ('chronic carriage' of hepatitis B) that may lead to chronic active hepatitis and eventually cirrhosis or hepatocellular carcinoma. Hepatitis B is transmited between adult individuals by unprotected sex or close contact with infected blood. Health-care workers or members of the emergency services are at increased risk. Long-stay diplomats or businessmen are also at increased risk as the possibility of giving or receiving urgent medical treatment or other close contact with infected individuals increases with time. Where the risk of exposure to hepatitis B is significant, immunization may be required.

A course of vaccine normally takes 6 months to administer. However, an accelerated course of vaccine can be given at 0, 1 and 2 months. The level of antibody protection should be measured 8 weeks after completion of the course for health-care workers, as boosting may be required. It is not routinely recommended that other occupational groups or travellers are tested for seroconversion. A holiday-maker to Oman who avoids sexual contact with the local population is highly unlikely to contract hepatitis B and immunization would not normally be advised.

JAPANESE ENCEPHALITIS

A woman is going on holiday to Bangkok, Thailand, for 2 weeks. She asks about immunization and whether it is necessary.

Japanese encephalitis is a flavivirus infection spread by the bite of culicine mosquitoes. It is endemic throughout South East Asia, mainly affecting rural communities. The natural reservoirs are wild birds (particularly waterfowl); the virus is spread by mosquitoes to an intermediate multiplier host, usually domestic pigs. Man is accidentally infected when virus is spread from the pig by a second mosquito. The net effect is that the infection is normally only seen in people who live and work in rural farming communities. It presents as an acute viral illness of short duration with marked neurological effects.

The vaccine is at present unlicensed but is available on a named patient basis. There have been a number of adverse reaction reports with this vaccine, and it should only be given after careful consideration of the risk of infection. Since the risk is greater in rural areas during the rainy season, the vaccine is normally recommended only for those individuals staying in areas of high transmission for a month or more. This woman is unlikely to require Japanese encephalitis immunization as she is only visiting for a short time and staying in a tourist area.

RABIES

A male member of a trekking expedition to the Himalayas asks for rabies immunization.
Rabies is found throughout the world and is a virus infection contracted via the bite or saliva of an infected mammal, normally a dog, cat or bat. Pre-exposure rabies vaccine is advised for individuals likely to be in close contact with animals in endemic areas. Human diploid cell vaccine (HDCV) is given in three doses on days 0, 7 and 28 by intramuscular injection into the deltoid. In travellers for whom post-exposure prophylaxis is likely to be available, 98 per cent of recipients will develop immunity after a two-dose course at days 0 and 28.

Post-exposure treatment of animal bites includes scrubbing the wound with soap and water, seeking local medical advice about the prevalence of rabies in the area and, if possible, identifying the suspect animal for a 10-day observation period. An assessment of likely rabies infection should be carried out and subsequent management with boosting doses of HDCV and human rabies-specific immunoglobulin (HRSI) may be required. The exact type of treatment will depend on the number of doses and quality of vaccine given pre-exposure within the last 2 years. In the previously non-immune individual, five doses of HDCV will be required on days 0, 3, 7, 14 and 30. HRSI will be required at a dose of 20 iu kg^{-1} body weight, with 50 per cent given intramuscularly and the remainder infiltrated around the wound site.

Due to the long incubation period of rabies infection (2–8 weeks), most travellers have enough time to reach medical care and ensure protective post-exposure treatment. In this particular expedition to the Himalayas, the trekkers will be passing through areas that have rabies-infected animals, and the ability to evacuate and treat individuals is not without difficulty. Rabies immunization is warranted.

TUBERCULOSIS

A diplomat is moving to New Delhi for 2 years with his wife and two children aged 5 and 7 years.
Tuberculosis is one of the main causes of infective mortality throughout the world and is caused by the bacterium *Mycobacterium tuberculosis*. Inadequate treatment and poor drug compliance have led to an increase in multi-drug-resistant tuberculosis, and this is particularly so in parts of Africa and the Indian subcontinent. The increasing numbers of HIV-positive cases has also worsened the control and prevention of tuberculosis throughout the developing world.

BCG is a live attenuated bacterial vaccine. In populations where there is low endemicity of tuberculosis, BCG vaccine has been shown to be protective. Trials involving indigenous populations of India and Africa demonstrated a far lesser protective effect with BCG. This is thought to be due to immune populations primed by natural environmental *Mycobacterium* species, causing BCG to have a reduced protective effect. In some countries, adults should routinely have had BCG as a child. This can be confirmed by the presence of a scar. For a child a prolonged period in an endemic area, such as India, warrants immunization after tuberculin skin testing.

TICK-BORNE ENCEPHALITIS

A camper is going to Bavaria on holiday.
Tick-borne encephalitis is a viral meningoencephalitis transmitted to man via a tick bite or, more rarely, through consumption of unpasteurized milk. Case fatality rate is 1 per cent and neurological recovery in survivors can be prolonged.

Infected ticks are predominantly found in thick, forested areas of Central and Eastern Europe and Scandinavia. It is important to know when the camper is going on holiday as the period of highest risk is late spring and summer, when tick nymphs and young adults are most numerous and active. The vaccine is at present unlicensed and is only available on a named patient basis. Insect repellents and covering exposed limbs help prevent tick bites, and offer additional protection against other tick-borne diseases such as Lyme disease. Vaccine should be given once a risk assessment has been done on the camper's likely exposure to ticks.

TETANUS

A student is backpacking through Africa.
Tetanus is a toxin-mediated disease caused by the anaerobic growth within tissues of *Clostridium tetani*. An effective toxoid vaccine has been available for many years. Current recommendations are that

all individuals should receive a primary course of three doses of tetanus toxoid as an infant. This is normally given as part of the diphtheria, tetanus and pertussis vaccine. A booster dose of diphtheria and tetanus toxoid is recommended 3 years after primary immunization (pre-school), with a further reinforcing booster of tetanus and low-dose diphtheria vaccine recommended for older children before leaving school. This five-dose course of tetanus toxoid is thought to maintain satisfactory protective antibody levels for life.

The management of 'tetanus-prone' or 'clean' wounds depends on the immunization status of the individual. All patients with tetanus-prone injuries are advised to have tetanus immunoglobulin, even if the last reinforcing toxoid dose was within 10 years. A student will probably have received all five doses of toxoid in childhood. Backpacking across Africa may lead to situations where tetanus-prone injuries could occur, and access to good quality tetanus immunoglobulin from a verified source cannot be guaranteed throughout Africa. It may be wise to consider a reinforcing booster dose of toxoid before departure.

DIPHTHERIA

A 45-year-old male teacher is undertaking voluntary work in Russia for 2 years.
Diphtheria is an upper respiratory tract disease caused by *Corynebacterium diphtheriae*. Severe pharyngeal inflammation can lead to respiratory obstruction and death. A toxin is produced by the bacterium during the illness, which is toxic to cardiac muscle and nerve tissues. The inactivated diphtheria toxoid vaccine has been available since 1942, and diphtheria is now seen rarely. Most adults under the age of 60 years will have received diphtheria vaccine as a child. Child vaccination programmes usually include diphtheria with tetanus and pertussis immunizations as a triple vaccine, or the double tetanus/diphtheria vaccine. Over the age of 10 years, reactions to diphtheria vaccine can be rather severe and low-dose diphtheria or low-dose diphtheria/tetanus vaccines are recommended in this age group.

It is difficult to predict how long immunity to diphtheria persists after primary immunization. There is no widely available serological test to measure diphtheria immunity and, due to its poor predicative value, the Schick test is no longer used. The whole of Eastern Europe and the countries of the former USSR have experienced a dramatic increase in the numbers of diphtheria cases in recent years. If the patient has not received a booster dose within the last 10 years, they should be given a low-dose diphtheria vaccine before departure.

MENINGITIS

A holiday-maker is off on a 10-day safari in Kenya.
Meningococcal infection is a severe, often devastating illness caused by the bacterium *Neisseria meningitidis*. There are several serotypes of this bacterium, but most illness is caused by groups B and C. The disease is spread by respiratory droplets and requires close contact such as prolonged living in the same household or kissing. In sub-Saharan Africa epidemics of *Neisseria meningitidis* group A occur mostly in the dry season.

A combination meningococcal polysaccharide A and C vaccine is recommended for visits longer than 4 weeks' duration, especially if living and working with local people or backpacking in isolated areas. A quadrivalent vaccine against meningococcal groups A, C, W135 and Y is recommended in the UK for pilgrims attending the Hajj in Saudi Arabia. The conjugate vaccine introduced recently protects against group C disease only, and, if required, the polysaccharide A and C vaccine should be given even if they have previously received the conjugate vaccine. A holiday-maker on a safari in Kenya will not be in exposed close contact with the local population and meningococcal immunization in this case is unnecessary.

POLIO

A 25-year-old woman is travelling to several South and Central American countries on holiday.
Poliomyelitis is an acute viral illness which can severely damage motor neurones and other nerve tissues. The majority of poliomyelitis infections are asymptomatic, resulting in a large number of apparently well individuals excreting virus particles in faeces or pharyngeal secretions. The virus may be present in faeces for greater than 6 weeks after the initial infection.

An inactivated vaccine (Salk) was introduced in the 1950s, followed by the live attenuated oral vaccine (Sabin) in the 1960s. Individuals born before these times may not have been immunized against poliomyelitis. A primary course of three oral poliomyelitis vaccines is recommended for infants from 2 months of age, with booster doses before school entry and before leaving school. Immunization has been successful throughout Western Europe with the disease virtually eliminated.

Reinforcing doses are only recommended for travellers going to high-risk areas. There have been no reported cases of wild-type poliomyelitis virus infection in any part of the Americas since 1991, and it is now considered eliminated from that region. The World Health Organization launched a global polio eradication initiative in 1988, since when the number of polio cases has dropped by over 95 per cent, from an estimated 350 000 in 1988 to 7094 in 1999. The 25-year-old woman should have received a primary course and school booster immunizations in the UK, and does not require reinforcing for a trip to South and Central America.

MALARIA

Malaria remains one of the most important infectious diseases in the world. An estimated 500 million individuals are infected annually, and more than 3 million die. Whilst the vast majority of the burden is borne by developing countries, a significant number of international travellers are affected. In the UK alone it is estimated that approximately 3.5 million people travel to tropical countries each year, resulting in an average of 2000 malaria cases per annum. In 1998, 15 deaths were reported, a figure that has remained more or less constant over the last 25 years. Detailed investigation of these cases has shown that the majority take few precautions to prevent malaria, and in those people most severely affected, the diagnosis is either delayed or missed altogether. Reducing the risk from malaria is relatively straightforward, and can be summarized as the 'ABC approach'.

A is for awareness

Travellers need basic education about the disease. For example, they must be told that the infection is spread by the bite of an infective mosquito, and that most vectors feed on humans between the hours of dusk and dawn. They need accurate information on the malaria risk posed by their particular destination. This may require a detailed travel itinerary, since malaria is not uniformly distributed in endemic areas, and is also seasonal in many parts of the world. An accurate source of up-to-date travel information is therefore mandatory for most travel health advisers.

Travellers should be advised that no precautions are totally effective, and that they may still develop the disease. The symptoms and signs that indicate possible malaria should be described, and they should be told to seek medical advice without delay if they become ill. The possibility of malaria remains for several months after return from an endemic area, and they should be asked to volunteer their travel history whenever they visit medical practitioners.

B is for bite avoidance

The simple truth is that malaria is spread by the bite of a malaria-carrying mosquito. It follows that if 'you don't get bitten, you don't get malaria'. The measures available to reduce bites can be divided into behavioural modifications and physical protection. Common sense precautions include limiting outdoor activity, such as 'drinks on the veranda' or the pursuit of nocturnal wildlife, during the hours of darkness when the malaria-carrying mosquitoes are active. If these cannot be avoided, then sensible clothing that offers a degree of protection against biting insects, such as long-sleeved shirts and trousers, should be worn.

Specific physical precautions include long-acting insect repellent creams, clothing impregnated with insecticide, and mosquito nets impregnated with insecticide. Bite avoidance would also include the use of insect-screened accommodation, together with knockdown insecticide sprays. Mosquito repellent coils and electrical vaporizing mats have been shown to be effective, but there is no scientific evidence to support the claims for electronic buzzers or similar devices. For long-term travellers, there can be attempts at reduction of local mosquito populations by environmental control. This may include drainage of standing water, the application of larvicide to mosquito breeding sites and the use of long-acting residual insecticides.

C is for chemoprophylaxis

Advisory committees on malaria prevention provide national guidance on the choice of antimalarials (Bradley and Warhurst 1997). It is important to recognize that there is international variation in advice. This results from pharmaceutical marketing strategies and national licensing differences, as well as differing opinions and idiosyncrasies. There is therefore no 'right or wrong' antimalarial for a given destination, merely one best suited to an individual traveller. Detailed discussion of individual antimalarial agents is beyond the scope of this chapter.

The spread of drug-resistant *Plasmodium falciparum* has led to a decline in usefulness of many drugs. Of the newer agents, mefloquine, in particular, has come under close examination over its adverse event profile. It remains extremely effective at preventing malaria in most parts of the world, but the safety concerns have led to increasingly poor compliance. Malarone, a combination of atovaquone and proguanil, has been introduced recently as a substitute for short-term travellers, but more clinical experience is needed. In practice, the main objective is to get the traveller to take any prophylaxis, not necessarily the best, and a compromise may be necessary. Relatively few travellers contract malaria as a result of 'breakthrough' on prophylaxis, but many more become sick because they have taken no medication. During pregnancy the patient should be advised not to travel to a region with malaria unless absolutely necessary. In such an event expert advice should be sought on prophylaxis.

D is for diagnosis

None of the measures outlined above can be guaranteed to be entirely effective, particularly in parts of the world like West Africa where malaria transmission is intense. Early diagnosis and treatment of cases when they occur are therefore important. Medical personnel should consider the possibility of malaria in any returning tropical traveller. Non-immune people with malaria can deteriorate quickly and cases are potentially a medical emergency.

SYMPTOMS OF AN INFECTION

Most travellers return to their country of origin in good health. Occasionally, a traveller will return with symptoms of an infection, which necessitates a visit to their medical practitioner. A proper history must be taken, including where they were, for how long they were there, what exactly were they doing whilst they were there, standard of living accommodation and food/water supply. A vaccination history and type of antimalarial prophylaxis should be noted. Any blood or body fluid contact and any sexual contacts should be documented. The presenting symptoms of any patient will vary depending on the nature of the disease and the type of patient infected, but generally include one or more of fever, diarrhoea, skin rash or genitourinary symptoms.

Malaria must be considered in all returned travellers with a fever, especially if they have been in or transited through a malarious area. Malaria prophylaxis is continued for 4 weeks after returning home. However, it should be remembered that no anti-malarial drug is totally effective, and that malaria can still develop despite continued prophylaxis. A malarial film is a simple and routine test, which is an essential requirement in the returned traveller with fever. Another common cause of fever is chest infection. Legionnaires' disease, which can be associated with hotel accommodation, should be considered in all travellers.

The need for laboratory investigations will depend on the history and clinical examination. However, illness in the recently returned traveller will probably require a blood culture, a mid-stream specimen of urine and a stool for culture and microscopy for ova, cysts and parasites. A full blood count should be included with particular attention to the white cells and any eosinophilia, which is an indicator of parasitic infection. Liver function tests and C-reactive protein are always useful. Viral and bacteriological serological tests can be requested. Diagnosis can be difficult and the early advice of a physician specializing in infectious diseases or a microbiologist may be appropriate.

REFERENCES

Anon. Tropical ulcers after sports injuries. [letter] *Lancet* 1992; **339**: 129–30.

Association of Port Health Authorities. *Code of Practice: on Dealing with Infectious Disease on Aircraft.* Runcorn, Cheshire: APHA, 1995.

Bradley DJ and Warhurst DC. Guidelines for the prevention of malaria in travellers from the United Kingdom. *CDR Rev* 1997; **7**: R138–51. [download from: www.phls.co.uk/advice/cdrr1097.pdf].

Connor MP and Green AD. Travellers diarrhoea and the use of single dose ciprofloxacin. *Lancet* 1995; **345**: 381–2.

Cossar JH and Reid D. Health hazards of international travel. *World Health Stat Q* 1989; **42**: 61–9.

Goldstein FW and Garau J. 30 years of penicillin-resistant *Streptococcus pneumoniae*: myth or reality? Editorial. *Lancet* 1997; **350**: 233–4.

Hargarten SW, Baker T and Guptil K. Fatalities of American travellers – 1975, 1984. In Steffen R, Lobel HO, Haworth J and Bradley DJ (eds), *Proceedings of the First Conference on Travel Medicine*. London and New York: Springer, 1989; 55–64.

Kenyon TA, Valway SE, Ihle WW, Onorato IM and Castro KG. Transmission of multidrug-resistant *Mycobacterium tuberculosis* during a long airplane flight. *N Engl J Med* 1996; **334**: 933–8.

Steffen R. Travel medicine. Prevention based on epidemiological data. *Trans R Soc Trop Med Hyg* 1991; **85**: 156–2.

Steffen R. Risk of hepatitis A in travellers. *Vaccine* 1992; **10** (Suppl): S69–72.

Stricker M, Steffen R, Gutzwiller F and Eichmann A. Casual sexual contacts of Swiss tourists in tropical Africa, the Far East and Latin America. In *Proceedings of the 2nd International Conference on Travel Medicine*. Atlanta: International Society of Travel Medicine, 1991; 220–1.

Wick RL and Irvine LA. The microbiological composition of airliner cabin air. *Aviat Space Environ Med* 1995; **66**: 220–4.

World Tourism Organization. *Global Tourism Forecasts to the Year 2000 and Beyond. Executive Summary.* New York: World Tourism Organization, 1999.

Zhi-Biao. Studies on the clinical manifestations, diagnosis and control of paragonimiasis in China. In Cross JH (ed.), *Emerging Problems in Food-borne Parasitic Zoonosis: Impact on Agriculture and Public Health.* Bangkok: Thai Watana Panish Press Co. Ltd, 1991; 345–8.

FURTHER READING: PUBLICATIONS FROM THE WORLD HEALTH ORGANIZATION

International Health Regulations, 3rd edn. Geneva: WHO, 1983.

International Travel and Health. Vaccination Requirements and Health Advice. Geneva: WHO, 2001.

Tuberculosis and Air Travel. Guidelines for Prevention and Control. Geneva: WHO, 1998.

Airsickness

JR ROLLIN STOTT

The sick bag in the seat pocket in front of every airline passenger is still a feature of modern commercial flying. To a large extent this is a legacy of the days when passenger aircraft were unpressurized and therefore limited to flying below 10 000 feet at which altitudes it was frequently necessary to fly through the turbulent air of the prevailing weather conditions. Present-day aircraft at cruising altitudes in excess of 30 000 feet may still encounter clear air turbulence, but are generally flying well above the atmospheric effects of the weather. The sick bag has gained alternative uses for the disposal of small items of rubbish, and the sequestering of items of food. In the hands of one enterprising bag designer, it can be used, if still pristine, as a postal bag for camera films so that on arrival at the airport the holiday snaps can be sent off for processing.

While it may be true that airsickness among passengers is much less a problem in present-day commercial flight, it has probably not entirely disappeared, though there are relatively few relevant studies to support this assertion. A survey conducted in 1946–47 gathered data from over a million air passengers flying in unpressurized aircraft, mainly DC3 and DC4 aircraft (Lederer and Kidera 1954). The authors reported that 'over three quarters of all cases of discomfort were caused by airsickness'. The overall incidence of airsickness was found to be 0.5 per cent, but it was noted that 'when motion sickness strikes in any one airplane the incidence is approximately 8 per cent of those on

board'. A comparison of the DC3 and DC4 showed that the incidence of sickness was greater on the smaller DC3 aircraft, which seated 21 passengers, as against 44 in the DC4.

The majority of the surveys carried out since that time has involved military operations that are of little relevance to the airline passenger. It is not surprising that meteorological flights at 500 feet into hurricane conditions provoked severe nausea and vomiting in about 20 per cent and some degree of malaise in 95 per cent of the aircrew involved. Airsickness was associated with the vertical motion of the aircraft, but the observation was made that it was not the 'bumpiest' conditions that provoked the most sickness but rather a lower, physically more comfortable, frequency of vertical oscillation at around 25 cycles min^{-1} (0.4 Hz). Studies under more controlled laboratory conditions have confirmed the inverse relationship between the incidence of motion sickness and the frequency of vertical oscillation and indicate that the peak incidence of sickness is found with sinusoidal motion at a frequency of 0.2 Hz.

A recent report (Turner *et al.* 2000) has gone some way to providing figures for the present-day incidence of airsickness. A questionnaire survey was carried out among 923 passengers on 38 flights within the UK. The survey involved two aircraft types, the Shorts 360, a 36-seat unpressurized aircraft of 12 290 kg maximum take-off weight with a cruising altitude of 7000 feet, and the British Aerospace ATP, a pressurized aircraft with a maximum take-off weight of 23 680 kg, seating 68 passengers and cruising at 15 000–20 000 feet. The duration of flights was short, ranging from 35 to 70 minutes. The survey found an overall incidence of nausea of 8.4 per cent, ranging on different flights from 0 to 34.8 per cent. The incidence of vomiting was 0.5 per cent. Asked what had been the worst they had felt during the flight, 0.4 per cent had felt 'absolutely dreadful', 1.6 per cent 'quite ill', and 14.2 per cent 'slightly unwell'. However, on individual flights the percentage of passengers reporting some degree of illness ranged between 0 and 47.8 per cent.

A direct comparison between this and the earlier study on the DC3 and DC4 aircraft is limited by a lack of gradation or definition in the earlier study of what constituted airsickness. However, given the similarity in size and flying altitude between the Shorts 360 and the DC3 and DC4 aircraft, a similar incidence of airsickness might be expected. Perhaps surprisingly, the recent study found no difference in the incidence of nausea or illness between the two aircraft types surveyed. It is possible that the relative brevity of the flights did not allow a significant advantage to accrue from the higher cruising altitude of the ATP aircraft.

Compared with sea travel, the motion environment of a commercial aircraft is extremely smooth. The survey by Turner et al. (2000) also involved measurement of triaxial accelerations within the aircraft. From these measurements the authors were able to calculate a motion sickness dose value (MSDV), an index of motion sickness incidence derived from laboratory studies using vertical oscillatory motion and measurements of the vertical component of motion aboard ships. This calculation involves weighting the measured accelerations, in order to retain only those frequencies that contribute to motion sickness (Figure 6.1), and integrating the squared weighted values over time. None of the flights yielded a value for MSDV greater than 10. By contrast, a series of measurements aboard cross-channel ferries yielded values for MSDV of up to 80. It is doubtful whether the results of this survey can be extrapolated to international short-haul operations, still less to long-haul intercontinental flights. These flights involve long periods at cruising altitudes where atmospheric turbulence is less and during which aircraft manoeuvres can be carried out more gently.

It could be predicted that the incidence of airsickness would be less, but data are lacking.

MOTION SICKNESS

Motion sickness gives rise to a sequence of symptoms and signs, the earliest of which may be a feeling of lethargy, yawning and a need for fresh air. Other early symptoms include light-headedness, dizziness and headache. Worsening nausea associated with pallor and sweating may eventually lead to vomiting. None of these symptoms is in itself specific for motion sickness. In circumstances in which the provocative motion stimulus is relatively mild, or in individuals who are less susceptible, the earlier symptoms may be the only evidence of motion sickness.

The apparent lack of purpose in vomiting in response to motion has led to the opinion, particularly among those who have never experienced motion sickness, that the condition is all in the mind. However, it has been known for over a century that the only individuals who are completely immune to the condition are those with total lack of function in the vestibular labyrinths of the inner ear. Bilateral labyrinthine deficiency is rare and the overwhelming majority of the population who have normal labyrinthine function can be made motion sick if the stimulus is sufficiently severe. However, there is a wide spread of susceptibilities to motion sickness, the physiological basis of which is as yet unexplained. From a theoretical point of view there are two essential questions:

- What is it about motion that leads to motion sickness?
- Why is the outcome nausea and vomiting?

From a practical point of view there is just one question: how can motion sickness be prevented? Theory and practice are not totally independent, however, and an understanding of the theory leads to practical measures for the prophylaxis of the condition.

The concept of sensory conflict offers the best explanation for why certain types of motion lead to motion sickness and others do not. The brain has to integrate information from various sensory receptors to arrive at a perception of orientation and motion with respect to the external environment.

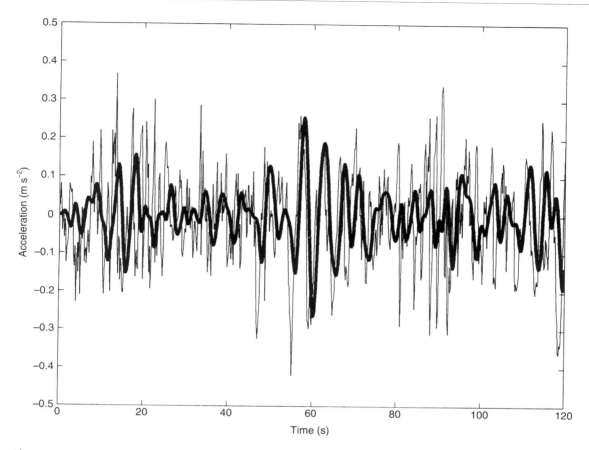

Figure 6.1 *Recording of vertical acceleration from a commercial aircraft during a 2-minute period of high-level turbulence (thin line). Superimposed is a version of the same record filtered to retain only the vibration frequencies liable to lead to motion sickness (thick line). The higher frequency oscillations evident at around 20 and 90 seconds through the recording contribute less to motion sickness than the lower frequency oscillations seen at around 60 seconds.*

While the eye transduces the visual environment, the vestibular system transduces the force environment. Because the visual environment is predominantly static and the force environment for pedestrian man is dominated by the force of gravity, constant in direction and intensity, certain sensory inter-relationships become the expected norm. During turning movements of the head there is an expect-ation that the visual world will remain stationary. However, we only perceive it as such if the field of view changes at a rate appropriate to the rate of turn of the head.

Similarly, tilting of the head out of the horizontal plane must result in an equivalently tilted view of the world to allow the brain to perceive it as static. Head tilt must also result in an appropriate change in the direction of gravity as sensed by the otolith organs of the inner ear. The sensed intensity of gravity is also expected to remain constant. Superimposed on the constant gravitational acceler-ation are the fluctuating vertical accelerations asso-ciated with locomotor activities. These fluctuations occur at the frequency of walking or running, about 1–3 Hz. Experimental studies of vertical oscillation indicate that motion sickness is not induced at these frequencies, but its incidence tends to increase as the frequency of vertical oscillation is reduced below about 0.8 Hz and reaches a maximum at about

0.2 Hz. A similar relationship of motion sickness with frequency is also found with horizontal oscillation, equivalent to the alternate acceleration and braking of a vehicle.

Whilst the concept of sensory conflict offers an explanation of the characteristics of motion that result in sickness, it has little to say about the relevance of the symptoms of nausea and vomiting to these types of motion. Another clinical feature of motion sickness is the output of stress hormones that accompanies the development of symptoms. For some reason, an abnormal motion environment evokes the declaration of a physiological state of emergency. Many animals when exposed to similar abnormal motion environments will also vomit. Even fish have been observed to vomit in response to motion. Neither these creatures, nor indeed humans, can have evolved this emetic mechanism as a purposeful response to types of motion that they could never have experienced in their evolutionary past.

On the other hand, vomiting *per se* has a more obvious evolutionary benefit if it results in the removal from the stomach of potentially toxic substances that the animal may have ingested. The more convincing explanation of the emetic response we call motion sickness is that the brain has evolved to use the constancy of the gravitational and visual environment as a form of self-calibration. If the expected inter-relationships between vestibular and visual sensory information are not found, this is interpreted as a malfunction of the brain itself. If such malfunction were the result of some ingested neurotoxin, then vomiting could be an appropriate response to eliminate any that still remained in the gut. The fact that certain motion environments generate patterns of sensory input that the brain detects as illegitimate and thereby trigger an emetic response now appears as an unfortunate coincidence.

AIRCRAFT MOTION

In aircraft, as in other means of transport, there are two components of the motion of the aircraft that may provoke motion sickness. One is determined by the external environment, specifically the turbulent air through which the aircraft is flying, the other by the way in which aircraft manoeuvres are flown by the pilot or the autopilot. Turbulent air can be generated at low level by winds blowing across surface features such as hills and mountain ridges. It also occurs from the meeting of air masses with different temperatures and water vapour content. When warm moist air is forced upwards by the influx of colder air, cumulus clouds are formed. In some conditions these can build into tall cloud columns (cumulonimbus), which may extend upwards to 30 000 feet or more, and are often associated with thunderstorms. The air in them is undergoing rapid vertical movement, which generates severe turbulence. Commercial aircraft can expect to be re-routed around such storm activity assisted by the aircraft's weather radar system, which detects regions of heavy precipitation where turbulence is likely to be most severe.

When flying at altitudes above the prevailing weather conditions, there remains the possibility that the aircraft will encounter clear air turbulence, often at the boundaries of high velocity horizontal air movements (jetstreams). Although the probability of clear air turbulence can be forecast, its precise location cannot be detected. The motion imposed on the aircraft by turbulence is predominantly a vertical oscillation but varies in character from a sensation akin to driving over cobblestones to a slow wallowing motion. On rare occasions, the downward motion of the aircraft may be so abrupt that objects and people encounter the roof of the aircraft cabin. Because the incidence of motion sickness caused by vertical oscillation is dependent on its frequency, so turbulence varies in its propensity to cause motion sickness. Whilst higher frequencies of vertical motion may be physically more uncomfortable, they are less likely to result in sickness, whereas frequencies of around 0.2 Hz, one cycle of motion every 5 seconds, will lead to nausea.

The way in which an aircraft is flown can also lead to airsickness. Many keen flying students with only moderate susceptibility to motion sickness have discovered that the over-enthusiastic demonstration of aerobatics in the early stages of training can be a nauseating and dispiriting experience. In passenger aircraft the only manoeuvres of any significance are turning manoeuvres. For aerodynamic reasons and also for considerations of passenger comfort and the stability of people and objects within the aircraft cabin, a change of aircraft heading is made by means

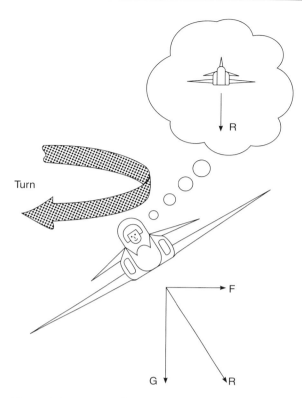

Figure 6.2 *In a coordinated turn, the aircraft is banked so that the combination of gravity (G) and the dynamic force associated with the change of direction (F) gives a resultant force (R) that no longer points to the centre of the earth but remains directed vertically with respect to the aircraft and feels like gravity to the occupants of the aircraft. To a passenger with no external view, the roll manoeuvre of the aircraft is not associated with any sense of tilt, either of self or of the visual world, as would normally be expected.*

of a coordinated turn (Figure 6.2). The combination of the radial inertial force that accompanies a change of direction of a moving object and the downward force of gravity creates a resultant force at an intermediate angle between the two forces. The aircraft is banked in the turn by an angle that leaves the resultant force directed at all times during the turn at right angles to the floor of the aircraft. The result of this is that throughout the turn the occupants of the aircraft are aware of no change in the direction of what they sense as gravity.

However, depending on the rate of turn demanded, the pilot has had to roll the aircraft by up to 30° to achieve this. Such a manoeuvre contravenes normal

terrestrial expectations in that rotation in roll would be expected to be associated with a change in the sensed direction of an invariant force of gravity and a tilted view of a static visual world. To the aircraft passenger with no view of the external world, neither of these expectations is fulfilled. In practice, this sensory conflict is minimized by keeping the rate of aircraft roll at or near to the threshold of perception for roll angular motion. Typical laboratory-measured perception thresholds are of the order of $2° \, s^{-1}$, though some individuals can detect velocities of $1° \, s^{-1}$. Under autopilot control in large commercial aircraft, roll rates are usually less than $3° \, s^{-1}$. In this way, changes of aircraft heading in the cruise can be achieved without most passengers being aware that any change has taken place. This, however, may not be possible for turns immediately after take-off or for turns in holding patterns or during aircraft positioning on the approach to land.

Another aspect of aircraft turns is the change in G force on the aircraft occupants during the turn. The combination of the radial force of the turn and the force of gravity produces a resultant force that is of greater intensity than gravity alone. For angles of bank of less than 10° this effect is negligible, at 20° the resultant force is 6 per cent greater than gravity and at 30° it is 15 per cent greater. Tilt head movements made in an altered G environment often provoke a sense of giddiness which with repetition may lead to nausea and vomiting. This effect is probably the major determinant of motion sickness during space flight, a condition which affects over 50 per cent of astronauts. In terms of sensory conflict, there is an expected agreement between the amount of angular head movement in pitch or roll as sensed by the semicircular canals and the amount of tilt with respect to the direction of gravity sensed by the otoliths. A changed gravitational intensity alters the neural signal from the otoliths for a given degree of head tilt and thus disturbs the normal canal–otolith relationship.

INDIVIDUAL SUSCEPTIBILITY

Susceptibility to motion sickness shows wide variation between individuals that cannot be explained by differences in tests of vestibular function or sensitivity to the detection of motion. There are only weak correlations between motion sickness susceptibility and a number of psychometric measures, which are consequently of little predictive value. Susceptibility changes with age. Questionnaire surveys from a variety of transport environments indicate that, while children below the age of 2 years are relatively immune, susceptibility increases until early adolescence and thereafter declines with age. Females are somewhat more susceptible than males. However, compared with the range of individual susceptibilities, these age- and sex-related differences in susceptibility are small.

Nauseogenic stimuli are likely to be additive so that an individual suffering from an illness characterized by nausea and vomiting may be made worse by encountering nauseogenic motion. Similarly, concurrent treatment with drugs whose side effects include nausea and vomiting can render an individual more susceptible to motion sickness. The same is probably true following radiotherapy. With continued exposure to the same nauseogenic motion, subjects tend to become increasingly tolerant. This is seen following repeated exposures (habituation) if these are separated by no more than a few days and also during a single period of exposure (adaptation). This ability to adapt to unfamiliar patterns of motion may well be the most important determinant of susceptibility in a particular motion environment.

There are a number of behavioural measures that can minimize the likelihood of airsickness. In roller-coaster-type flight manoeuvres it has been shown that individuals who kept the head upright became less airsick than those in whom the head was held tilted forwards towards the floor. The benefit of fixing the head relative to the shoulders by the use of a collar has been shown in relation to airsickness induced by parabolic flight manoeuvres in which periods of 0 G alternate with periods of 2 G. These findings suggest that when a passenger aircraft encounters turbulence or is executing turns at higher angles of bank, those with a susceptibility to motion sickness should avoid head movement and keep the head upright resting against the head cushion of the seat. These prophylactic measures are most relevant at the start and end of a flight when turns are more frequent and often at greater angles of bank. Once in the cruise, apart from the possibility of encountering a prolonged period of clear air turbulence, discordant motion stimuli are infre-

quent and there is less likelihood of developing airsickness.

There is laboratory evidence of the benefit of mental distraction. Subjects undergoing nauseogenic motion who were instructed to concentrate on the motion that they experienced became unwell more rapidly than those who were given a mental arithmetic task to perform. In the survey of Turner et al. (2000), respondents to a questionnaire were asked to indicate their predominant activity during the flight. The highest incidence of nausea was found in the group who reported doing nothing whilst the lowest was found in the group who gave reading as their principal activity. Unfortunately, these observations do not necessarily imply a causal connection but there is no denying the distracting qualities of a good book. For some individuals flying is an activity that provokes a degree of anxiety. The survey also found that among those who said that they disliked flying, the incidence of illness and nausea was three times greater. Again, it is not possible from this finding to determine whether a fear or dislike of flying is a contributory factor to symptoms that could be described as motion sickness or whether previous motion illness aboard aircraft leads to a dislike of flying. Some travellers susceptible to motion sickness claim benefit from the use of elasticated bands that apply pressure to a point near the wrist, the Nei-Kuan point of Chinese acupuncture, though laboratory controlled studies have not shown an effectiveness greater than placebo.

MEDICATION

For those in whom behavioural measures are insufficient, there are several drugs available for the prophylaxis of motion sickness. The airsickness survey found a higher incidence of nausea among the 2.7 per cent of passengers who had taken anti-motion sickness medication than those who had not. It would be perverse to conclude from this that anti-motion sickness medication causes motion sickness. Rather, there is a degree of anticipatory behaviour that leads those with a susceptibility to motion sickness to take prophylactic medication. However, it does indicate that such medication is not always effective and may also suggest that the anticipation of becoming motion sick contributes to its likelihood. There should be no need for the use of prophylactic drugs in children below the age of 2 years, nor should it be assumed that if an older child requires medication for travel sickness in cars and coaches there will necessarily be a similar need during travel by air.

Motion-induced nausea and vomiting is unresponsive to a number of drugs that are conventionally used against emesis in a clinical setting. Drugs such as metoclopramide, domperidone, chlorpromazine and other phenothiazines such as prochlorperazine, are all without effect in motion-induced nausea and vomiting. Likewise, the $5HT_3$ antagonists, such as ondansetron, that are valuable antiemetics following cytotoxic chemotherapy are similarly ineffective in motion sickness. The beneficial effect of tincture of belladonna, whose active ingredients are atropine and hyoscine (scopolamine), was first described in sea-going passengers in 1865. Hyoscine, the more effective of the two constituents, was not fully investigated until World War II when it was used to protect against motion sickness in troop transport by air and sea. It remains the most researched drug, though not necessarily the most appropriate. In an oral dose of 0.3–0.6 mg, hyoscine reaches a peak activity within 1 hour and has a plasma half-life of about 4 hours. Side effects are frequent, including dry mouth, light-headedness and drowsiness. Hyoscine has also been shown to impair short-term memory. With repeated doses, impairment of visual accommodation may become evident, particularly in hypermetropes.

Laboratory studies using oral hyoscine indicate wide individual differences in its degree of efficacy and also in the incidence of side effects. Hyoscine is also available in the form of a dermal patch that delivers approximately 1 mg over a 72-hour period. Following application it may take 6–8 hours to build up an effective level of drug. The use of these patches in children has been associated with serious toxicity and they are therefore contraindicated below 10 years of age. In both childhood and in the elderly, there is a reduced therapeutic margin for hyoscine, which renders it less appropriate for motion sickness prophylaxis in these groups.

Some of the older antihistaminics that have good CNS penetration are also effective in the prophylaxis of motion sickness. In this group are cinnarizine, cyclizine and promethazine. The time to peak activity for these drugs is longer than that for hyoscine. In a laboratory study of cinnarizine no prophylactic benefit was found at 1 hour after ingestion whereas benefit was evident at 5 hours. The adult dose of cinnarizine 30 mg (half this dose in the age group 5–10 years) should therefore be taken at least 2 hours before a flight and can be repeated every 8 hours if required. Cyclizine may be marginally more effective than cinnarizine. It is taken in a dose of 50 mg (25 mg if aged 5–10 years) at least 2 hours before flight and further doses at 8-hourly intervals if necessary. Promethazine, a phenothiazine derivative, possesses in addition to its antihistaminic activity significant anti-muscarinic activity. It tends to be more sedating than the other antihistaminics and has a longer duration of action of about 24 hours, which makes its use inappropriate for all but the longest flights. It is taken in a dose of 25–50 mg (half this dose in childhood) 3–4 hours before flight. Because of its slow onset and long duration of action, 25 mg may be taken on the night before a morning flight.

A further group of drugs that has shown some prophylactic benefit in laboratory studies is the centrally acting sympathomimetics, amphetamine and ephedrine. These drugs are seldom, if ever, used alone but have been used in conjunction with hyoscine or promethazine principally to counter their sedative side effects. Although the anti-motion sickness properties of amphetamine may be slightly greater than ephedrine, its use for this purpose is seldom justified on account of the possibility of drug dependence. The combinations of ephedrine 30 mg with either hyoscine 0.6 mg or promethazine 50 mg have been shown to be highly effective in more demanding motion environments than are likely to be encountered in commercial flight.

The prophylactic benefit of any drug is most necessary at the start of motion exposure before there has been any opportunity for adaptation. It is therefore important to follow the manufacturer's recommendations concerning the time of ingestion, and better to take medication too early than too late. It is also important to give consideration to the duration of action and sedative side effects so that unwanted effects do not add risks, for example, to car driving before or after the journey. Sufferers from motion sickness may need to try several of the available drugs to find the one that is most suitable.

REFERENCES

Lederer LG and Kidera GJ. Passenger comfort in commercial air travel with reference to motion sickness. *Int Rec Med Gen Pract Clin* 1954; **167**: 661–8.

Turner M, Griffin MJ and Holland I. Airsickness and aircraft motion during short-haul flights. *Aviat Space Environ Med* 2000; **71**: 1181–9.

FURTHER READING

Benson AJ. Motion sickness. In Ernsting J, Nicholson AN and Rainford DJ (eds), *Aviation Medicine*. Oxford: Butterworth-Heinemann, 1999; 455–71.

Motion Sickness: Significance in Aerospace Operations and Prophylaxis. Lecture Series 175. Neuilly-sur-Seine: AGARD/NATO.

7

Sleep disturbance and jet lag

ANTHONY N NICHOLSON

Individuals undertaking long air journeys may have little restful sleep, and after the journey they will have to cope with the adaptation to a new time zone (jet lag). Though for some, disturbed sleep and jet lag will be no more than inconveniences as they adapt, at leisure, to the new time zone, there may be significant problems for those involved in business and commerce. These problems are influenced by the timing and direction of the flight. The timing of scheduled flights takes into consideration the opening hours of airports, particularly when sited near to centres of population, the local diurnal variation in temperature which can be relevant to take-off loads, and the working hours of the local engineering maintenance staff. Putting these and other considerations together, it is the practice for many north–south and south–north schedules, as between Europe and South Africa, to operate overnight and land early in the morning. Similarly, most long-haul eastward and some westward flights operate overnight and land the next day, though many westward flights, with the lengthening of the day brought about by the time zone change, tend to depart and land within daylight hours.

It is, therefore, inevitable that passengers on many long-haul flights will be flying overnight and, to be as refreshed as possible the next day, sleep during the night is necessary. Essentially, the likelihood of adequate sleep overnight depends on the nature of the sleeping environment. A near upright back to the seat (Nicholson and Stone 1987) and limited space in a noisy cabin are not conducive to rest, whereas spacious seats which recline and provide support to the legs in quiet cabins provide a more favourable environment (Figure 7.1), although air turbulence may be a problem. In-flight beds are ideal. For those who have to cope with less than ideal accommodation, it may be just as well to accept the likelihood of a journey with little or no sleep, and then to occupy the hours with a meal, reading and, if available, in-flight entertainment.

If the accommodation is conducive to rest, it is useful to have a strategy that will ensure some hours of sleep. It is wise to consider having the evening meal on the ground. Such a strategy is particularly appropriate when the journey does not exceed 7 or 8 hours, as across the Atlantic, as the period available for rest is unlikely to be more than 5 hours. With longer single-sector flights as to Europe from the west coast of the USA, South America, South Africa and the Far East, the period for rest will be several hours longer, though the latter part of the flight may well be in daylight. With the ever-changing schedules of worldwide operations, it is not possible to provide simple advice that will ensure the best possible sleep. Careful reading of the schedule and consideration of the time-zone change, whether advanced or delayed, are necessary to identify the most favourable time to rest and then other matters can be arranged around that interval of time. If the passenger is not fully adapted

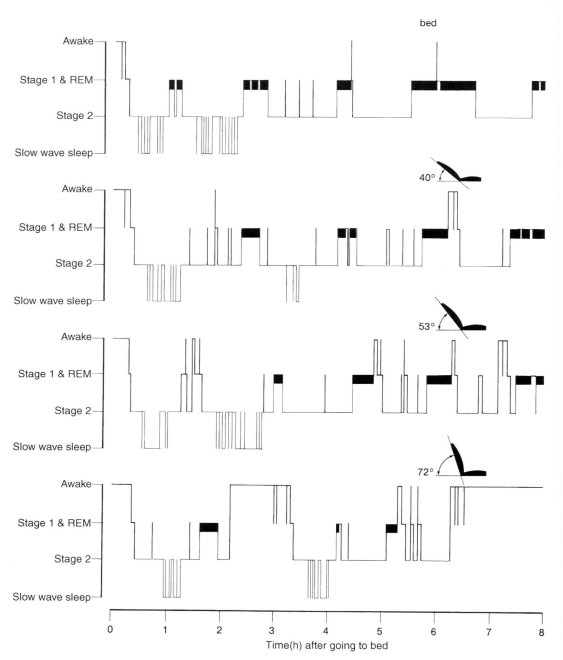

Figure 7.1 *Hypnograms of an individual sleeping in bed and in a chair with three different back angles. Lying down is the usual position when sleeping, but the airline passenger when travelling overnight may have to cope with a near upright posture when trying to sleep. Sleep in seats with different back angles is shown in the figure and compared with sleep in a bed. Sleep-onset latency does not differ significantly between the three positions and does not differ markedly between the three positions and lying in bed. However, total sleep time is reduced in the chair with a back angle of 72° with the horizontal compared with that in bed and with the other two seats. There is prolonged awake activity and more awakenings. Less restful sleep is more apparent as the back angle from the horizontal increases. (Reproduced from Nicholson and Welbers 1987).*

to the time zone of the departure airport, it will be necessary to modulate the calculations accordingly.

IN FLIGHT

Whether an hypnotic should be used during an overnight flight is problematical, and, in any case, they should not be ingested with alcohol. Hypnotics will assist in obtaining several hours of sleep, and there are now available several short-acting drugs which are free of residual effects on performance and vigilance after about 6 hours from ingestion. These are temazepam (10–20 mg), zolpidem (5 mg) and brotizolam (0.125–0.25 mg). There is also an ultra-short-acting hypnotic which provides an hour or two of sleep, though how useful an ultra-short-acting drug would be has yet to be established. Other hypnotics are available, but the recommended dose range may not be free of residual effects. The duration of action may extend beyond that of a short period of rest in flight and lead to a 'hangover'.

A low dose of a short-acting hypnotic may be useful for a healthy adult occupying an in-flight bed, but caution should be exercised in prescribing an hypnotic, especially if the passenger has cardiovascular or pulmonary disease, limited mobility or predisposition to thrombosis. With cardiovascular or pulmonary disease, depression of breathing induced by an hypnotic, together with the hypoxic environment of the cabin, may compromise even further the low oxygen saturation of the blood, whilst passengers with restricted mobility may remain motionless for several hours with subsequent difficulties in moving. Passengers with a history of thrombosis or even with a predisposition to thrombosis, who remain motionless, could suffer an embolism. Indeed, even healthy individuals could suffer from deep vein thrombosis or a pulmonary embolus as thrombosis could be precipitated by the risk factors inherent to the in-flight environment. The best advice may well be that in no circumstances should an hypnotic be used to assist sleep in flight except, possibly, for a healthy adult using an in-flight bed.

Sleep apnoea

Passengers with sleep apnoea, except those with only mild snoring and limited daytime somnolence but certainly if they normally use equipment which provides continuous positive airway pressure (CPAP), may need assessment prior to a flight. Sleep apnoea is characterized by respiratory disturbances during sleep and intermittent desaturations of the blood. Both could be exacerbated by the hypoxic environment of the cabin and, as little is known of the potential aggravation of sleep apnoea in an hypoxic environment, it would be wise to consider certain options. All patients with significant sleep apnoea intending to fly should have their oxygen saturation measured during sleep and wakefulness.

Those with marked apnoea and/or desaturations who would like to sleep in the cabin should consider using their CPAP equipment. They should ascertain whether the equipment is compatible with the on-board electrical installations and whether the airline will accept the carriage and use of the equipment in-flight. Battery-powered equipment may be more suitable. Probably the best advice to an intending passenger with sleep apnoea is to travel when possible during the day and avoid sleeping overnight. Some patients with sleep apnoea have impaired pulmonary function apart from their sleep-related respiratory disturbances, and so their in-flight oxygen exchange may be prejudiced by multi-pathology. Such patients should be referred to a respiratory unit for assessment prior to the flight.

POST-FLIGHT SLEEP DISTURBANCE

Once the flight is over, the passenger will have to cope with the process of adapting to a new time zone if the journey has involved a significant east–west or a west–east translation. The body clock of the passenger will be in advance of local time after a westward flight and behind local time after an eastward flight. This will mean that when the passenger goes to bed at local time after a westward flight, sleep will have been delayed by, say, at least 5 hours, whereas when the passenger goes to bed at local time after an overnight eastward flight, the rest period will be earlier than that demanded by the natural rhythm of the body. Trying to sleep after time-zone changes can, therefore, be problematical. Immediately after a daytime westward journey the passenger will fall asleep quickly as sleep has been delayed, but will tend to wake within a few hours as wakefulness ensues as if they were in their home time zone (Figure 7.2).

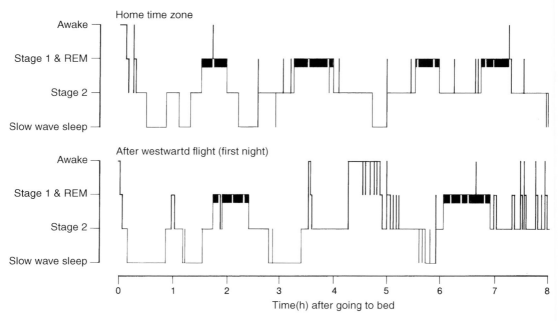

Figure 7.2 *Sleep after a westward flight from Europe across the North Atlantic with a time zone change of 5 hours and a similar delay to the first local rest period. Passengers tend to fall asleep quickly and sleep more deeply. There is some degree of sleep deprivation, although the short sleep latency is also related to the delay in going to bed, which is well within the night of the natural rhythm for sleep and wakefulness of the home time zone. There is less restful sleep during the latter part of the new local night as the passenger tries to sleep toward the local time of rising, which is around midday of the home time zone. After a westward flight, the usual sleep pattern is established within a couple of days. (Reproduced from Nicholson and Welbers 1987).*

Fortunately, difficulty with sustaining sleep after a westward journey usually lasts only a day or perhaps two, but it can be helpful to those who are particularly disturbed by such journeys to take an hypnotic at the usual local time for rest. It is uncertain whether an ultra-short-acting hypnotic taken only on wakening during the middle of the local night could be an alternative strategy.

Disturbed sleep after an eastward journey is a more complex issue (Figure 7.3). The journey may well have been overnight and, so, if no rest has been taken during the first day in the new time zone, the passenger will be tired when the local time for rest arrives. It is, therefore, likely that, though the period of rest may be several hours before the natural time for sleep, they will sleep well throughout the first night in the new time zone. This can be somewhat misleading. It is the next two, three or even four nights when sleep is likely to be impaired with the passenger still attempting to sleep at a time when the body clock is promoting wakefulness. There can also be a problem with maintaining vigilance

during the latter part of the day. This may be associated with inadequate sleep over several days, particularly if the individual is working during the early part of each day when the body clock is demanding sleep. In addition, loss of the diurnal increase in arousal during the day due to generalized depression of the circadian rhythm, which controls variations in alertness, may also be a significant factor.

Hypnotics

As suggested above, hypnotics can ensure good sleep during the process of adaptation to transmeridian journeys. As far as a westward flight is concerned, disturbed sleep is usually a problem for only a day or two, but sleep disturbance is likely to persist after an eastward flight. After an eastward flight an hypnotic with the potential to sustain sleep, yet free of residual effects and of accumulation on daily ingestion, is appropriate and is likely to be more useful than an

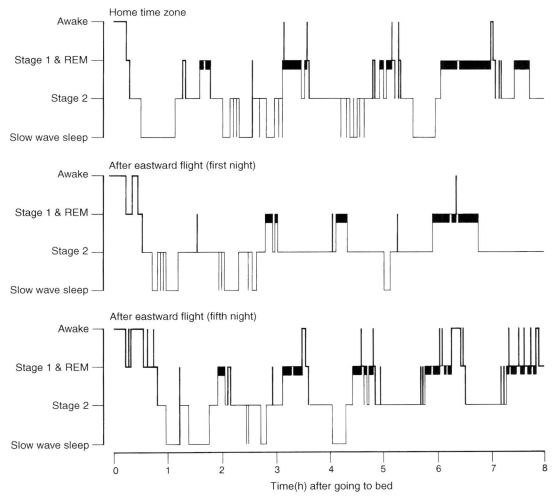

Figure 7.3 *Sleep during the first night after an overnight eastward journey. Sleep may be even better than before the flight – especially if the passenger has not slept on the aircraft or during the day on returning to the new time zone. Subsequently, with the sleep period being advanced compared with the new time zone, sleep latencies are prolonged, and sleep can be disturbed for several days. (Reproduced from Nicholson and Welbers 1987).*

ultra-rapidly eliminated drug. Brotizolam is particularly useful (Nicholson *et al.* 1986) and its effects on sleep duration after time-zone changes are illustrated in Figure 7.4.

Adaptation to a new time zone after an eastward journey may not involve a simple advance of the body clock to the new local environment. This is especially so after journeys across more than six time zones when the body clock may not move toward the new time zone by simply reducing the 6-, 7- or 8-hour lapse. It may adapt by 'going westwards' and, therefore, crossing up to 16 time zones. In the circumstances of a westward shift of the body clock after

an eastward flight, the process of adaptation may take many days, and an hypnotic can be very useful.

The extreme case of adaptation is an inversion of the day–night cycle, after journeys such as those between Europe and the Antipodes and between the west coast of the USA and the Middle East. The process of adaptation will take many days and, certainly in the case of Europe to the Antipodes, the body clock may shift in a westward direction across Asia or in an eastward direction across the Americas (Nicholson 1998). Whichever strategy is adopted, the ensuing sleep disturbance is likely to be marked. An hypnotic can be a valuable means of ensuring sleep after such a journey,

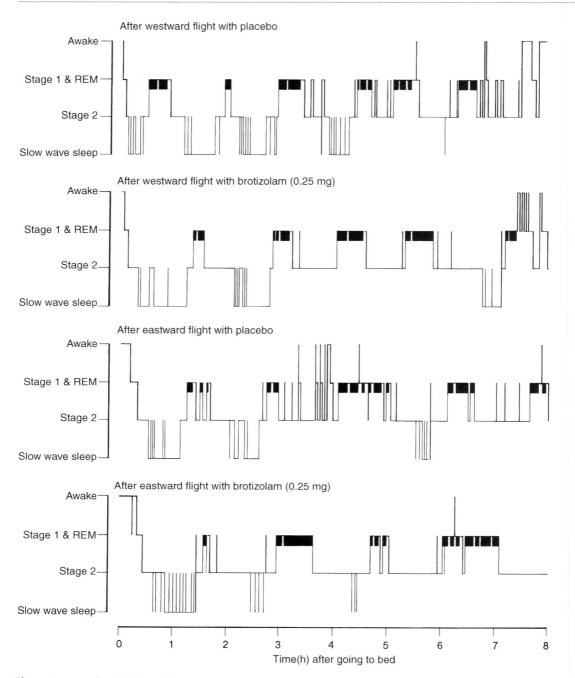

Figure 7.4 *During the first night after a westward flight, brotizolam (0.25 mg) increased total sleep time and there was less awake activity. It was particularly useful for the latter part of the night. On the first night after an eastward flight, the 19-hour delay to the period for rest had led to good quality sleep without the need for an hypnotic. However, brotizolam (0.25 mg) was particularly useful for subsequent nights and sustained sleep through the night. (Reproduced from Nicholson and Welbers 1987).*

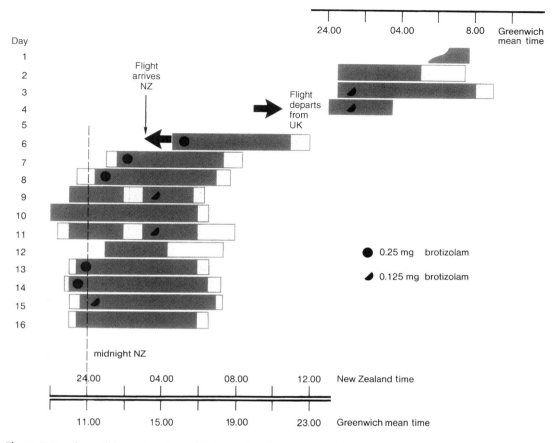

Figure 7.5 *The usefulness of an hypnotic (brotizolam 0.125–0.25 mg) in adapting to a new time zone can be seen from the sleep diary of a journey from London to New Zealand. The total length of each bar indicates the time spent in bed with the darker part reported by the individual as time asleep. The passenger used a small dose (0.125 mg) and had a good night's sleep at home prior to departure and some sleep during the initial part of the flight. On arrival in New Zealand, 0.25 mg brotizolam was ingested and this led to a restful period of sleep. Over the next two nights the rest period was moved toward local time and 0.25 mg brotizolam ensured good-quality sleep each night. The body clock had not yet aligned to the local time zone and rest without the hypnotic over the next three nights failed to provide sustained sleep. Indeed, the individual even used 0.125 mg half-way through some rest periods (about 0400 hours New Zealand time) in an attempt to gain some sleep. However, with two further nights with 0.25 mg and another night with 0.125 mg, all with good sleep, the adaptation process was complete. With an inversion of the day–night cycle, sleep disturbance will persist until the circadian rhythm is realigned and, as in this context, an hypnotic is most appropriate, but may be needed for several nights. (Reproduced from Nicholson and Welbers 1987).*

and it may be needed for several nights. An interesting adaptation to such a journey is described in Figure 7.5.

ADAPTATION TO THE NEW TIME ZONE

Whether the process of adaptation to a new time zone can be accelerated is a topic of continuing debate.

There are various approaches, and these include - shifting, prior to the flight, the diurnal rhythm of the home time zone toward that of the destination, and exposure to intense lights at appropriate times either during the flight or after landing. Shifting the diurnal rhythm to that of the destination has practical difficulties, and if it is the intention of the passenger to continue with their day-to-day routine at home, as far as possible, before they depart, it is unlikely that an anticipatory shift in the body clock can be achieved. Exposure to bright lights will ensure, as quickly as possible, the shift of the body clock to the new time zone, but here again it involves the passenger in a routine that may not be convenient. For example, exposure to bright light early in the morning will aid the advance and avoidance of light until, say, midday will aid in the delay of the circadian rhythm. Light-emitting goggles can be used during the flight together with eye shades, but such an approach has to be carefully planned and, again, may not be compatible with the routine of the aircraft.

Melatonin

Another question is whether a drug could quicken the adaptation process and many passengers report the usefulness of melatonin. Much has been written about melatonin, but only when more knowledge has been gained about its pharmacological activity will it be possible to advise on any role in this context. Early subjective work reported that passengers benefited from the use of melatonin, but this could have been due to an improvement in perceived well-being, possibly some form of mood modulation induced by the drug, rather than any alignment to a new time zone. Melatonin may well have some effect on circadian activity, but it may not be strong enough in its own right to realign the rhythm with a new time zone (Czeisler 1997). It could, together with a strong zeitgeber such as light, speed the response. However, if an effective strategy were possible, it would demand careful planning of ingestion times. In this context it has been taken during the day in an attempt to accelerate an adaptation to a new time zone, but this may be hazardous because of its immediate sedative effect.

Melatonin (5 mg) certainly possesses hypnotic activity somewhat similar to that of a low dose of a benzodiazepine, such as temazepam (20 mg), but this is only evident when the intrinsic levels of melatonin are low, such as during the day – assuming the circadian rhythm is aligned to the local time zone (Stone et al. 2000). Further, ingestion of melatonin at certain times may actually disturb sleep. Indeed, the uncertainty of the hypnotic effect of melatonin at any particular time of the day during worldwide travel clearly presents problems as to the appropriate time of ingestion. It must also be appreciated that melatonin can modify endocrine activity, and that it has not undergone the development process required of drugs approved by agencies that control medicines and ensure their safety. It is also worth noting that many bodies that regulate aviation, as well as the airlines, have advised against the use of melatonin by air personnel.

Essentially, all passengers involved in critical activity on reaching a new destination should appreciate that for a day or two they may not be able to carry out their duties in the usually accomplished manner. Those who profess to be unaffected by a time-zone change are usually not called upon to undertake analytical work. They may be carrying out a representative function or merely be in attendance, though in a senior capacity, and so have no need to exercise their skills. Such individuals may have gained little insight into their shortcomings in such circumstances. Certainly, critical decision making based on information that is only made available at the new destination should be delayed for a couple of days when the passenger will have had, at least, the benefit of good sleep – with the help of a hypnotic, if necessary. For most mortals, taking off a shoe and banging on the lectern is unlikely to be the successful opening of a critical negotiation.

CONCLUSION

Disturbed sleep is the overriding, though not the only adverse feature of long-haul flights. It is particularly acute when the accommodation does not facilitate sleep and when the time-zone change leads to a persistent desynchronization of the need to sleep from the local rest period. The use of hypnotics in-flight should be restricted to the healthy passenger, and passengers less healthy, even in spacious accommodation, should avoid their use, as should all passengers flying in confined cabins. It is during the adaptation to the new time zone after the flight when hypnotics are useful.

REFERENCES

Czeisler CA. Commentary: evidence for melatonin as a circadian phase shifting agent. *J Biol Rhythms* 1997; **12**: 618–23.

Nicholson AN. *Neurosciences and Aviation Medicine: a Century of Endeavour.* Kohimarama, Auckland: International Academy of Aviation and Space Medicine, 1998.

Nicholson AN. Disturbed sleep in aircrew: clinical considerations. In Ernsting J, Nicholson AN and Rainford DJ (eds), *Aviation Medicine*, 3rd edn. Oxford: Butterworth Heinemann, 1999; 217–31.

Nicholson AN and Stone BM. Influence of back angle on the quality of sleep in seats. *Ergonomics* 1987; **30**: 1033–41.

Nicholson AN and Welbers IB (eds), *Postgraduate Medical Services 8: Transient Insomnia.* Ingelheim am Rhein: Boehringer Ingelheim International GmbH, 1987.

Nicholson AN, Pascoe PA, Spencer MB, Stone BM, Roehrs T and Roth T. Sleep after transmeridian flights. *Lancet* 1986; **ii**: 1205–8.

Stone BM, Turner C, Mills SL and Nicholson AN. Hypnotic activity of melatonin. *Sleep* 2000; **23**: 663–9.

APPENDIX

Explanation of sleep patterns depicted in Figures 7.1–7.4

The electroencephalogram, together with electro-oculograms and the sub-mental electromyogram, are used to define the various stages of sleep, and these provide information on sleep quality and quantity. Wakefulness is characterized by alpha and/or low-voltage mixed-frequency activity. It is usually accompanied by a relatively high-amplitude electromyogram with blinks and eye movements. The change from waking to drowsy (stage 1) sleep is associated with a general slowing of activity and by a decrease in the amount, amplitude and frequency of the alpha rhythm. The appearance of spindles and K complexes signals the onset of sleep (stage 2). The deeper stages of sleep (stages 3 and 4) involve slow wave activity. Rapid eye movement (REM) sleep is characterized by episodic eye movements and low-amplitude myographic activity.

The healthy adult passes quickly from waking through the stages of sleep to slow wave sleep and the first period of REM sleep occurs around 70–90 minutes after sleep onset. The first third of the night is dominated by slow wave activity (stages 3 and 4) and the latter two-thirds by the cyclical appearance of REM sleep. In the healthy adult, there are only a few awakenings during the night. A more detailed account of the sleep process is given in the third edition of *Aviation Medicine* edited by Ernsting, Nicholson and Rainford (Nicholson 1999). In Figures 7.1–7.4, the time spent in each sleep stage is depicted. Dark bars indicate REM sleep.

8

Obstetrical and gynaecological incidents

GEOFFREY VP CHAMBERLAIN

The number of airline passengers increases each year and so does the number of women flying world wide. These are, of course, at risk from obstetrical and gynaecological problems. Relative familiarity with such matters is likely to be restricted to those who practise in the specialty and to general practitioners, yet all medical practitioners will have an obligation to provide assistance should a difficulty arise during a flight. In the case of an obstetrical emergency, it is quite possible that a midwife may be on board, and in this event most practitioners would do well to defer to their expertise and experience, although specialist advice may be available through the airline if it is linked to a ground-based advisory service. The advice of a medical practitioner will be sought if a diversion is under discussion, though in all cases the final decision will rest with the captain.

Of particular relevance to the unborn child is the relative hypoxia of the cabin. The cabin environment and the effects of the reduced pressure on oxygen carriage and delivery are discussed in detail elsewhere. Essentially, the cabin altitude can reach 8000 feet and this leads to a much reduced partial pressure of oxygen in the cabin compared with sea level. The effect on haemoglobin saturation of the mother is limited due to the sigmoid nature of the oxygen dissociation curve. However, although the partial pressure of oxygen in the blood of the mother is reduced from about 100 mmHg (13 kPa) to around 60 mmHg (8 kPa), transport of oxygen to the fetus is relatively unaffected. This is due to the greater affinity of fetal haemoglobin for oxygen with the dissociation curve displaced to the left and the relatively high concentration of haemoglobin in the fetus, i.e. 16 g dl^{-1}

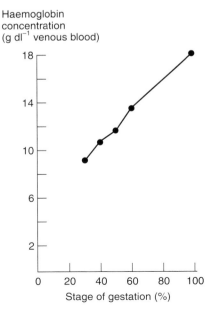

Figure 8.1 *Haemoglobin concentration of the fetus at various stages of gestation.*

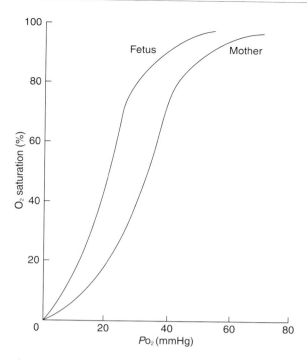

Figure 8.2 *Oxyhaemoglobin dissociation curves for human maternal and fetal blood. (Reproduced from Chamberlain 1996).*

compared with $12\,g\,dl^{-1}$ in the healthy mother (Figures 8.1 and 8.2).

PREGNANCY

Pregnant women undertaking a flight on a commercial aircraft must follow certain guidelines. Generally they are not allowed to fly on an international flight after 32 weeks of gestation, though this restriction may be eased to 36 weeks for domestic flights. Many airlines require a note from the obstetrician or midwife containing the stage of gestation and appropriate details. It is wise to certify the gestational age as, if there is any doubt, she will be referred to the airport medical officer whose obstetrical expertise may not be recent, and who may be inclined toward the safe side, perhaps refusing permission to fly. The wearing of loose coats or frocks does not fool the astute flight attendant either at the booking-in desk or at the entrance to the aircraft. A certificate

from the doctor or midwife should take into account the dates of the return flight, which may be a few weeks later to ensure eligibility to fly at the later stage of gestation. It may be wise to contact the airline itself rather than to rely on the interpretation of the airline guidelines by the travel agent.

As well as these formal certificates, the record of the antenatal care, so far, should be carried. This should include details of any drug treatment using the recommended international non-proprietary names. Some preparations may not be available abroad so a supply of drugs sufficient to last for the visit should be taken. Enquiries should also be made of the town or region of the country being visited, particularly about its obstetrical facilities. In many countries, facilities are limited and the expected help may not be available in the event of pre-term labour. Further, enquiries should be made about insurance to cover obstetrical events on the aircraft and after arrival at the foreign destination.

Pre-flight

If pre-booking is allowed, an aisle seat should be sought, but if not pre-booked this should be requested when arriving at the airline desk. Seat belts are compulsory, even in pregnancy, and they should be worn low on the abdomen just above the pelvis. This is a safe position for both mother and baby. Gas in the intestines can expand in the low pressure of the cabin and so food that contributes to such gases should be avoided for a day or two before the flight. Jet lag occurs in the pregnant as well as the non-pregnant passenger, and can be troublesome for those who travel west to east over several time zones. Pharmacological treatments for jet lag are inappropriate in pregnancy. It is better to prepare for the flight with exercise and, perhaps, attempt to align sleep schedules to those of the destination, though it is uncertain whether this will be effective. Some dehydration may occur while travelling, and in consequence, reasonable quantities of non-alcoholic drinks may be taken.

The advice of the medical adviser, whether the general practitioner or a consultant obstetrician, should be sought in good time to decide whether it is wise to take the flight and, even more important, whether it will be wise to fly back a few weeks later when further into the pregnancy. Prognosis cannot be precise so it must be expected that advisers may range on the side of caution. Generally, between 14 and 28 weeks of pregnancy there should be no reason why a fit woman without obstetrical complications in a past or in the current pregnancy should not fly in a pressurized cabin. After this time, flying becomes less advisable as each week of gestation goes by. The need to fly should be reviewed. Usually the journey is less important than the safety of the pregnancy and the peace of mind resulting from being near to good and familiar care in the event of an early birth.

Any condition that reduces the placental bed afferent blood flow, and hence fetal oxygenation, is a contraindication to flying as the fetus could be at jeopardy. This is difficult to quantify for any individual but anaemia, pre-eclampsia or a history of antepartum haemorrhage are reasons to think very carefully whether the air journey should be undertaken. In the event of going against considered advice, the general practitioner should give serious thought to advising the medical officer of the airline about the potential problem. Supplementary oxygen could be provided if ordered in advance, but, in general, it is inappropriate. Any pregnant woman needing oxygen would, in any case, be in a high-risk group and should not fly.

Miscarriage

Some 15 per cent of women miscarry in the first 12 weeks of pregnancy. They usually know they are pregnant, and start to bleed with mild uterine contractions. This can come on at any time and in any place. Usually, the bleeding is not very heavy and can be treated conservatively, resting in a seat. Collection of the blood and clots will be of help to the gynaecologist who sees her when the aircraft lands. Ergometrine 500 µg with oxytocin 5 units (1 ampoule of Syntometrine) may be given intramuscularly if there is heavy bleeding. This causes the uterus to contract down, but the medical practitioner must bear in mind that this is blind treatment. There is little point in trying to decide if the miscarriage is threatened or will be inevitable on the aircraft. Inevitable miscarriages usually bleed more heavily than threatened ones, and a cervical examination, unless the examiner is skilled, would be difficult and could even provoke more bleeding. Try to keep everybody else from getting excited (particularly if the husband or relatives are on board) and ride it out with ground-based advice.

Antepartum bleeding

Antepartum bleeding is rare and occurs in less than 1 per cent of all pregnancies, but could occur by chance in a late pregnancy while flying. The differential diagnosis is between a low-lying placenta and an abruption or separation of a normally sited placenta. The former is painless and, although reported as recurrent, the next bleed may not present for a few days. Nothing can be done on the aircraft, but it is important to ensure prompt attention at a hospital with ultrasound facilities on arrival. Abruption of the placenta is more serious. There is acute abdominal pain and shock. The uterus is often very hard. The few case reports of abruption on board aircraft seem to have occurred during landing. Indeed, as the plane decelerates, the forces may cause the uterus to flatten against the abdominal wall. As deceleration continues, there may be shortening of the long axis of the uterus with shearing of the placental attachments (Matzkel *et al.* 1991).

Thromboembolism

Pregnancy and the puerperium are higher-risk times for venous thromboembolism. Flying increases the risk still further. Air passengers tend to be confined with their knees sharply flexed and with, sometimes, a ridge of upholstery in the seat pressing against the upper part of the popliteal vein. This is particularly so when pregnant women are strapped into their seats. Distension of abdominal gases in the viscera may also contribute to the adverse effects on the venous system. Preventative measures include isometric leg exercises, but walking is probably better. Those at risk should choose an aisle seat. It should always be remembered that deep vein thrombosis may not appear for hours or even days after the journey is over. The chapter on thromboembolism deals with these issues in more detail.

Anaemia

Anaemia is common in pregnancy, a time of maximum utilization of iron stores. Should the level of haemoglobin be below 9 g dl^{-1}, it is probably unwise to fly for, in addition to any pathological process, there is the hypoxia of the cabin. The mean thickness of the villous membrane of the placenta is significantly less in anaemia. Compensatory changes may maintain placental function, but the pregnant woman with significant anaemia should not fly on commercial aircraft unless there is an overriding reason. Those with sickle cell anaemia must be protected from low oxygen levels, and this condition is dealt with in a later chapter. However, when pregnant, it is wise not to fly for anything other than very short periods as the low oxygen partial pressures could precipitate a crisis. This may manifest itself with pain in the gut or the bone. It is a difficult condition to treat without analgesia. Extra oxygen is imperative to prevent further episodes, although it does not relieve the thrombosis.

Diabetes

The placenta may also have a reduced surface area for gas exchange in patients with poorly controlled diabetes. The potential effect of this on the fetus when the oxygen saturation is reduced even further by the reduced pressure of the cabin needs careful consideration (Reshetmickvo *et al.* 1958). Babies who have intrauterine growth restriction are likely to be suffering from a lack of the dilatation of the placental bed arteries, which normally occurs in pregnancy. Hence, afferent blood supplies to the placental bed are limited and growth substances are also reduced. Should such a placental system be subjected to a lower ambient oxygen, this would result in a reduced oxygen supply to the fetus. In consequence, the woman with known intrauterine growth restriction of any degree should not fly.

PRE-ECLAMPSIA AND ECLAMPSIA

Pre-eclampsia is common in pregnancy with an incidence of about 5 per cent. Among its manifestations are poor perfusion of the placental bed and a reduced terminal villus surface (Mayhew 1988). It is a condition where the hypoxia of the cabin could affect the oxygenation of the baby. Furthermore, there is some evidence that placental lactate could be increased by hypoxia and this, too, could lead to an exacerbation of the process (Schumacher *et al.* 1999). Pre-eclampsia is a contraindication to flying. Eclampsia is exceedingly rare, about two in a thousand pregnancies, and is nearly always preceded by pre-eclampsia with raised blood pressure and proteinuria detected at the antenatal clinic.

Should a woman who is far into pregnancy have a fit on the aircraft she should be laid on her side and her airway cleared of any obstructions such as false teeth. She needs sedation. Eclampsia can be well treated by intramuscular magnesium sulphate (probably unavailable), but since the doctor may not make this precise diagnosis, any other sedative would be helpful. Very rarely would women who have been perfectly normal before boarding the aircraft suddenly develop eclampsia. The warning condition, pre-eclampsia, is unlikely to draw itself to the attention of any doctor on the aircraft, although a severe headache, itching of the mask area of the face or abdominal pain due to stretch of the liver capsule in severe pre-eclampsia are the usual features. All these are best dealt with by rest and handing over as soon as possible on landing. This is a condition in which serious consideration should be made to shortening of the flight.

UNEXPECTED LABOUR

Unexpected labour and delivery on board an aircraft is worrying for all concerned. Labour itself usually has some length. If there are early contractions and the aircraft is close to its destination, the flight should be allowed to proceed. However, taking the worst scenario, the woman may go into labour and deliver in the course of a long-haul flight with no possibility of a diversion. The contractions of early labour are usually fairly painless and might hardly be noticed; by the time it is realized what is happening labour may be well established. Try to move the woman to a quiet part of the aircraft. This may be difficult in an overcrowded flight, but in a long-haul aircraft it may be possible to use the cabin attendants' rest area. The back row of the more spacious cabins can sometimes be re-seated to provide a reasonable confinement space and blankets can make screens. This is important, not only for decency, but to reassure the mother that she will not be viewed by strangers during childbirth. As mentioned before, if a midwife is on board, she should deal with the situation as she will be more familiar with a delivery than most doctors.

A swift assessment should be made, checking that the woman is not in too much pain. The blood pressure should be measured and the abdomen examined to assess uterine contractions. These are regular hardenings of the uterus, which are usually fairly easy to palpate, though in a plump woman this can be difficult. An attempt should be made to assess the frequency of the contractions and how long they last. In early labour, contractions may be 15 minutes apart, but as labour progresses they become more frequent and by the end of the first stage of labour, just before full dilation of the cervix, they occur every 1–2 minutes. Early in labour, contractions are not very strong and they do not last very long, but as the labour progresses they extend their duration and painfulness.

If the woman has not ruptured her membranes spontaneously (there is not a trickle of clear fluid), it is wise to try and maintain them intact, for once they rupture, labour tends to speed up. A vaginal examination in labour requires some experience. It is a useful procedure if undertaken by a doctor in the field of obstetrics, or by a midwife as it provides information on how far labour has progressed. A woman who is 2 cm dilated with a partially taken up cervix has a much longer labour ahead of her than one who has a thin, flat cervix which is 8 cm dilated. Normally, delivery will not commence until 10 cm of dilatation has been achieved when no cervix can be felt at all. For those not used to vaginal examinations, this is hard to determine for the cervix is flat and pressed against the descending fetal head.

It may be difficult for those with little experience to hear the fetal heart, though it can be heard with an ordinary binaural stethoscope. A fetal stethoscope is not essential. It is useful to remember that the first monaural stethoscope was a rolled-up tube of cardboard and the same can be done on board an aircraft. If, however, the doctor is not used to fetal heart auscultation, he may not hear it – especially in a noisy aircraft. If he does succeed, the fetal heart beat should be counted and the rate recorded just after a uterine contraction.

It is to be hoped that by this time contact will have been made with the ground-based advisory service and that an experienced obstetrician will be available to give advice. The aircraft captain should be informed that a birth on board is likely, and this will give him the opportunity to assess, in consultation with the ground-based medical adviser, the options for a diversion in the event of an untoward event. Such consultation is immensely reassuring, particularly if the medical practitioner is not familiar with obstetrics. If it is decided that the aircraft should divert to allow the delivery on land, the pain of labour should be relieved as much as possible. Few analgesics are actually carried and most of the proprietary ones offered by other passengers are not very effective during labour. They are nearly always in tablet form and as gut mobility in labour is reduced, absorption would be slow. Various breathing techniques can be very helpful, and these may have been learned during antenatal classes. If that is so, the techniques learned should be reinforced, beginning rather like coaching a boat crew, getting the patient to breathe deeply and slowly in a controlled fashion during the contractions.

DELIVERY

If the process of labour has progressed too far for a diversion, the doctor must make preparations for the delivery. In most cases nature is best and the baby will be delivered normally. The less the amateur obstetrician does the better. Obstetricians have learned this over the years and are happy to be in attendance without actually doing anything. It is wise to clean the perineum with antiseptic solution and, in the absence of a midwife or anyone else with experience, the doctor should put on rubber gloves and prepare to receive the baby. The woman can often provide guidance as she feels the baby coming down the canal. Soon the bulging of the head separating the labia will be evident. This should be allowed to proceed without interference. The head will crown, as the maximum diameter passes through the ring of tissues at the forchette and labia. Now it is helpful to steady the head gently with the flat of one hand so the head does not pop out too vigorously, for such decompression can be damaging. The last minutes of delivery should be guarded, remembering what the labour-ward sister taught. After the head has been born, it will rotate to allow the shoulders to enter the pelvis. Usually the baby will be delivered thereafter without any assistance. If the shoulders do not come down, one can try pushing the head gently into the aircraft seat so that the anterior shoulder can be released, but this will not be necessary in most cases. Once the shoulders are delivered, the delivery is soon over. The captain of the aircraft should be informed, with the caution that all potential problems are not over.

The baby is still connected by the umbilical cord. The baby is held head down to drain fluid from the nasopharynx, and in most cases the infant will cry within 30 seconds. If the baby does not cry, gentle stimulation by patting the soles of the feet may help. The baby is then wrapped in a warm blanket as soon as possible to avoid cooling. If the baby is breathing well, the head should be kept down and, very soon after drainage of fluids from the nasopharynx, the baby should be given to the mother who may want to put the baby to the breast. This is an extremely good way of making sure that the last stage of labour, the delivery of the placenta, follows swiftly as the oxytocin released stimulates this process.

POST-PARTUM CARE

Invariably, the attention of others helping at the birth is paid mainly to the baby, but the doctor must look after the mother as well and see to delivery of the placenta. The baby is separated from the mother by tying the umbilical cord in two places about 3 inches (7.5 cm) apart, using any string or catgut available and cutting between the ties with a pair of scissors. The ties prevent bleeding from either the baby or the placenta. The former could be dangerous; the latter is messy. A few airlines are now carrying in their emergency kit Syntometrine, a mixture of ergometrine maleate (500 µg) and oxytocin (5 iu). This helps the uterus to contract and stop bleeding. If it is available, it should be given to the mother intramuscularly as the shoulders are delivered so that the placenta will come out easily with little blood loss. Many airlines, however, do not carry Syntometrine and in its absence the delivery of the placenta must be awaited. A hand on the top of the uterus may detect uterine contraction. When the placenta starts to come away, the umbilical cord will lengthen and a little blood will appear. The placenta can then be gently guided out. No attempt should be made to pull on the cord; it should be allowed to come away spontaneously.

One may have to wait up to 20 or 30 minutes, but usually the placenta will deliver itself. When it does, it should be checked to make sure that it is complete and kept for inspection by an obstetrician when the aircraft lands.

There may be some blood loss at delivery, commonly 200–300 ml. Provided it is less than 0.5 litre it is not a major problem; it just needs mopping up and measuring if possible. The woman should stop bleeding very soon after delivery. After childbirth, there may be a small trickle of blood either from the uterus or from a tear. Unless this is excessive, the latter is best dealt with by pressing a sterile sanitary towel against the area and holding it in place by a hitch around the waist and a thong between the legs tied to the hitch. In the absence of an oxytocic drug it would be meddlesome to try and prevent further uterine bleeding, although someone with experience may rub the uterus, hoping to make a contraction and stop any bleeding due to uterine laxness. Pressure on the perineum may stop bleeding from a tear. Suturing should not be attempted unless bleeding is uncontrolled – a very rare occurrence. The woman is made comfortable by removing any sodden sheets or napkins, and allowed to lie comfortably across three seats with the baby being nursed wrapped in a blanket.

It should be reassuring to the amateur obstetrician that nearly always delivery is normal, is not accompanied by major bleeding and the placenta is delivered spontaneously. This is the case in 90 per cent of cases, particularly in those who have had a child before. Bleeding will be rare while giving birth in-flight for the mother is likely to be producing a slightly smaller baby than usual and will have a short labour and spontaneous delivery due to the very limitations of the journey. All these factors can be reassuring to those attending. Desperate measures like bimanual compression of the uterus are not going to be helpful when carried out by the amateur accoucheur. Indeed, such measures could be very distressing, causing even deeper shock. Probably the major contribution that any doctor attending such an untoward event can do is to stop other people from panicking. Doctors, after all, have probably seen some deliveries, at least in their student days; they know roughly the course of events, and can stop others from interfering or raising the stress level. Childbirth is a natural event, which is sometimes assisted by doctors, but often proceeds without any medical help and nearly always ends up quite successfully.

The major problem that might occur when oxytocic drugs are not given is a post-partum haemorrhage. Here a major loss (500–1000 ml blood) might take place and this is a serious problem. An intravenous set is provided in many aircraft medical kits and there would be no harm in setting up a drip; however, it should be remembered that airlines will probably only provide one unit of intravenous fluid and this has to last the rest of the journey. It would only provide temporary refilling of a hypovolaemic vascular system, and the advice to the pilot to divert should be exercised if bleeding continues.

THE BABY

Most babies cry and start respiration within 30 seconds of delivery. This can be delayed by a minute or so. The baby should be dried vigorously with a warm towel and wrapped up. If respiration has not occurred within 2 minutes, then gentle inflation of the lungs is indicated. A laryngoscope or endotracheal tube is unlikely to be available, but one can try mouth-to-mouth respiration. The baby is placed on a firm surface with the head extended over a smooth roll of towel in the neutral position and starting with the resuscitator's mouth at right angles to that of the baby's lips. Two or three mouthfuls of air (cheek pressure only) may be given swiftly, trying to see if the anterior chest wall inflates. If it does, continue. If there is no heart beat palpable, then external cardiac massage may be helpful at this stage. This is done with the two fingertips placed over the midline of the lower sternum and continued at a rate of two sternal compressions (2 cm in depth for a term baby) every second with the mouth-to-mouth respiration every third compression, seeing that the chest moves with each inflation. A stethoscope can be used to listen for heart sounds. If cardiac resuscitation must be performed, it must be remembered that one is dealing with a baby and not an adult with a thick sternum and ribs.

Problems with pregnancy may occur in places where the life of the mother or fetus is at risk because of the lack of facilities, and where travel by road could take many hours or days. In this context, air transport has improved the outcome for mother and baby

enormously and staff skilled in both aviation medicine and obstetrics are available. Indeed, with such organizations, women are often transferred for 3 or 4 hours with various obstetrical conditions (Elliot *et al.* 1996). Pre-term labour and its threatened equivalent are probably the commonest causes for using air transport, but patients with pregnancy-induced hypertension, pre-eclampsia and the HELLP syndrome (haemolytic anaemia, elevated liver function tests, low platelets) have also been transported as well as those with trauma to the abdomen in pregnancy.

GYNAECOLOGICAL INCIDENTS

In-flight emergencies of gynaecological origin threaten less than the obstetrical ones. Any patient who has had a laparoscopic or open gynaecological operation should not fly for at least a week afterwards to ensure that there are no gases left inside the peritoneal cavity to cause swelling and discomfort. Anyone who has heavy periods would do well to avoid air travel at this time. Dysmenorrhoea may be worse in-flight for a mixture of psychological and stress reasons. It is best treated by rest and analgesia. It is remarkable what a plethora of pain-relieving pills are available from passengers when a call goes out for help in providing pain-relieving medication. Some may and others will not help. By the time the physician has worked his way through those available, the plane will have landed and the problem can be passed on to a ground-side gynaecologist.

Many gynaecological problems can be encountered in flight. Abdominal pain of gynaecological origin can occur at any time. Twists of an ovarian cyst can happen in the young during air travel and rupture of ovarian cystadenomas has been reported. Both these conditions will eventually need surgery. There is usually time for the patient to arrive at the destination, although arrangements should be made for an ambulance and medical help to meet the plane with an escort straight to a hospital where definitive treatment can be provided. Both torsion and rupture of the cyst have similar symptoms. There will be a sudden sharp pain in the lower abdomen. There is often no other history but on examination there will be a varying degree of tenderness and rigidity. The medical practitioner must assess the seriousness of the situation in consultation with the ground-based medical adviser. Rarely does a vaginal examination help. It is an emergency and the question is how much shock is occurring with the pain in the abdomen. Few flights need to be diverted, but the facilities at the destination should be alerted.

Ectopic pregnancies can occur in women who are unaware of being pregnant, and they occur at a rate of one per one hundred pregnancies. An ectopic pregnancy can rupture at any time and must be considered in any woman with sudden severe lower abdominal pain, particularly if she has had a short period of amenorrhoea. A pregnancy test, if available, could prove valuable. A small number exsanguinate rapidly into the abdominal cavity and are at risk of dying. If the on-board doctor in consultation with his medical colleagues on the ground consider that a woman is deteriorating rapidly, intravenous fluids should be used and a diversion requested to the nearest airport capable of coping with this situation. However, this applies to few ectopic pregnancies. Most ectopic pregnancies can wait until the next morning's operating list, and so it is probable that a passenger can last the rest of the flight.

As well as pain, dysfunctional uterine bleeding can be affected by the stress of travel and the anticipated pleasure or anxiety of what will happen on arrival. If a woman is starting to pass clots of blood, this is an indication that she is overwhelming her own fibrolytic system in the uterus and that the blood loss is heavier than usual. Such loss is not usually enough to cause concern. Consultation with the land-based medical service may advise an early landing, with diversion of the aircraft, but this is rare.

CONCLUSION

The author was once travelling on an aircraft when the call went out: 'Is there a gynaecologist on board?' This is the only time the author has been called for his specialty and he was curious enough to respond. The steward took him to the back of the plane where a large lady was wheezing and gasping for breath. The author talked her down to a normal respiratory rate. It then transpired that she had attacks of asthma and a cold, on top of which she felt that the air conditioning had made her short of breath and

had panicked herself into hyperventilation. Just about to leave, the author suddenly remembered the wording of the call and asked why she thought a gynaecologist was required. Very shyly she replied: 'I am 8 weeks pregnant.' Such misallocation of symptoms is commonly made by patients and there is no reason why this should not happen in-flight as it does in the surgery or consultation room.

Emergencies in obstetrics and gynaecology are rarely seen in-flight but when they are, doctors or nurses of any specialty should respond. They can give help according to their ability and with the medical kit provided by the airline. By far the most difficult problem is childbirth and this chapter aims to help all those whose primary work is not in this field. Provided one keeps calm, and keeps others calm, events usually transpire happily.

ACKNOWLEDGEMENTS

My thanks are due to Mrs Audrey Warren, Labour Ward Superintendent, Singleton Hospital, Swansea, for commenting on the text and to my secretary, Mrs Caron McColl, who prepared the manuscript. I am also grateful to the many flight attendants I have worked with over 30 years.

REFERENCES

Chamberlain G. *Lecture Notes in Obstetrics.* Oxford: Blackwell Sciences, 1996.

Elliot J, Foley M, Young N *et al.* Air transport of obstetric critical care patients to tertiary centres. *J Reprod Med* 1996; **41**: 171–5.

Matzkel A, Lurie S, El Chalal U and Blickstein I. Placental abruption associated with air travel. *J Perinat Med* 1991; **19**: 317–20.

Mayhew T. Thinning of intervascular layers of the placenta. *Obstet Gynecol* 1988; **8**: 101–9.

Reshetmickvo O, Burton G and Teleshova O. Placentinal histomorphology and morphometric diffusion capacity of the villious membrane in pregnancies complicated by maternal iron deficiency anaemia. *Am J Obstet Gynecol* 1958; **173**: 724–7.

Schumacher B, Olson GL, Saade GR *et al.* Simulated airplane flight increased plasma lactate in fetal rabbits. *Undersea Hyperb Med* 1999; **26**: 67–73.

9

Infants and children

MARTIN P SAMUELS

More and more infants and children travel by air, or journey to high altitude destinations. Most are healthy, but some may seek treatment for severe illness or injury. Unfortunately, information on infants and children undergoing airline flights is sparse and limited to case reports and observational studies. This is because problems in flight have been considered to be rare occurrences, and practitioners generally do not deal with large numbers of children travelling by air. There are also logistical problems in undertaking studies in-flight. However, there is a greater body of data in children regarding problems at high altitude, though related to altitudes higher than those experienced during commercial airline flights. Nevertheless, the information has increased our understanding about the effects of hypoxia in flight. This chapter addresses the effects of altitude, their relevance to children with acute and chronic medical conditions who undertake flights, and the management of children who become ill during flight.

PHYSICAL EFFECTS OF ALTITUDE

There are a number of environmental changes that arise from altitude, including changes in atmospheric pressure, partial pressure of oxygen (Po_2), humidity,

temperature and radiation (particularly over the polar areas). Additional effects include fatigue, vibration, noise and motion. Of these it is the fall in oxygen levels that is associated with the potentially most serious consequences. The varying oxygen content of the atmosphere at different altitudes is given in Table 9.1. At sea level, barometric pressure is 760 mmHg (~100 kPa), and the partial pressure of oxygen (Po_2) of 160 mmHg (~21 kPa), i.e. 21 per cent of barometric pressure. Aircraft usually cruise at altitudes of 30 000 – 40 000 feet above sea level, where the atmospheric Po_2 is usually ≤40 mmHg (5 kPa). This would result in a lethal level of hypoxia, and so aircraft cabins are pressurized to 5000–8000 feet above sea level. At the maximum cabin altitude of 8000 feet, the atmospheric pressure is 565 mmHg (75 kPa), giving an atmospheric Po_2 of 118 mmHg (15.7 kPa). This is equivalent to 15–16 per cent of the ambient oxygen available at sea level.

Serious effects of altitude hypoxia do not usually arise until atmospheric pressure drops to that at about 10 000–12 000 feet, although there is a large variability in the response to hypoxia between individuals. Aircraft operate with maximum cabin pressures of 8000 feet, although this may on occasions be exceeded. In one study the median cabin altitude was 6214 feet, but a maximum of 8915 feet was recorded. Newer generation aircraft

Table 9.1 *Barometric pressure and partial pressures of oxygen at altitudes*

| Altitude | | Barometric pressure | | Atmospheric P_{O_2} | | Inspired P_{O_2}* | |
metres	feet	kPa	mmHg	kPa	mmHg	kPa	mmHg
Sea level		100	760	21	159	20	150
1 000	3 280	90	674	18.9	142	17.4	132
2 000	6 560	80	596	16.8	125	15.4	115
3 000	9 840	70	526	14.7	111	13.4	100
5 000	16 400	54	405	11.3	85	10.0	75
8 000	26 240	36	267	7.6	56	6.2	46
10 000	32 800	26	198	5.5	42	4.2	32

*Inspired oxygen pressure is calculated from: oxygen fraction in inspired air × [atmospheric pressure – saturation pressure of water at 37 °C (6.28 kPa/47.1 mmHg)].

may operate at higher altitudes than older aircraft, with a greater risk of hypoxia (Cottrell 1988). It is, therefore, useful to be familiar with the potential risks to infants and children at altitude, even though the cabin altitude is limited and subclinical effects may only become manifest in the setting of other illness.

DIFFERENCES FROM ADULTS

Infants and children have a range of anatomical and physiological differences compared with adults, which increases their susceptibility to hypoxia. These apply particularly to newborns and infants in the first 12 months of life (Table 9.2). Newborns start life with high pulmonary artery pressures, which fall in the first few weeks of life as a result of a fall in pulmonary vascular resistance. This occurs simultaneously with closure of the arterial duct and foramen ovale. However, there remains a relative increase in the proportion of muscularized peripheral arterioles for some months, which can result in marked rises in pulmonary vascular resistance in response to hypoxia. Pre-term newborns also lack surfactant, which makes them more prone to atelectasis and hypoxia. It would not be appropriate for low-birth-weight infants to travel at altitude, except as part of a medical transfer.

In infants, the rib cage is more compliant, and so negative pleural pressures are less effective, contributing to falls in lung volume particularly during active sleep when chest wall muscle tone is reduced. Infants and young children have fewer alveoli than older children and adults, and so during the first few months of life, there is a disproportionate growth in the alveolar region, compared with the airways. Upper and lower airways are smaller

Table 9.2 *Factors increasing the susceptibility of infants and young children to hypoxaemia*

- Hypoxia produces inhibition of respiratory drive (up to 1–2 months of age) – greater tendency for infections to present with apnoea / hypoventilation
- Reduced surfactant (pre-term newborns) – this makes atelectasis and hypoxia more likely
- Higher proportion of the pulmonary vascular bed with muscular arterioles (early infancy) – rises in pulmonary vascular resistance occur more readily leading to hypoxia and right to left shunting
- Lung volume at end expiration is similar to closing volume (early infancy) – small airway closure, and hence non-ventilated units, occur more readily
- Smaller upper and lower internal diameters of the airways – reductions in diameter from, e.g. oedema, reduce patency sooner
- Reactivity of airways, and response to hypoxia prominent in infancy
- Upper respiratory infections may reduce lower airway patency (in infancy)
- Fewer alveoli (early childhood) – increases the susceptibility to mismatches between ventilation and perfusion
- More compliant rib cage, providing less support of lung volume

in diameter, with airway conductance falling from birth to 2 months of age. In the setting of upper or minor respiratory infection, airway patency is reduced, increasing the tendency to airway closure, ventilation–perfusion mismatch and hypoxaemia. Airway (alveolar) hypoxia in infants (arising from falls in inspired Po_2, respiratory infections or chronic lung disease) can cause bronchoconstriction. In infancy, lung volume at end expiration is similar to closing volume, so that during active sleep, feeding and crying when lung volume falls, the number of ventilated units may fall.

Airway (alveolar) hypoxia in infants arising from falls in inspired Po_2, respiratory infections or chronic lung disease can cause pulmonary vasoconstriction, there being greater pulmonary vascular responses to inspired hypoxia in older infants than in newborns. Up until 4–6 months of age, there is still fetal haemoglobin present. This shifts the oxygen dissociation curve to the left, so oxygen is given up less readily to the tissues. At any given Po_2, the haemoglobin oxygen saturation (Sao_2) is higher, consistent with the higher values reported in neonates at 10 000 feet (3100 metres) compared to values at 4 months of age.

Many of the above factors may contribute to an increased tendency to ventilation–perfusion mismatch in early life, with the result that infants and young children are particularly susceptible to hypoxaemic episodes with illnesses and airway hypoxia. The adverse effects of chronic hypoxia are well documented, particularly in early infancy and those with chronic lung disease. These include poor weight gain, pulmonary hypertension, rise in airway resistance and apnoeic–cyanotic episodes. The importance of these factors in the healthy infant who sustains shorter periods of hypoxia, as occurs during airline flights, is unknown. Nevertheless, there are some data that have examined the short-term effects of hypoxia in infancy.

PHYSIOLOGICAL EFFECTS OF ALTITUDE

The effects of altitude, both acute and long term, are summarized in Table 9.3. Children have been studied in the high altitude regions of the world (>10 000 feet (>3000 metres)), and they have been shown to have higher minute ventilation, tidal volume, expiratory duration, vital capacity, lung compliance, pul-

Table 9.3 *The physiological effects of high altitude*

	Acute effect	Found in indigenous
Respiratory		
Arterial Po_2 and oxygen saturation	↓	↓
Minute ventilation	↑	↑
Carbon dioxide	↓	↓
Oxygen consumption/CO_2 production	↓	→
Lung volumes (vital capacity, residual volume)	↑	↑
Lung compliance		↑
Peak flow/forced expiratory volume in 1s	↓	
Lung gas transfer (DLCO)	↓	↑
Nocturnal arousals/less active sleep	↑	
Periodic breathing	↑	
Cardiovascular		
Heart rate	↑	→
Cardiac output	↑	→
Pulmonary artery pressure	↑	↑
Pulmonary vascular resistance	↑	
Capillary leak	↑	
Erythropoietin and red blood cell production	↑	↑
Neurological		
Cerebral blood flow	↑	
Intracranial pressure	↑	
Body growth		
Birth weight	↓	
Post-natal growth	↓ *	

Comparisons are related to sea level values: →no difference; ↑ increased; ↓ reduced.
Data relate to children where it exists.
*May be accounted for by factors such as socioeconomic deprivation.

monary diffusing capacity, oxygen extraction, haematocrit and haemoglobin levels, and an increased tendency to pulmonary hypertension and to maintain pulmonary vascular reactivity.

Infants and children also have lower Sao_2 levels, dependent on altitude (Table 9.4). At sea level, normal Sao_2 levels have been defined. Measurements in quiet sleep (when motion is minimal and a steady state is more reliably obtained) are 96–100 per cent in healthy infants and children. Hypoxaemia at altitude can be a useful predictor of illness severity, and is strongly associated with mortality in acute illness.

Upon exposure to hypoxia, the usual response is to increase minute ventilation, mainly as a result of increased tidal volume. Newborn infants, born at

Table 9.4 *Summary of normal Sao$_2$ levels at different altitudes*

Altitude (metres)	Age studied	Sao$_2$ (%) mean/median	range
Sea level	2–16 years, mean 8 years	99.5	96–100
	2 months–5 years	98.7	96–100
1610	< 48 hours old	93.0	79–98
	3 months old	92.2	86–97
1670	7 days–36 months	95.7	89–99
2640	5 days–24 months	93.0	84–100
2800	3–670 days	91.7	88–97
3100	6 hours–4 months	86.5	81–91
3658	< 24 hours	Immigrants	76–90
		Indigenous	86–94
3750	2–60 months	88.9	81–97
4540	0.5–72 hours		57–75

Values given are those in (quiet) sleep.

either full term or pre-term, show a characteristic biphasic response, with a transient increase in ventilation followed by a decline by 3–5 minutes. This decrease in ventilation may persist for some time after the reinstitution of normoxic breathing. The biphasic response is short lived, usually disappearing after a few weeks of age, but may persist longer in infants born pre-term, making them prone to greater degrees of hypoxaemia in relation to ambient hypoxia.

In infants, exposure to 15 per cent oxygen for 6 hours at sea level produces hypoxaemia, with a median fall in Sao$_2$ of 4.9 per cent. The response is highly variable, and is not predicted from the baseline variables of oxygenation, respiratory rate, or pattern. There is a decrease in regular breathing pattern (equated to quiet sleep), more time is spent in periodic breathing, and a decrease in prolonged apnoeic pauses. The latter is opposite to the effect noted in pre-term newborns, where increased apnoea occurs. Episodic desaturation occurs much more frequently, but infants are not aroused by the hypoxaemia. Clearly, hypoxaemia, though not clinically evident, may occur in infants at cabin altitudes.

It is not possible to predict the degree of hypoxaemia or any systemic effect in infants from exposure to current cabin altitudes without undertaking some pre-exposure challenge test. This knowledge is important for those with an already identified medical condition, though it is those who are healthy on long-haul flights who might most benefit from knowledge of their individual response.

ASSESSMENT OF RESPONSE TO HYPOXIA

A key question is when should oxygen therapy be administered. For example, should a healthy child who has Sao$_2$ levels below the normal range at any given altitude receive additional inspired oxygen? On the ground, oxygen has been given to infants without pulmonary disease so as to maintain Sao$_2$ $\geq$90 per cent at 5280 feet (1610 metres) and $\geq$88 per cent at 9190 feet (2800 metres). These altitudes are within those of the aircraft cabins. In an attempt to determine whether children should receive additional inspired oxygen in-flight, they can be exposed to a hypoxic environment similar to that of the flight cabin. In one study in children aged 11–16 years with cystic fibrosis, the response to 15 per cent oxygen was measured before a flight to a high altitude destination (5900 feet (1800 metres)). The test identified those at risk of desaturation below 90 per cent. However, there is little information on the effect of such an hypoxic environment for the several hours of a transcontinental flight.

In the presence of respiratory problems and in those receiving oxygen, it is advisable to use oxygen therapy to maintain levels of Sao$_2$ in the higher end of the relevant normal range. This is most easily achieved by titrating the oxygen supply against pulse oximetry measurements. In spontaneously breathing children, the flow rate of oxygen can be increased according to the Sao$_2$ level, whereas in ventilated patients, the fractional inspired oxygen concentration may be increased to account for the hypoxia at altitude. This was done in the 4907-mile transfer from Vancouver to London of a 6-year-old boy for heart–lung transplantation (MacNab *et al.* 1990). The aircraft operated at a low altitude with maximum cabin altitude of 3700 feet to ensure Sao$_2$ levels of at least 80 per cent.

CLINICAL EFFECTS OF HIGH ALTITUDE

Acute mountain sickness, high-altitude pulmonary oedema and high-altitude cerebral oedema may occur at altitudes above 8000 feet. Acute mountain sickness presents with headache, nausea, vomiting, anorexia, weakness and insomnia and symptoms may occur 12–24 hours after arrival at altitude and worsen over the next 2–3 days. However, although such problems are not thought to occur after long-haul flights, it is useful to be aware of the symptomatology as mild versions could possibly occur in susceptible children. Studies in high-altitude regions have identified a number of factors which increase susceptibility to the effects of hypoxia. These are young age, exercise, recent infections and rapid ascent as well as genetic susceptibility, state of hydration and any underlying illness. There are also two physiological responses which when depressed may contribute to the effects of hypoxia. These are a poor ventilatory response and loss of normal diuresis at altitude.

SUDDEN INFANT DEATH SYNDROME

There is uncertainty as to whether the effect of high altitude hypoxia is related to sudden and unexpected infant death (Niermyer and Moore 1998). Epidemiological, pathological and clinical evidence links hypoxia to sudden death, for example, severe hypoxaemic episodes can lead to sudden death (Southall *et al.* 1990). There is also a high prevalence of hypoxaemia in pre-term infants who have suffered cyanotic episodes receiving resuscitation, or near death events (Samuels *et al.* 1992). In addition, infants who are at risk of subclinical hypoxaemia, i.e. pre-term infants, those with respiratory infections, and those who have suffered apparent life-threatening events, have increased risk of sudden infant death.

Nevertheless, despite evidence linking altitude-related hypoxia and sudden death, the altitude of aircraft cabins is clearly not sufficiently high to cause major problems. In one enquiry into deaths during infancy, air travel was documented. There were 130 cases of the sudden infant death syndrome and 528 controls (Ward Platt *et al.* 1998). None of the infants who died had flown. Sample size may have been too small to discount absolutely a relation between air travel and sudden infant death, but any possibility of infants dying during the first few days after a long-haul flight is unlikely, and so there is no reason on this evidence to make any recommendations that infants should not fly. Essentially, flying appears to be safe for healthy children in the first year of life, though care must be taken with the use of sedatives and when undertaking flights with current respiratory infections.

AIR TRANSPORT

The potentially adverse effects of air travel, other than hypoxia, are highlighted by the problems faced by sick neonates and children when transported over large distances to specialized units. These include expansion of trapped gases, stress from noise, vibration and motion, and decreased temperature. Gases expand at altitude [100 ml at sea level becomes 130 ml at 6000 feet (1830 metres) and 400 ml at 10 000 metres], and this may have adverse effects on gases in body cavities, such as the pleural space, gut and middle ear. Without anticipation and management of these problems, severe discomfort, pain and ill health may occur. In children with severe respiratory illness or those receiving mechanical ventilation, life-threatening complications can follow, including tension pneumothorax, pneumomediastinum and pulmonary interstitial emphysema. Abnormal air collections, such as may occur in the pleural space, should be drained before transport by air or may preclude air transport altogether.

Lower environmental temperatures can occur at altitude, which means that small or exposed infants may lose heat easily. Careful attention should be paid to temperature regulation, particularly in sick infants, as hypothermia and shivering increase oxygen consumption, and may aggravate metabolic acidosis and hypoglycaemia. Humidity also falls with altitude, and this may pose problems for those who regularly produce sputum. In sick children, who are transported with mechanical ventilation, it is possible to provide additional humidity in inspired gases. This will assist temperature control and fluid balance and help to ensure that the tenacity of secretions is optimum.

ADVICE FOR FLYING

There is little published data to help with guidance on the suitability of flying or travel to high altitude for medical conditions other than those where hypoxia is a risk factor. For example, advice on the timing of travel after surgery, particularly when air has entered a body cavity, is predominantly down to the views of individual practitioners. If there are concerns whether the health of an infant or child could be impaired during or after an airline flight, an opinion from a paediatrician should be sought to ensure the child is healthy. In young infants some reassurance may be gained by normal Sao_2 levels at sea level, although these do not necessarily predict the response to an altitude related hypoxia.

Some airlines produce their own literature to help in planning the needs of the healthy infant and child going on a flight. Their key advice is given in Table 9.5. An issue with long flights, in addition to keeping infants and children occupied and happy, is changes in time zones. Generally, it is simplest to adjust as soon as possible to the new time. This may mean extending waking hours or going to sleep sooner than usual. Any medications given regularly should also be adjusted to the new time zone. In chronic conditions such as epilepsy or asthma, taking half to one dose more or less than normal to account for the increase or decrease in hours on the day of travel may be appropriate.

Some practitioners have advised the use of sedation for children travelling long distances by air, or indeed other modes of transport. Whilst some patients have enjoyed a more peaceful journey, the effects of sedation are not always predictable in children. Some respond by fighting the effects, which can make their behaviour all the more difficult. It is preferable that, if such medication is to be given in-flight, that the parents have had some experience beforehand. Sedating antihistamines, such as promethazine (10–25 mg) and trimeprazine (2.5–5 mg), or choral hydrate (30–50 mg kg^{-1}), have been used in this setting. However, it is not advisable to give such medication to children under age 2 years. Indeed, in infants, the use of phenothiazine medication has been associated with sudden infant death. With children it is always advisable to carry some basic first aid items including simple analgesics, plasters, oral rehydration sachets, antiseptic wipes, emollient or barrier cream, sunscreen lotion and insect repellent.

Although a newborn infant, normal on examination, may appear well enough to fly, it is advisable to delay airline travel for the first few months of life. Theoretically, at least, exposure to the hypoxia of the cabin could trigger an hypoxaemic episode. There are anecdotal reports of life-threatening episodes and sudden infant death occurring on or shortly after airline flights, particularly long-haul flights, though there are currently no data that show whether such events occur with a greater or lesser frequency in airline flights compared with being on the ground. Essentially it is not possible to state whether sudden death could be precipitated in susceptible infants. However, newborn infants, particularly in the first 6–8 weeks of life, are more likely to present with illness in a sudden or unexpected way. They may fail to show the usual early signs of an infection such as fever, but present with episodes of apnoea (aggravated or brought on by hypoxia), and have a greater tendency to cardiorespiratory failure. The susceptibility to illness is an even greater problem for the pre-term infant, and for infants with chronic lung or cardiac disease. Infants with active respiratory infections should avoid travel, as even an apparently minor cold may be associated with subclinical hypoxaemia.

If the child is already receiving oxygen for part or all of the day, oxygen will be needed in flight. If there is a respiratory problem that could be associated with hypoxaemia and the child is not already receiving oxygen therapy (Table 9.6), an assessment should be undertaken to decide whether oxygen should be used in flight. An infant or a child susceptible to

Table 9.5 *Airline advice for travellers flying with infants and children*

In advance of flight

- Have valid passports and visas
- Ensure necessary immunizations obtained
- Obtain a letter of certification for medicines
- If health problems exist, obtain details of medical history and current drugs from the doctor
- Take out adequate health insurance
- Book any special dietary needs, or children's mini meals
- Book the use of carry cots
- Consider the use of papoose-type baby carriers for boarding and disembarking
- Carry a change of clothing in the hand luggage
- Carry toiletry/first aid items in the hand luggage, e.g. toothbrush and paste, emollient/chap stick, wet wipes/cloth, simple analgesics

During flight

- Feed babies, offer drinks or give sweets to suck during ascent and descent to prevent/relieve middle ear discomfort
- Offer drinks regularly on longer flights to counteract the dry air on board
- Carry sufficient feeds (plus extra water), as well as snacks for children
- Carry sufficient medications in hand luggage to last longer than the flight
- Take some favourite toys/games to help occupy the child
- Use sleep wear/bedtime toys to encourage sleep routine

hypoxaemia should have their saturations estimated during the flight by pulse oximetry, and be provided with oxygen according to the saturation levels.

Airlines require that oxygen is booked in advance, and so intending passengers should ideally undergo some form of hypoxic challenge in advance. However, this may not be possible and it may be necessary to give an opinion with only an assessment of sea level saturations. A short period of measurement while awake has limited predictive value and may easily underestimate the potential degree of desaturation. In infants and those with respiratory problems, saturation levels are usually lowest after a few hours of sleep, particularly in REM sleep when the ribcage muscle tone is low and lung volumes fall. Only a sufficiently long period of measurement in a normoxic environment is likely to be useful in pre-

Table 9.6 *Medical conditions with increased risk for hypoxia-related problems*

Chronic lung disease

- of prematurity
- cystic fibrosis
- reactive airway disease

Sleep-related upper airway obstruction

Chest wall conditions

- muscle weakness, e.g. muscular dystrophy
- restrictive lung disease, e.g. scoliosis and other rib cage disorders

Infections

- respiratory: upper and lower

Haematological

- sickle cell diseases

Cardiac conditions

- increased pulmonary blood flow, e.g. ventricular septal defect, patent arterial duct
- pulmonary hypertension
- heart failure
- cardiomyopathy
- arrhythmias

Neurological

- seizure disorder with respiratory effects
- cerebral palsy, with truncal weakness/chest deformity
- brainstem disorder (with bulbar effects or sleep disordered breathing)
- raised intracranial pressure

dicting saturations at altitude. Where there is doubt, it is a safer option to arrange for oxygen to be available, even if not ultimately used.

The decision that oxygen might be needed in-flight should lead to a request, well before the intended flight, to the airline to provide oxygen. The pre-flight assessment will have helped to determine the amount of oxygen needed to maintain adequate SaO_2 for, perhaps, several hours. Arrangements should also be made to ensure that supplies of oxygen are available before and after the flight.

MEDICAL EMERGENCIES IN-FLIGHT

Medical emergencies in infants and children in flight are fortunately uncommon. Although a flight may have a medical practitioner on board, it is essential that the parents of children with known medical conditions are clear about how to deal with potential problems. These are usually no different from those that may occur everyday, but the stress of long-distance travel and changes in the physical and temporal environment increase the likelihood of a deterioration in many established conditions. Consultation with the paediatrician is advised prior to long flights, particularly where the stability of the child's condition is less than optimal, or where clinical deterioration has potentially serious or life-threatening consequences. For children with known medical problems, parents should ensure that there is enough medication for at least twice the duration of the flight. In addition, if equipment or drugs are carried, it is helpful to have a letter from the family doctor which explains the need for these, and when they are to be used. If a child shows signs of being seriously ill, then the captain must be informed about the likely natural history. The condition of a child can change quickly and repeat assessments should be undertaken. Progression of illness with signs of respiratory, circulatory or neurological failure, despite basic treatment, may well warrant a diversion.

THE SERIOUSLY ILL CHILD

There are a number of clinical signs that are important in assessing the severity of an illness in an infant or child. As far as breathing is concerned, tachypnoea may occur from fever, pain, respiratory or circulatory failure (Table 9.7). Chest wall recession indicates increased respiratory effort, but the intensity of stridor or wheeze does not indicate the degree of airways obstruction. Grunting (expiratory noise indicating attempts to keep open the airways/alveoli) can also occur with acute abdominal emergencies and raised intracranial pressure. In infants, the use of their accessory muscles may cause head bobbing. Nasal flaring and pallor are also important signs. These signs of respiratory distress may not be seen or heard when there is muscle disease, depression of consciousness or extreme fatigue.

Heart rate (Table 9.7) and pulse volume are relevant signs as far as the circulatory system is concerned. Capillary refill can be assessed by pressing on the sternum or on skin that is level with the heart for 5 seconds. The blanched skin should start to re-perfuse within 2 seconds in a war environment. Blood pressure in children is usually normal until there is severe shock (Table 9.7).

The level of consciousness is an important assessment. This can be done using the AVPU scale:

- **A**lert,
- responds to **V**oice,
- responds to **P**ain, and
- **U**nresponsive.

The posture of children who are unwell becomes more hypotonic while decorticate or decerebrate postures are, of course, signs of serious dysfunction. Dilatation, unreactivity and asymmetry of the pupils are of serious import.

Knowledge of what is normal for a child at any particular age is valuable in assessing changes. Children who are seriously ill are usually quiet, pale and inattentive. They may not recognize their parents. Severe respiratory, circulatory or neurological problems warrant diversion of the aircraft. The clinical condition of a child can change quickly. Regular and repeat assessments of an ill child are helpful. Even giving an antipyretic/analgesic, such as paracetamol, to a child with fever can dramatically improve their colour and degree of alertness.

SPECIFIC CONDITIONS

Respiratory

With severe breathing difficulties, priorities include assessment and adequacy of the airway, the provision of high-flow oxygen (use of a facemask, preferably with a reservoir bag, at as high a flow rate as possible, e.g. 10–15 l min^{-1}), and if respiratory effort is poor, assisted breathing with a mask and self-inflating bag,

Table 9.7 *Clinical measurements by age*

Age (years)	Respiratory rate (breaths per minute)	Heart rate (beats per minute)	Systolic BP (mmHg)
< 1	30–40	110–160	70–90
1–2	25–35	110–150	80–95
2–5	25–35	95–145	80–100
5–12	20–25	80–120	90–110
>12	15–20	60–100	100–120
Weight estimates	**(kg)**		
Pre-term	1–2.5		
Term	3.5		
5 months	7		
1 year	10		
> 1 year, weight (kg) = 2 × (age + 4)			
e.g. 6 years	20		

Note: drug doses are calculated up to a maximum 40 kg.

or mouth-to-mouth/mouth-to-mask. In less severe cases, consideration needs to be given to specific treatment of the underlying causes (see below). Stridor indicates upper airway obstruction (e.g. croup, foreign body); wheeze occurs with asthma and bronchiolitis; marked tachycardia, pallor and hepatomegaly indicate heart failure; and fever suggests pneumonia. Change in conscious level may reflect respiratory depression of central origin or severe respiratory failure. The use of a pulse oximeter is helpful to guide the need for additional oxygen therapy.

With moderate to severe respiratory distress due to asthma and bronchiolitis, high-flow oxygen should be given (use of a facemask with a reservoir bag and as high a flow rate as possible, e.g. 10–15 l min^{-1}, provides close to 100 per cent oxygen). Bronchiolitis is commonest in the first few months of life, and whilst there is no specific treatment, attention should be given to ensuring adequate oxygenation and hydration, and clearance of upper airway secretions (particularly from the nose). Inhaled adrenaline may be found to help in some circumstances. The use of inhaled bronchodilators and systemic steroids (oral prednisolone 0.5 mg kg^{-1} or intravenous hydrocortisone 4 mg kg^{-1}) is usually unhelpful in the first few months of life, but may be tried in infants from around 9–12 months. Nevertheless, in severe cases, it would be reasonable to use systemic steroids and intramuscular adrenaline 5–10 μg kg^{-1}.

Exacerbations of asthma should be treated with an inhaled bronchodilator given every 30 minutes to 4 hours, depending on response and severity. In severe cases, a continuous bronchodilator may be given, in addition to oxygen. This can be provided with the patient's usual inhaler, or alternatively with an aerosol inhaler via a spacer device (commercial spacers include the Aerochamber or Volumatic, or use a large plastic bottle or cup, with the inhaler sealed in one end, and the other end on the face). Give 2–10 sprays as needed, with one spray being followed by four to five inhalations, and repeat as needed. Rises in heart rate may occur with bronchodilators, but may also indicate increasing respiratory distress. Oral prednisolone 0.5 mg kg^{-1} should also be given (a less effective option is 5–20 inhalations of the usual inhaled corticosteroid dose). The patient with asthma should include in their travel medications a short course of steroids, as well as their usual maintenance therapy.

The inhalation of a foreign body is a problem common in pre-school children, and should be suspected if there is a sudden onset of respiratory difficulties with coughing, gagging or stridor. If these symptoms are due to a respiratory infection (croup, epiglottitis), or the child is still breathing adequately, physical methods of clearing the airway may lead to respiratory deterioration or arrest, and should be avoided. If the diagnosis of foreign body is clear-cut or apnoea has occurred, then the foreign body may be removed by blows on the back and thrusts to the chest in infants or by back blows, abdominal thrusts or the Heimlich manoeuvre in infants over 1 year of age. Depending on the size of the child, these can be done with the child laid over the lap, supported in a sitting position or supine on the floor.

In croup and upper airway obstruction, oxygen should be provided. It is important to avoid upsetting the child as this may precipitate respiratory arrest. As most causes of upper airway obstruction involve some degree of inflammation and mucosal oedema, it is helpful to give steroids (dexamethasone 0.15 mg kg^{-1} orally or 0.5–1.0 mg kg^{-1} prednisolone orally) and nebulized (or inhaled) adrenaline 2–5 ml. In severe cases, as intubation is impractical, it may help to give intramuscular adrenaline 10 μg kg^{-1}.

Children with cystic fibrosis and other chronic respiratory conditions should be assessed for hypoxaemia, in case they need oxygen therapy in flight. A short-term reading of baseline Sao$_2$ in air and when awake is not a good predictor of the likely Sao$_2$ levels at altitude, and such patients should undergo a preflight simulation test with a hypoxic gas mixture. This more accurately predicts the response to the hypoxia in the aircraft cabin and at altitude (Oades et al. 1994). Children with chronic suppurative lung disease should have their lung function optimized before travel, if necessary with a course of antibiotics and physiotherapy. Travel medications should include high-dose antibiotics.

Hypoxia will seriously aggravate the condition of children with heart failure or pulmonary hypertension. Airline travel would usually be advised against, or if undertaken, oxygen is likely to be essential. Children with right-to-left shunts may have moderate to severe arterial hypoxaemia, but in most cases their airway/alveolar oxygenation will be normal, and with additional oxygen therapy there may be little effect on their arterial oxygen levels. It is important that advice is sought from a cardiologist prior to arranging airline travel.

Gastrointestinal

In diarrhoea and vomiting it is necessary to assess any degree of dehydration (Table 9.8). The signs may indicate loss of total body fluid and must not be confused with shock (tachycardia, weak pulse volumes, prolonged capillary refill, cool/mottled peripheries, altered mental status and pale colour). If dehydration is mild, or not even present, then it is only necessary to ensure the child is given regular fluids (with calories) to maintain hydration. Ideally this should be given orally, providing small and frequent drinks. Based on body weight, this can be estimated per hour as 4 ml kg^{-1} for the first 10 kg body weight, 2 ml kg^{-1} for the second 10 kg body weight, and 1 ml kg^{-1} for each subsequent kg body weight. For example, a child of 8 years, with an estimated weight of 24 kg (see Table 9.7), would need 40 ml + 20 ml + 4 ml = 64 ml fluid per hour.

If there is >5 per cent dehydration, it is necessary to ensure that the child takes an oral rehydration solution, or some fluid that contains salt (salted rice water, a salted yoghurt, vegetable or chicken soup). In addition, fluid should be replaced with 50 ml kg^{-1} over 2–4 hours if there is moderate dehydration (poor skin turgor, sunken eyes, dry mucous membranes) and 100 ml kg^{-1} in severe dehydration. If vomiting has occurred, a teaspoon every 5 minutes is given, increasing as tolerated. Drinks sweetened with sugar should be avoided as these can cause osmotic diarrhoea and hypernatraemia. Fluids with stimulant, diuretic or purgative effects, for example, coffee and some medicinal teas or infusions, should also be avoided. Consider replacing each watery or loose stool passed with 10 ml kg^{-1} and each vomit with 2 ml kg^{-1}. If this is not tolerated, the condition is more severe or there is evidence of shock (tachycardia, weak pulse volume, prolonged capillary refill, altered mental status and pale colour), fluid replacement should be given intravenously – initially as a bolus dose of 20 ml kg^{-1} normal (0.9 per cent) saline or Hartmann's solution. In an emergency, vascular access can be obtained by the intraosseous route, using a large bore needle (14–18 G).

Shock

Management of shock is more of a priority than that of dehydration. Shock has numerous causes, including gastroenteritis, septicaemia, gut surgical emergencies, anaphylaxis, heart failure and diabetes. Treatment will require ongoing fluid replacement and treatment of the underlying cause, for example, antibiotics for septicaemia, adrenaline (10 μg kg^{-1} intramuscular) for anaphylaxis, and diuretics for heart failure.

Seizures and loss of consciousness

Hypoxia, sleep disturbance, the excitement of travel, and caffeine found in cola drinks and chocolate may increase susceptibility to fits. In known epileptics on long westbound flights where the day is prolonged, an extra dose of anticonvulsant may be given. Children with uncontrolled epileptic fits should travel with some medication for stopping a seizure, such as rectal diazepam or paraldehyde. During a major convulsion, the priorities are maintenance

Table 9.8 *Symptoms and signs of dehydration*

Sign/symptom	Mild (< 5%)	Moderate (5–10%)	Severe (>10%)	Notes
Dry mouth	+/−	+	+	Dry in mouth breathers
Reduced skin turgor	−	+/−	+	Check different sites
Tachypnoea	−	+/−	+	From fever, or acidosis
Tachycardia	−	+/−	+	From fever, pain or shock
Less urine output	+	+	+	Unseen if stools very loose

Other signs include sunken eyes and anterior fontanelle (in infants <1 year).

of the airway, provision of oxygen and avoidance of accidental injury. After a convulsion, the recovery position should be used to help maintain an adequate airway, and oxygen provided. If convulsions do not stop spontaneously after 5–10 minutes, quick-acting anticonvulsants should be used, such as rectal diazepam 0.5 mg kg^{-1}, rectal paraldehyde 0.4 ml kg^{-1} (made up with the same volume of olive oil or normal saline), intravenous lorazepam 0.1 mg kg^{-1} or intravenous diazepam 0.25–0.4 mg kg^{-1}, and repeated if necessary. Attention should be given to the adequacy of breathing, and checking a blood sugar, particularly in known diabetics. Febrile convulsions are common in pre-school children – usually from viral infections (although even meningitis can present in this way) but are short-lived tonic–clonic convulsions. If fever is present, measures should be taken to cool the child, including removing layers of clothing and administering an antipyretic such as paracetamol 10–15 mg kg^{-1} or ibuprofen 5–7 mg kg^{-1}.

The conscious level of a child can be assessed rapidly with the AVPU scale. Responsiveness to pain or worse is a situation where there may be associated effects on the airway and breathing, so oxygen therapy should be considered. The main immediately treatable causes of coma should be considered. A blood sugar stick test should be undertaken and if hypoglycaemia is found (<3 mmol l^{-1}), intravenous dextrose 10 per cent 5 ml kg^{-1} should be given. A fever or purpuric rash may indicate meningococcaemia and high-dose antibiotics should be given. On returning from a tropical country, malaria is a possibility and quinine may be useful. If there are signs of raised intracranial pressure (posturing, abnormal pupillary responses with dilatation, abnormal breathing patterns, bradycardia and raised blood pressure), prop the head up 20 degrees and, if available, give mannitol 0.5–1.0 g kg^{-1} intravenously. Induce hyperventilation with a facemask and bag to lower carbon dioxide levels.

Close control of diabetes is necessary to avoid hypo- or hyperglycaemia. For hypoglycaemia, give sweet drinks or food, intravenous dextrose 10 per cent 2–5 ml kg^{-1}, or glucagon 20 µg kg^{-1} intramuscularly. Diabetic ketoacidosis is recognized by rapid breathing, acetone on the breath, marked diuresis and dehydration. This should be treated with oxygen therapy and plenty of fluids given. If shock exists, fluids will need to be given, preferably intravenously (normal saline or Hartmann's solution 20 ml kg^{-1} over 20–30 minutes). Regular maintenance fluids should be given (as for 'diarrhoea' above), plus extra for any dehydration given over 8–12 hours. This can be calculated as deficit (litres) = per cent dehydration × body weight (kg) – see Tables 9.7 and 9.8 for calculating this on age and clinical signs. Extra insulin will be needed: when given as an intravenous infusion, a rate of 0.05–0.1 unit kg^{-1} h^{-1} reduces the blood sugar. An equivalent dose can be calculated to give subcutaneously every 2–4 hours, with checks on blood sugar. Do not omit to give a source of calories, particularly once blood sugar levels are below 12 mmol l^{-1}.

Fever and the irritable child

There are numerous reasons for the irritable and screaming child, from behavioural problems to severe pain, fever or meningitis. A calm approach is necessary using historical pointers and observation to determine the problem. Sedation is not usually needed, although sleep may follow the administration of analgesic/antipyretic medication (see below). Earache on descent or ascent may be missed and drinks or sweets may relieve any pressure maldistribution across the eardrum.

Children with fever look and feel miserable, but are mostly aware of their parents. The main cause is infections, most of which are fortunately self-limiting of viral origin. Some produce transient, blanching rashes (a purpuric rash should be considered to be meningococcaemia and antibiotics given), or may be associated with other non-specific symptoms such as central abdominal pain, diarrhoea, listlessness, delirium and anorexia. Pre-school children may have febrile convulsions with a fever. These are short, generalized tonic–clonic convulsions. Recurrence is common, so there may be a history of this response. Children will determine themselves their own level of activity, but small and frequent drinks should be offered, and antipyretics/analgesics, such as paracetamol 10–15 mg kg^{-1} or ibuprofen 5–7 mg kg^{-1}, used for high fever or pain. The decision as to whether to use antibiotics is generally based on recognition of a specific source of infection with a likely bacterial origin, e.g. meningitis, urinary infection or pneumonia, or if symptoms and signs are non-specific, the degree of fever, listlessness and pallor.

Otitis media

There are concerns about the risks of flying with acute or chronic serous otitis media (glue ear). The danger is of either air in the middle ear not escaping as expansion occurs on ascent, or of air not entering the middle ear on descent because of Eustachian tube dysfunction. The failure to equilibrate pressures in the middle ear is more likely in children with adenoidal hypertrophy, and recurrent otitis media. Middle ears that are filled entirely with fluid are probably less likely to cause problems, than those where there is a fluid–air interface (Weiss and Frost 1987). Because air travels more easily from the ear to nasopharynx, descent of the aircraft is potentially a time for more problems. If the Eustachian tube does not vent, the tube may block because of the higher atmospheric pressures (Brown 1994). In children with recent or chronic otitis, simple manoeuvres, such as swallowing, drinking liquids and Valsalva manoeuvres during ascent and descent may help avoid such problems. Where there is a higher level of concern, nasal decongestants have been used 1–2 hours before take-off, and 30 minutes before descent.

Sickle cell disease

Children with sickle cell disease are at risk from sickling crises during flight. This particularly applies to patients with splenomegaly and relatively higher blood viscosity (from near normal haemoglobin levels). Patients with HbSC and sickle cell thalassaemia are more at risk, and oxygen therapy has been recommended at altitudes over 7000 feet (Green *et al.* 1971). These recommendations suggested that for classical sickle cell disease, where the spleen was known to have previously auto-infarcted, travel in pressurized aircraft should not pose a problem. If a child with sickle cell disease or trait suffers a problem with acute chest, abdominal or bone pain, or a cerebrovascular event, then attention should be paid to providing additional inspired oxygen,

adequate hydration and warmth. Pain relief with intravenous/intramuscular morphine 100–200 μg kg^{-1} (25–100 μg kg^{-1} under 1 year of age) should also be given.

Anaphylaxis

Anaphylaxis may arise from allergy to certain foods, especially nuts, shellfish, eggs, dairy products, and medications such as penicillin. Early symptoms include a burning sensation in the mouth, itching of lips, mouth and throat, angio-oedema, urticarial rash, conjunctivitis, nausea or abdominal pain, cough, wheeze and stridor. This may progress to respiratory distress, shock and cardiorespiratory arrest. Management includes removal of the allergen, if possible, oxygen therapy, and intramuscular adrenaline 10 μg kg^{-1}. Other medications that may be useful include nebulized adrenaline (for upper airway obstruction), inhaled salbutamol (for lower airway obstruction), oral prednisolone 1 mg kg^{-1} or intravenous hydrocortisone 4 mg kg^{-1}, and oral antihistamine.

REFERENCES

Brown TP. Middle ear symptoms while flying. Ways to prevent a severe outcome. *Postgrad Med* 1994; **96**: 135–42.

Cottrell JJ. Altitude exposures during aircraft flight. Flying higher. *Chest* 1988; **92**: 81–3.

Green RL, Huntsman RG and Serjeant GR. The sickle-cell and altitude. *Br Med J* 1971; **4**: 593–5.

Macnab AJ, Vachon J, Susak LE and Pirie GE. In-flight stabilization of oxygen saturation by control of altitude for severe respiratory insufficiency. *Aviat Space Environ Med* 1990; **61**: 829–32.

Niermyer S and Moore LG. No known mechanism links hypoxia and sudden infant death syndrome. *Br Med J* 1998; **317**: 675–6.

Oades PJ, Buchdahl RM and Bush A. Prediction of hypoxaemia at high altitude in children with cystic fibrosis. *Br Med J* 1994; **308**: 15–18.

Samuels MP, Poets CF, Stebbens VA and Southall DP. Oxygen saturation and breathing patterns in preterm infants with cyanotic episodes. *Acta Paediatr* 1992; **81**: 875–80.

Southall DP, Samuels MP and Talbert DG. Recurrent cyanotic episodes with severe arterial hypoxaemia and intrapulmonary shunting: a mechanism for sudden death. *Arch Dis Child* 1990; **65**: 953–61.

Ward Platt M, Fleming PJ, Blair PS, Leach CEA and Golding J. Danger to babies from air travel must be small. *Br Med J* 1998; **317**: 676.

Weiss M and Frost JO. May children with otitis media with effusion safely fly? *Clin Pediatr* 1987; **26**: 567–8.

10

Breathlessness and chest pain in-flight

ANDREW RC CUMMIN

Medical practitioners called to an unwell passenger may well have not practised in the relevant field for decades, and, even if they have, they will not have access, in flight, to their usual tools for diagnosis. Yet the practitioner may well be expected to know what is wrong and what advice to give and, for the sake of the patient, they may well have to assume an air of confidence. Some conditions may not cause too much concern even for the rustiest of practitioners. A patient collapsing to the floor following a simple faint tends to cause public consternation but, although the patient may initially look very unwell, calm assessment is all that is required to allow enough time to pass for nature to take its course and effect a prompt full recovery for which the doctor may be able to take some credit. But some conditions will alarm even the experienced medical volunteer. Amongst these are chest pain and breathlessness.

BREATHLESSNESS

Breathlessness is a common symptom that may be caused by a wide range of conditions, each requiring different treatment. The cause of breathlessness occurring in-flight is likely to fall into one of three main categories: respiratory disease, cardiac disease, or psychogenic causes. Amongst the other possible causes and one that might be exacerbated by air travel is anaemia. Despite the variety of conditions that may cause breathlessness, the sen-

sation is essentially the same whatever the cause. Attempts to identify descriptors of breathlessness that will distinguish one cause from another have not met with success (Elliott *et al.* 1991). Nevertheless, there are features in the history that may help. Unfortunately, breathless patients find it difficult to talk and on an international flight there may well be language difficulties. The patient, their relatives and cabin crew seek treatment rather than diagnosis. Desperate patients may clutch the doctor's arm and beg for relief while anxious relatives may distract the doctor by demanding that something is done. But proper treatment cannot occur without diagnosis and the most important aid to diagnosis is a thorough history. It is important, in these circumstances, to appear calm and gently persevere with obtaining as full a history as practicable.

One of the most important factors in diagnosing the cause of breathlessness is the time course of the onset of the shortness of breath. Breathlessness occurring in-flight is likely to be of rapid onset and this can be very helpful diagnostically as breathlessness occurring suddenly has only a limited number of likely causes. Common causes of breathlessness of rapid onset include pneumothorax, pulmonary embolism and pulmonary oedema. Some patients with asthma have sudden severe attacks and pneumonia may also cause breathlessness developing over as short a period as an hour.

The age of the patient will alter the likelihood of some diagnoses. A young patient with sudden breathlessness is likely to have asthma. Older patients may also have sudden asthma attacks, though in the second half of life asthma tends to be less labile. Pulmonary oedema is much more likely in the elderly or those with pre-existing heart disease. Pneumonia may affect any age, as may pulmonary embolism, but the latter is seen mainly in those aged over 40. Typically, spontaneous pneumothoraces are seen in tall young men, but, when secondary to underlying lung disease, older age groups are affected. Smoking substantially increases the risk of pneumothorax.

Pulmonary embolism

There are reasons to believe that air travel may predispose to venous thromboembolic disease. According to Virchow's triad, alterations in blood flow, damage to the vessel wall, or changes within the blood itself can affect susceptibility to thrombosis. Immobility related to air travel tends to cause venous stasis in the deep veins of the legs, and it is possible that the vein walls may be damaged by pressure resulting from cramped seating. The hypoxia of flight is potentially a factor that might alter coagulation factors, but it is unlikely that dry cabin air has a significant effect. These issues are the subject of current research which has followed publicity relating to a number of deaths from pulmonary embolism following long flights (Lapostelle *et al.* 2001). Assuming air travel does predispose to pulmonary embolism, it is likely that its effects will not be seen until towards the end of a long flight or some time after the flight is over. It is worth bearing in mind that many passengers may have had a long journey by coach before their flight. The history may help identify this and other predisposing factors such as recent surgery, trauma, malignancy, pregnancy and the use of oral contraceptives. Some 80–90 per cent of patients with pulmonary emboli have some predisposing factor, but most will not have clinical evidence of deep venous thrombosis.

Pulmonary embolism should be considered in all cases of sudden unexplained shortness of breath. The clinical picture depends on the size of the embolus. A large embolus obstructing a major pulmonary artery results in intense dyspnoea, cyanosis and shock. If the patient survives, there may be a cardiac type of chest pain, making distinction from myocardial infarction difficult. Examination may reveal a raised jugular venous pressure. However, this may not help in the differential diagnosis and it is unlikely that auscultation on board an aircraft will help either. Patients with massive pulmonary emboli tend to be as comfortable lying flat as sitting, in contrast to those with heart failure, but this is not an observation that is readily made in the confines of an aircraft cabin. One issue is clear. The patient is severely ill and the medical practitioner should recommend diversion to a well-equipped hospital. In the meantime, the patient should be given high concentrations of oxygen. Apart from this, there is little else that can be offered on board an airliner. The diagnosis is unlikely to be secure. Intravenous fluid would normally be indicated, but the quantities available are unlikely to make much difference and might be harmful if the problem was in fact a cardiac one.

Small pulmonary emboli present quite differently. Whereas large thrombi may obstruct major arteries, causing a profound effect on the pulmonary circulation, small emboli pass to the periphery of the lungs and may cause a cone-shaped infarct. In these patients dyspnoea is variable, but pleural involvement may cause a pleuritic pain. In some patients there will be haemoptysis. Whereas patients with large pulmonary emboli may be difficult to distinguish from patients with myocardial infarction, those with small pulmonary emboli may present in a similar way to pneumonia. Fever, tachycardia, dyspnoea and a pleural rub may occur with both pneumonia and pulmonary emboli. None of this is much help in making a confident diagnosis on board an aircraft. The best approach is to explain the situation to the captain and, where possible, make use of ground-based advice. Try to form an opinion on just how ill the patient is and base advice on this. Pleuritic pains do not necessarily have a serious cause and neither the patient, other passengers, or the airline would welcome an unnecessary diversion. Quite often patients, having been informed of the situation, will want to proceed to their expected destination – a risk they are more able to take than their medical advisor. Interim treatment should include oxygen and analgesia.

Asthma

Asthma is believed to be becoming commoner and is a likely cause of acute breathlessness occurring in flight, especially in the younger age groups. It is the most common potentially life-threatening condition seen on aircraft (Dowdall 2000). Usually the patient will be a known asthmatic, often young, and will know the cause of their symptoms. However, it would be wise to keep an open mind about the diagnosis, and stay alert to the possibility that there might be some other cause of the breathlessness. A coexisting pneumothorax is easy to miss. Sometimes the patient will have some idea of what may have precipitated the attack, but this is not necessarily the case. Attacks can be very sudden, especially in the young, but quite often there has been a progressive deterioration over some days. Patients reliant on bronchodilator inhalers may develop symptoms when they have run out of inhalers and this may be particularly likely in those who have been travelling abroad or who simply forgot to put an inhaler in their hand luggage. Generally, the patient complains of shortness of breath and tightness in the chest with wheezing. Dyspnoea may be intense. Inspiration is short and gasping while expiration is prolonged. Even on an aircraft some wheezing should be audible, though in severe attacks the chest can be silent.

An attack of asthma can vary from an episode that is quite mild to a situation which is life threatening. If the diagnosis is clear, it is important to try and estimate the severity of the attack because the question of diversion will need a decision. The patient will not find talking easy, but it is important to establish whether severe attacks in the past have required admission to hospital. Any patient who has required mechanical ventilation is in a high-risk group. Many patients measure their own peak flow so it might be worth seeing if they have their meter. If so, the peak flow should be measured and the patient asked what their best value is. Above 75 per cent of this value is a mild attack, 50–75 per cent moderate, 33–50 per cent severe and below 33 per cent is life threatening. Many patients cannot be bothered with peak flows and the likelihood is that this luxury will not be available and it will be necessary to rely on other observations. One of these can be made while taking the history. Patients who cannot complete sentences in one breath are at the severe end of the spectrum. A respiratory rate of 25 per minute or above is also a sign of severity as is a pulse rate above 110 per minute.

Cyanosis may be apparent, hypoxia is likely and oxygen in high concentration is indicated. The patients easiest to help are those who have forgotten their inhaler. A suitable β_2-agonist bronchodilator inhaler from the medical kit or from another passenger is likely to bring about a rapid improvement. Patients who have their bronchodilator inhaler will invariably have used it – usually to excess. Frequently they will complain that it is no longer working – another index of severity. Although patients are cautioned against using excessive doses of inhaled β-agonists, it is worth remembering that the dose of salbutamol (albuterol) in one puff from a standard inhaler is just 100 μg, whereas the dose often given via a nebulizer is 5 mg. In the absence of a nebulizer, it would be reasonable to give large numbers of puffs from an inhaler containing a short-acting agonist instead. Patients with severe asthma may not be able to manage an inhaler effectively and ideally should use a suitable spacer. If none is available, it may be possible to improvise by pushing a standard inhaler through the base of a paper cup. It is important to continue to administer oxygen while giving the bronchodilator.

Corticosteriods are an essential part of the management of severe asthma. Some patients carry an emergency supply. Oral prednisolone 30–60 mg or intravenous hydrocortisone 200 mg should be given, but will take some hours to bring about improvement. If there is no improvement and a fellow passenger has an anticholinergic inhaler such as ipratropium, this could be added. Side effects are very uncommon. Again the dose often given in a nebulizer is many times the usual inhaler dose. Passengers may also offer tablets containing a xanthine such as aminophylline or theophylline. Serum theophylline levels are critical. Oral preparations are often formulated so as to be slowly absorbed and are not really suitable for acute use.

The best advice is to focus on treatment with oxygen, inhaled bronchodilators and corticosteroids. If there is no improvement, inhaled bronchodilators can be repeated at frequent intervals. As for diversion, this will depend on the severity of the patient's condition, whether or not improvement is taking place and the options available. The doctor's role is to read the situation as accurately as possible so that the aircraft captain can make the best overall decision. Many factors need to be taken into account. Putting down at an airport remote from modern medical facilities is not necessarily in the patient's best interest and it would be sensible, where possible, to involve the patient in the decision.

Pneumothorax

Pneumothorax is a condition in which there is the potential for dramatic interactions between the pressure cabin environment and the pathophysiology affecting the patient. Spontaneous pneumothorax typically occurs in fit young men who tend to be tall and thin. In those over 40, pneumothorax is most likely to be caused by underlying lung disease, usually emphysema. In patients with asthma, a pneumothorax may easily be mistaken for an acute asthma attack. As is usual in cases of breathlessness, the history is all-important. Usually the presenting symptoms are sudden – often instantaneous chest pain and shortness of breath. The chest pain tends to be located on the affected side of the chest, but may be felt in the shoulder or neck or even be central. Many of the physical signs will be difficult to elicit on board an aircraft. There will be decreased movement on the affected side accompanied by hyper-resonance and absent or diminished breath sounds. Vocal resonance is usually diminished. Hyper-resonance is difficult to detect at the best of times and detecting differences in breath sounds will be difficult on board a noisy aircraft. Perhaps the easiest sign to pick up will be the decreased movements. Decreased movements show that there is pathology on that side and this is crucial information.

A large pneumothorax causes an immediate fall in oxygen saturation. This will be particularly marked in an aircraft at altitude and oxygen in high concentrations is indicated. The volume of air in the pleural space will vary with the ambient pressure and will expand if the cabin pressure falls. If a pneumothorax is suspected, the captain should be informed immediately. It may be possible to fly at a lower altitude and increase the cabin pressure or at least avoid the cabin pressure falling further. Falling cabin pressure could create a tension pneumothorax in which air expanding in the pleural cavity compromises the function of the other lung and the heart. Dyspnoea will worsen, there will be increasing tachycardia, and the trachea and apex beat will become displaced away from the affected side. Pallor, sweating and anxiety indicate an urgent need to release the air.

A tension pneumothorax is a life-threatening emergency. An aircraft is no place to have to deal with such a problem, but there is no alternative. It may be possible for the captain to increase the cabin pressure and this may buy a little time while the medical practitioner confirms the diagnosis. Chest drains have been inserted on the wrong side during medical evacuations – a disastrous situation if only one drain is available. On board an aircraft an inexperienced practitioner may well be best advised to do nothing unless he is absolutely certain of the diagnosis. Nevertheless, in an emergency, any available needle or cannula inserted into the affected side of the chest can be life saving. A convenient site is the second intercostal space in the mid-clavicular line. The air under pressure in the pleural space may make a sound as it escapes and the patient will improve rapidly. In one celebrated case, an underwater seal using a bottle of mineral water was used, but an underwater drain is difficult to build and manage in-flight. A simpler, but equally effective solution is to use a finger cut from a rubber glove. Cut a small hole in the end of the finger and tie the base tightly around the cannula. This acts as a valve. As air leaves the chest, the finger of the glove inflates and the air escapes. Air is prevented from entering the chest as the finger of the glove collapses when the pressure within the chest falls.

A small pneumothorax occurring on board an aircraft is difficult to diagnose with confidence. The defect in the lung following a small pneumothorax may close spontaneously and treatment might not normally be required. However, a small pneumothorax occurring on board an aircraft could easily develop into a larger pneumothorax either spontaneously or as a result of falling pressures. If a small pneumothorax is suspected, the wisest course of action would be to administer high concentrations of oxygen, advise diversion and explain to the captain the need to maintain cabin pressure, if this is practicable. Meanwhile, the patient must be observed carefully, and preparations made to deal with the situation should a tension pneumothorax develop. Fortunately, as the aircraft descends the volume of the air in the pleural space will lessen, and the patient will tend to improve.

Pulmonary oedema

Pulmonary oedema occurring in flight is most likely to be cardiogenic with myocardial ischaemia heading the list of causes. It may occur in a passenger with known heart disease who perhaps has missed their diuretics before the flight or it may occur as a result of an acute cardiac event. Patients who have had problems before may have had episodes of paroxysmal nocturnal dyspnoea and may suffer from orthopnoea. A history of cardiac chest pain, palpitations or worsening ankle oedema may be relevant or there may be a history of renal failure suggesting the possibility of fluid overload. In an acute attack of left ventricular failure the patient complains of sudden breathlessness, and there may be a cough and sometimes some wheezing. When severe, there may be spink frothy sputum. The patient is gasping for breath, anxious, pale, sweaty and cyanosed. The pulse is rapid and the blood pressure can be high. Auscultation of the lungs reveals crackles, but there may be wheezes too. A gallop rhythm is characteristic, but none of these signs is specific and many will be difficult or impossible to elicit on an aircraft.

High concentrations of oxygen should be given. A loop diuretic such as frusemide (furosemide) may well be available in the medical kit. If so, the standard dose should be given intravenously. If not, the patient may have some tablets. Glyceryl trinitrate may also be available and may help while the diuretic takes effect. Even severe cases may respond well to treatment, although in those with an initially low blood pressure, the prognosis tends to be poor. Some attention should be given to the underlying cause. Acute myocardial infarction is a possibility even if there has been no chest pain. The underlying cause needs to be considered if a diversion is a possibility, and an electrocardiogram, if available, might help with this decision.

Pneumonia

The most likely form of pneumonia to present in otherwise healthy travellers on board an aircraft is pneumococcal pneumonia. This illness may start with a nasopharyngeal infection followed by fevers and rigors. There may be pleuritic pain and a cough in addition to breathlessness. The cough may become productive of purulent sputum, which can be bloodstained. The patient will look ill and cyanosis is common. There will be signs of consolidation over the affected lobe. These include decreased movement, dullness to percussion and, initially, basal crackles. There may also be a pleural rub and later bronchial breathing may develop. None

of these signs would be easy to detect on board an aircraft and, as is so often the case, the best clues to the diagnosis will probably come from the history. Many other organisms may cause pneumonia but *Streptococcus pneumoniae* is the most likely causative organism. There are some differences in the typical clinical picture depending on the causative organism, but there is too much overlap for this to be of much help in determining the choice of antibiotics. The previously well passenger with pneumonia falls into the category of community-acquired pneumonia and the choice of antibiotics is based on the most likely possibilities.

A patient with suspected pneumonia should be given high concentrations of oxygen. The exception might be the patient who also has chronic obstructive pulmonary disease when high concentrations of oxygen might decrease respiratory drive. If antibiotics are available, a case could be made for starting them on board the aircraft if the patient is very ill, and the flight still has a considerable way to go. Pneumonia has a high mortality, especially in those over 60 with other underlying disease. The choice of antibiotic will depend very much on what is available and whether there is any history of penicillin allergy. It would be reasonable to use amoxicillin, cefuroxime or erythromycin, but a practitioner unfamiliar with the antibiotics on offer should take the advice of ground-based medical services.

Inhaled foreign body

Listed in most textbooks as a rare cause of acute difficulty in breathing is the 'café coronary'. This deserves a special mention because rapid treatment is life saving and it is perhaps more likely to witness the event on a plane than in day-to-day practice. Typically the victim, while eating and engaged in happy conversation or laughing, suddenly chokes and becomes cyanosed. The usual cause is a lump of meat impacted in the larynx. If several sharp slaps between the shoulder blades with the patient leaning forward do not help, Heimlich's manoeuvre must be carried out immediately. The patient must be moved towards the aisle so that the doctor can put their arms round from behind. A fist is then placed over the xiphisternum and the other hand is placed over the fist. A sharp jerking movement under the sternum may then dislodge the food.

Acute exacerbation of breathlessness

It is important to establish that the breathlessness is really of sudden onset. Patients with exacerbations of chronic obstructive pulmonary disease (COPD) may present with apparent shortness of breath that has, in fact, occurred on a background of chronic shortness of breath. These patients have usually been smokers for many years. Such patients, even when 'well', may have a very limited exercise tolerance. It is essential to obtain this history. Patients become so used to poor exercise tolerance that the information will not normally be volunteered. The patient should be asked whether they can normally manage stairs and how many steps they can climb before resting. A small deterioration perhaps brought about by an infection may be the cause of their apparently acute dyspnoea. Pulmonary function becomes just marginally worse but, because it was already so poor, severe breathlessness now occurs at rest. Recurrent episodes are characteristic – another feature to look for in the history.

If everything fits, an exacerbation of COPD may be the diagnosis, but it is important to realize that any of the other causes of acute shortness of breath may coexist. Indeed, the patient may well be predisposed to pneumothorax, pneumonia and pulmonary embolism. However, the likelihood of rupture of an emphysematous bulla does not appear to be increased by a routine flight. On examination there may be cyanosis, signs of hyperinflation of the chest and expiration may be prolonged. Patients with exacerbations of COPD will be hypoxic and oxygen is indicated. There is a theoretical risk of giving too high a concentration of oxygen, but this situation is difficult to manage without access to arterial blood gases.

Psychogenic breathlessness

Many passengers are made anxious by the stress of air travel and there is always the possibility that this may precipitate psychogenic breathlessness. Such patients may appear anxious and may have the sensation that they cannot get enough air into their lungs. Hyperventilation will cause symptoms such as tingling in the fingers and lightheadedness, which may reinforce any anxiety. The symptoms of hyperventilation are similar to those brought about by hypoxia when a subject breathes air at altitudes of between 15 000 and 20 000 feet. Small aircraft have been lost as all on board have lapsed into unconsciousness following unrecognized loss of cabin pressure. This possibility should be considered first. Oxygen should be given before appraising the situation. Psychogenic breathlessness is a diagnosis of exclusion. Any patient who is breathless on an aircraft is likely to feel anxious and conditions such as pulmonary embolism may cause the patient to hyperventilate. Central cyanosis would be an indication of something more serious than uncomplicated hyperventilation, but this is a difficult sign, especially if the lighting is poor. If the problem really is psychogenic, calm reassurance with instructions not to over-breathe should help. If necessary, rebreathing from a paper bag can relieve the symptoms of hypocapnia.

CHEST PAIN

In the appraisal of the patient with breathlessness the history is crucial. The same is true for the patient with chest pain. Similarly, the duration of chest pain is an important part of the history. Pain that has been present for days is seldom pleuritic and pain that has been present for days is less likely to have an important cause. Pain presenting on a flight is likely to be a pain that the patient does not recognize and of recent onset. This makes it more likely to have an organic cause. Pain of very sudden onset may be due to a pneumothorax or, if following coughing, a cough fracture. The age of the patient is also important. For example, an otherwise fit young woman is very unlikely to suffer myocardial infarction, but could have pericarditis. The quality of the pain may help in determining its cause. Oesophageal pain may have a burning quality whereas pleural pain is sharp or stabbing. The pain of myocardial ischaemia tends to feel constricting or tight.

The chest is a large structure and it is important to identify the exact location of the pain. Broad categories are lateral chest pain and anterior chest pain. Some pains are well localized whilst others are felt more diffusely or radiate. Local inflammation or trauma tend to cause well localized pains. Examples would include pain from a fractured rib, intercostal muscle pain or pleurisy. These are often felt laterally and tend to be worse on coughing or deep breathing. While they may be difficult to distinguish from one another, they are quite different from the typical pain of cardiac ischaemia which is not affected by breathing, has a tight or heavy quality and tends to be central with radiation to the neck, jaws or arms.

Angina pectoris tends to be brought on by exertion, but exercise may also worsen pleuritic pains – though the two are not usually confused. On the other hand, the pain of pleurisy is difficult to distinguish from a simple muscular pain. Sometimes in muscular pain or pain arising from the ribs, a tender spot can be found over the affected area. Pleurisy close to the diaphragm may cause pain referred to the neck or shoulder, but often the patient can point to one spot where the pain is worst and here it is worth listening to see if there is a pleural rub, though on a noisy aircraft this would be difficult. Pericardial pain may be similar to that of pleurisy, perhaps because it is sometimes accompanied by pleurisy. Typically, it can be relieved by sitting forward. Sometimes the pain of pericarditis is more like that of myocardial infarction with which it can be confused.

In addition to cardiac causes, central chest pain may arise from a dissecting aortic aneurysm. The pain is very severe and is usually mistaken for that of myocardial infarction, though in contrast with myocardial infarction, the pain tends to be maximal from the moment of onset. Sometimes pain is felt between the scapulae. Oesophageal pain is also usually felt in the centre of the chest, but is not usually so severe. It may have a deep location and be associated with reflux of acid into the mouth. Antacids may give relief.

Management in-flight

What should be the approach to a passenger with chest pain? The first point to remember is the importance of taking a thorough history. An interpreter should be used, if necessary, though histories taken in this way lack the nuances that can be so helpful. Particular attention should be paid to the exact details and time course of the presenting complaint, listening carefully to the patient and trying to determine the origin of the pain, looking out for the features described above. The cabin crew should be asked to provide some privacy for the patient to be examined. Failure to examine young female passengers on board aircraft has led to avoidable mistakes. The doctor should take a general look at the patient and try and determine how ill they appear. This is important. Is the patient bright and cheerful with just a little discomfort or pale and sweaty with cool peripheries and a tachycardia? It is important to try to examine all the systems, not forgetting to have a good look at the legs. Even if competent with a stethoscope, the medical practitioner may hear very little over the noise of the aircraft.

If the patient is in the second half of life, has had a typical cardiac-type pain and looks ill, has cool peripheries and is pale and sweaty, then myocardial infarction must be assumed. If an electrocardiogram is available it may help confirm the diagnosis, but if the history is typical it should not change the diagnosis. The most dangerous time after a heart attack is now. The patient is at risk of ventricular fibrillation. If there is a defibrillator on the aircraft, it should be brought to the patient at once. The cabin crew will have been trained in its use. Oxygen is given in high concentrations, about 300 mg aspirin administered and the effects of glyceryl trinitrate tried. Any available analgesic should be administered. There is still a differential diagnosis and antacids would be worth a try. The situation should be conveyed to the captain. As time passes the risk of ventricular fibrillation lessens. An early landing would be ideal, but if hours must pass before this is possible the time of greatest risk will be over. The patient might even be safer on a plane with a defibrillator than without in a remote airport. Without a defibrillator the patient will be at great risk and there may be many other possible complications. The decisions that need to be made are difficult. The captain will need the best assessment of the situation. Ground-based advisors may be able to help.

Quite often chest pains do not fit the textbook descriptions. This puts the medical practitioner in a difficult position. What should be done if the patient is elderly and has a vague central chest pain? No doctor can say that such a patient has not had a heart attack. Here an electrocardiogram might help if it were to show evidence of acute myocardial infarction, but it is more likely that it would be normal or show a non-specific abnormality. Trying some treatment might help. If the pain went away following antacids, this would be reassuring. Failing this, the response to glyceryl trinitrate might be helpful. All the doctor can do in such a situation is convey a level of uncertainty to the captain and make use of ground-based advice.

Lateral chest pains are in some ways less worrying. Pain from a rib or intercostal muscle requires only simple analgesia. Pleural pain is of rather more concern as it is often a result of bacterial infection of the underlying lung or it can be viral. Sometimes, as outlined above, it may result from pulmonary infarction. Unless there are other features to help, it will be difficult to distinguish between these possibilities. Whatever the underlying cause, the risks are less immediate than those related to a pain of possible cardiac origin and if the patient is otherwise well, reassurance, analgesia and oxygen may be all that are immediately necessary.

CONCLUSION

This chapter has been written for the many medical practitioners who fly, but rarely, in their daily practice, see a case of breathlessness or chest pain. Aircrew, in common with the public, may have unreasonable expectations of medical practitioners in this situation. Doctors have been called while an aircraft is on the tarmac and asked to appraise a passenger's fitness to fly. Quick decisions have led to mistakes. It is unreasonable to expect a doctor to be able to cast their eyes over someone that has caused concern to the cabin crew and declare them fit or otherwise. In such a situation, it is wise to advise that the patient is taken off the plane and properly assessed.

Once in the air, the medical practitioner may be on their own, and though they may lack familiarity with acute medicine, they could still be the most able person to deal with the problem. It is important to focus on the history as it is usually much more helpful than examination which, in any case, has limitations on board an aircraft. The information should be conveyed to the captain and advice sought from ground-based services. Breathlessness and chest pain can be difficult to diagnose and manage even for the experts (Pearson *et al.* 1980).

REFERENCES

Dowdall N. 'Is there a doctor on the aircraft?' Top 10 inflight medical emergencies. *Br Med J* 2000; **321**: 1336–7.

Elliott MW, Adams L, Cockcraft A *et al*. The language of breathlessness. Use of verbal descriptors by patients with cardiopulmonary disease. *Am Rev Respir Dis* 1991; **144**: 826–2.

Lapostelle F, Surget V, Borron SW *et al*. Severe pulmonary embolism associated with air travel. *N Engl J Med* 2001; **345**: 779–83.

Pearson SB, Pearson EM and Mitchell JR. How easy is it to diagnose and treat breathlessness? *Lancet* 1980; **2**: 1368.

Passengers with pulmonary disorders

ANDREW RC CUMMIN

Over the past 50 years there has been an exponential increase in the number of airline passengers. In 1949, just 30 million passengers travelled by air. Now each year there are around one and a half billion. People used to fly largely out of necessity, but today tourism accounts for more than 500 million arrivals per annum. The elderly with increasing disposable incomes now frequent the airways and the disabled, infirm and terminally ill also feel they have the right to travel. Some severely ill patients may have to fly to get the treatment they need. Chest diseases, both acute and chronic, are common, so the average doctor may expect to receive a large number of enquiries from respiratory patients about their fitness for air travel. The number taking advice would probably be much greater, but for the commonly held belief that the pressure in a modern aircraft is equivalent to sea level. The aim of this chapter is to outline the potential problems facing patients with chest disease who wish to travel by air. From the limited information available and from first principles, some guidance is offered on the medical assessment and management of these patients.

CABIN ENVIRONMENT

Commercial aircraft cruise at altitudes of up to around 40 000 feet or in the case of Concorde up to 60 000 feet. The ambient pressure at 40 000 feet is just 140 mmHg (18.7 kPa) and at 60 000 feet 54 mmHg (7.2 kPa). These pressures are insufficient to maintain adequate oxygenation while breathing air. For this reason and to prevent decompression sickness, airliners are pressurized. Pressurization to an equivalent of sea level (760 mmHg or 101 kPa) would be ideal physiologically, but this would place excessive demands on the design of the pressure cabin and the pressurization equipment with adverse consequences on weight and fuel consumption. Higher cabin pressures also make aircraft more vulnerable to structural failure. The optimum level of cabin pressurization is a compromise between the physiological needs of the passengers and the engineering and economic requirements. In practice, for most flights, passengers are exposed to a pressure equivalent to an altitude of 5000–8000 feet (632–565 mmHg or 84.3–75.3 kPa). This produces a level of hypoxia that can be tolerated safely by healthy passengers.

Air for pressurization is drawn from outside the aircraft. The temperature of this air at cruising altitudes is extremely cold (below −50° C) and very dry. As a result, cabin humidity tends to be very low, typically 10–20 per cent, and even lower on the flight deck where the airflow is greater (10–15 per cent). Average values tend to be below the minimum value needed for comfort. The energy required to pressurize and condition the cabin comes from the aircraft engines. As engines have become more efficient, an increasing proportion of the fuel consumption has been required to maintain pressurization. To improve economy, recirculation systems have been developed so that in most modern aircraft 50 per cent of the air is recycled. Recycled air is passed through high-efficiency particulate air (HEPA) filters, which remove micro-organisms as well as particulate matter and gaseous tars from tobacco smoke. Air entering the aircraft is bled from the engines at extremely high temperatures, so is essentially sterile.

Hypoxia

The most important difference between the environment within an airliner and that of a bus or a train relates to the pressure within the cabin. The pressure in a vehicle at sea level will be around 760 mmHg (101 kPa), whereas the pressure in an aircraft will change and may fall to as low as 565 mmHg (75.3 kPa, equivalent to 8000 feet), rising again on descent. Cabin altitudes approaching 9000 feet have been recorded during scheduled commercial flights. Cabin pressures may be lower in more modern aircraft. Potential consequences follow from both the low cabin pressure and from changes in pressure. The concentration of oxygen in air entering the aircraft does not vary with altitude and is always about 21 per cent. But when cabin pressure is low the partial pressure of oxygen will be reduced. The partial pressure of oxygen in the air entering the trachea when the cabin pressure is 565 mmHg (75.3 kPa, equivalent to an altitude of 8000 feet) is 109 mmHg (14.5 kPa) compared with 149 mmHg (20 kPa) at sea level (Figure 11.1). By the time the air has reached

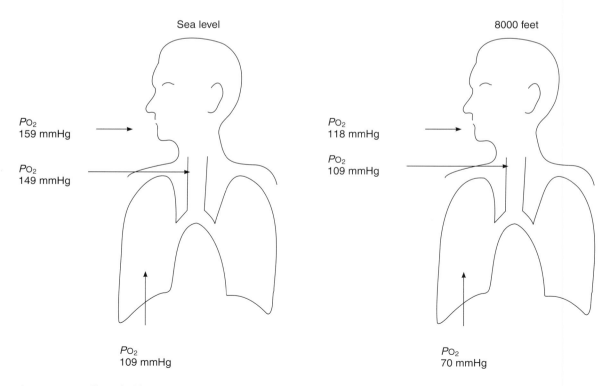

Sea level

Po_2 159 mmHg

Po_2 149 mmHg

Po_2 109 mmHg

8000 feet

Po_2 118 mmHg

Po_2 109 mmHg

Po_2 70 mmHg

Figure 11.1 *Effect of altitude on the partial pressure of oxygen in the ambient air and in air entering the respiratory tract.*

the alveoli, the partial pressure will have fallen to around 70 mmHg (9.3 kPa) as gas exchange takes place. The arterial P_{O_2} will be even lower (because of the alveolar-arterial gradient), perhaps as low as 55 mmHg (7.3 kPa) in a healthy passenger. This corresponds to an arterial haemoglobin saturation approaching 90 per cent and is not a problem for the healthy traveller. In patients with diseases affecting gas exchange, the arterial P_{O_2} may be much lower. Lower values fall on a steeper part of the oxygen dissociation curve, causing potentially severe desaturation. In healthy travellers, the fall in alveolar P_{O_2} may be partially offset by increased ventilation in response to hypoxia, but the response is modest and variable. Some patients may not have the capacity to respond to hypoxia in this way.

Pressure

Changes in pressure may cause problems due to the consequences of Boyle's law. When cabin pressure falls from 760 mmHg (101 kPa) to 565 mmHg (75.3 kPa, equivalent to 8000 feet), air expands by more than 30 per cent. Gas in body cavities expands even more because of the presence of water vapour. It is expansion of air in the middle ear that causes the familiar popping sound as the aircraft ascends. Exactly what happens depends on the nature of the body cavity. If the air is in an essentially solid structure such as the middle ear or a paranasal sinus, the expanding air tends to open up ostia or ducts so that the air is readily vented and ascent usually causes few problems. Descent is more likely to cause symptoms as ostia or ducts venting air spaces tend to close as the air contracts (Figures 11.2, 11.3). The resulting low pressure within a structure that cannot collapse may result in severe pain. For this reason, the maximum rate of increase in cabin pressure is usually limited to 1 kPa min^{-1}. If, on the other hand, the air is in a compliant viscus, such as the gastrointestinal tract or the lung, descent will not cause symptoms, as soft structures will simply lose volume. Problems are more likely on ascent when the air expands. Expansion of gas in the gastrointestinal tract has little effect on healthy passengers but can cause distress to patients with respiratory disease. Expansion of air in a lung bulla is also a potential cause of problems if communication with the airways is poor. A large bulla could expand, causing pressure on

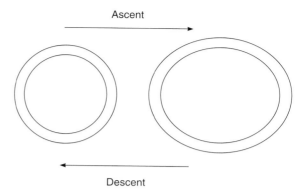

Figure 11.2 *Air in a soft viscus is free to expand and contract. Contraction is unlikely to cause any problems but expansion may cause symptoms as a result of pressure on neighbouring structures or excessive tension in the wall.*

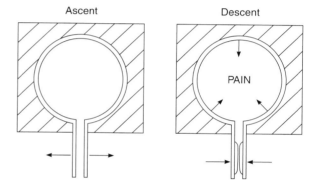

Figure 11.3 *Air within a solid structure can usually be vented easily on ascent as the pressure within the venting duct is higher than the ambient pressure, tending to keep the passage open. If the venting duct is partially obstructed, perhaps as a result of an infection, problems may occur on descent as the ambient pressure becomes progressively higher than the pressure within the duct, causing obstruction which becomes increasingly difficult to relieve.*

surrounding structures, or it might rupture, causing a pneumothorax or cerebral artery gas embolism. Similarly, air in a pneumothorax is free to expand by compressing the lung and mediastinum.

CHRONIC OBSTRUCTIVE PULMONARY DISEASE

Chronic bronchitis, emphysema and poorly reversible chronic asthma are amongst the disorders embraced by the term chronic obstructive pulmonary disease (COPD). Symptoms can be mild, but some patients become severely disabled and some are chronically hypoxic. Even when their illness is severe, patients with COPD may wish to travel by air. Some airlines suggest that a sufficient pre-flight assessment is ensuring that a patient can walk 50 metres without severe breathlessness. Evidence to support this approach is limited. Though many patients with lung disease travel by air, it is unclear what proportion suffer ill effects. Patients with advanced disease can suffer severe in-flight complications (Kramer *et al.* 1995) and arrhythmias occur in patients with stable COPD exposed for relatively short periods to modest hypoxia (Gong *et al.* 1984). It is possible that patients with COPD may be adapted so that they can tolerate hypoxia. Normal people can certainly adapt. It is well known that mountaineers can climb to the top of Mount Everest (29 028 feet) without oxygen supplements whereas an unadapted resting man acutely exposed to the same altitude would rapidly lose consciousness. However, unlike normal climbers, patients with obstructive lung disease may not be able to increase their ventilation in response to altitude.

What, then, should be our approach to the patient with COPD who wishes to fly? A thorough history including that of previous air travel is essential. Exercise tolerance will give some idea of the severity of the disease. Patients with symptoms interfering with daily living and those who have required hospital admission after an exacerbation are potentially at risk. This group will have a forced expiratory volume in one second (FEV_1) below 50 per cent of normal. Radiological evidence of emphysematous bullae, especially in patients who have had a previous pneumothorax, may imply that the patient is vulnerable to the effects of pressure changes. A chest radiograph taken shortly before travel will exclude acute abnormalities such as consolidation of the lung or a pneumothorax.

There is some correlation between FEV_1 and hypoxia at altitude, but tests, such as carbon monoxide transfer factor (Gong *et al.* 1984) and exercise studies (Schwartz *et al.* 1984) add little information. Measurement of arterial blood gas pressures at rest is potentially the most helpful in predicting altitude hypoxaemia, but in-flight measurements do not correlate well with arterial gases unless they are performed shortly before the flight (Schwartz *et al.*

1984). A pre-flight arterial Po_2 of below 50 mmHg (6.6 kPa) has been suggested as the value below which oxygen supplements should be provided in-flight (British Thoracic Society 1997a). This equates to a resting arterial Po_2 of around just 35 mmHg (4.7 kPa) at 8000 feet (Gong *et al.* 1984), which many believe to be too low (Sinha 1998). A figure of 70 mmHg (9.3 kPa) is claimed to be adequate 'in most cases' (Aerospace Medical Association 1996), but ideally this should be measured within hours of flight. Some patients with resting sea level arterial Po_2 values of above 70 mmHg (9.3 kPa) have had falls in arterial Po_2 to below 40 mmHg (5.3 kPa) when exposed at rest in a hypobaric chamber to a simulated altitude of 8000 feet (Dillard *et al.* 1989). Similar falls have been observed during flights in unpressurized aircraft to an altitude of just 5415 feet (Schwartz *et al.* 1984).

The arterial Po_2 at any altitude can be predicted more accurately by including more variables. Various equations and nomograms are available, but it is still not possible to predict the arterial Po_2 at altitude for an individual patient – or even a healthy subject. One reason for this is that exposure to altitude increases the hypoxic stimulus to breathe, tending to increase ventilation and lessening the fall in arterial Po_2. Two factors make this unpredictable. Hypoxic sensitivity varies from one individual to another, and patients with COPD have a variable capacity to increase their alveolar ventilation in response to this stimulus. Hypercapnic patients are likely to be particularly vulnerable (Lien and Turner 1998). A further difficulty is that the pathophysiology underlying the initial hypoxia may vary from one patient to another, and this may alter the effect of altitude. Equations and nomograms do not predict arterial Po_2 during in-flight exertion or sleep, and are not suitable for patients with hypercapnia or on long-term oxygen (Lien and Turner 1998).

Hypoxic challenge test

Uncertainties about the way in which individual patients may respond to altitude have led to the development of hypoxic challenge tests. Exposure to hypobaric hypoxia would be the most realistic test, but this requires a hypobaric chamber. It is the low partial pressure of oxygen rather than the low total pressure that matters, and this can be simulated at ground level by adding nitrogen to the inspired gas. This may even be a slightly more severe test than exposure to low pressure as some COPD patients find their breathing feels easier at altitude (Schwartz *et al.* 1984). Patients should be tested at the worst level of hypoxia that they are likely to encounter on the flight. For most flights, the maximum likely cabin altitude will be about 8000 feet. This is equivalent to breathing 15 per cent oxygen at sea level. Before starting the test, it is important to check that the patient's arterial haemoglobin saturation is adequate while breathing room air, otherwise the test itself may be hazardous. In some laboratories, patients breathe from a premixed cylinder of 15 per cent oxygen. An alternative is to use pure nitrogen delivered through a 40 per cent Ventimask (Vohra and Klocke 1993). Gradually decreasing the inspired oxygen concentration by bleeding nitrogen into a flow-past system in an incremental fashion may be safer but requires an oxygen analyser. Patients must be monitored with a pulse oximeter and electrocardiogram throughout. When the oximeter reading is stable, an arterial blood sample should be taken for estimation of blood gas tensions. Conventional advice is that if the arterial P_{O_2} falls below 55 mmHg (7.3 kPa), supplemental oxygen must be 'considered' (Aerospace Medical Association 1996).

Unless the proposed flight is very short, the patient is likely to need to walk to the toilet or take a nap, both of which may cause a further fall in arterial P_{O_2} with a profound effect on arterial saturation. Walking will also increase the myocardial oxygen demand. Particular risks apply to the patient with coexisting ischaemic heart disease. Patients with COPD are frequently elderly male smokers and are quite likely to have coronary artery disease. This is another reason for carrying out an hypoxic challenge. The effects of hypoxia on an individual's symptoms or electrocardiograph cannot be predicted from equations or nomograms. Arrhythmia during hypoxic challenge in this group of patients is well recognized and of clinical concern (Gong *et al.* 1984).

Exercise test

If there are no symptoms or changes in the electrocardiogram at rest during the hypoxic exposure and the arterial saturation remains above 85 per cent, the patient should then be asked to stand and walk for-

wards and backwards for several minutes to simulate walking to the lavatory. If at any stage during the test the arterial saturation falls below 85 per cent or the patient develops any untoward symptoms or significant abnormalities in the electrocardiogram, the patient must sit and rest while oxygen is added to the inspired gas. The test can then be repeated while the patient breathes oxygen (usually via nasal cannulae). Two or three litres per minute of oxygen will make up for the fall in partial pressure of oxygen at altitude, but lesser amounts may often be sufficient to maintain an arterial P_{O_2} above 50 mmHg (6.6 kPa). In theory, there is a risk to giving too high a flow as some patients with hypercapnia may be reliant on an element of hypoxia to drive their breathing. This is another aspect of the problem that can be assessed during exposure to simulated altitude. In general, it is probably best to err in the direction of too much rather than too little oxygen. COPD is characterized by intermittent exacerbations and there is always the possibility that the patient may not be quite as well as on the day of travel (Figure 11.4).

BULLAE AND PNEUMOTHORAX

The potential danger of flying with a pneumothorax was dramatically illustrated when a 39-year-old woman boarded a Boeing 747 after falling off a motorcycle on the way to the airport. After more than an hour into the flight she developed respiratory distress and a deviated trachea. Fortunately, it was possible to insert a chest drain. Patients who have recently suffered a spontaneous pneumothorax should have a chest radiograph to check that there is no residual air in the pleural space. Smoking substantially increases the risk of a first spontaneous pneumothorax, especially in men and all patients must be urged to stop. Most airlines will accept them as passengers provided that 6 weeks have elapsed since resolution of the pneumothorax. However, patients remain at risk of a recurrence. Those that have had more than one pneumothorax are at such a high risk of recurrence that they might best be advised to undergo surgical pleurodesis before flying. The incidence of pneumothorax amongst the general population tends to rise a couple of days after a fall in barometric pressure (Bense 1984), suggesting that changing pressure during air travel might precipitate a pneumothorax.

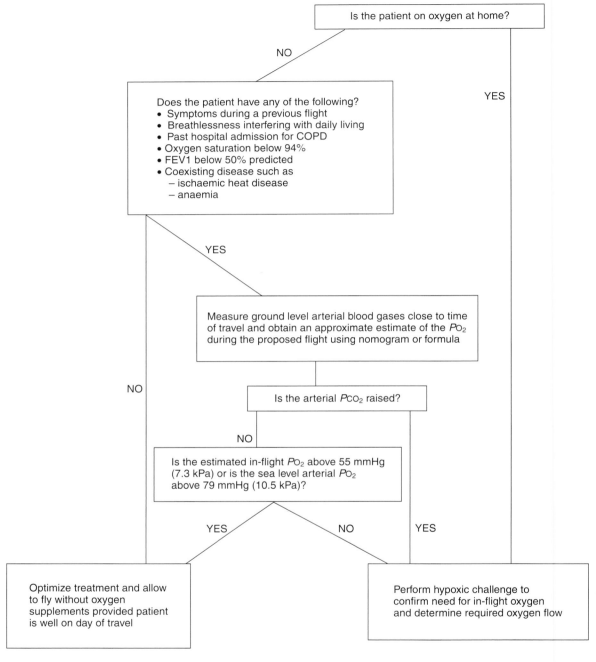

Figure 11.4 *Proposed algorithm for the assessment of patients with COPD who wish to travel by air.*

However, the incidence of spontaneous pneumothoraces in flight is low.

Some patients, particularly those with COPD, are known to have thin-walled bullae or lung cysts, but these are not usually a problem (Aerospace Medical Association 1996). The fact that the cystic spaces are filled with air indicates that they communicate with the airways – though they are not necessarily well ventilated. Potential problems result from the fall in cabin pressure with expansion of air within these spaces. In general, the air can be vented quickly enough to prevent rupture and the development of a pneumothorax or cerebral artery gas embolism. Nevertheless, cerebral artery gas embolism may have caused the death of one young aeroplane passenger in whom the only pathological finding was a lung bulla (Neidhart and Suter 1985). Where there is concern, ventilation scans will give some indication of how well the airspace communicates with the airways. Hypobaric exposure in a chamber can be used to test the effect of a fall in pressure, but is rarely necessary.

DIFFUSE PARENCHYMAL LUNG DISEASE

A wide range of conditions, including cryptogenic fibrosing alveolitis and sarcoidosis, may cause diffuse parenchymal (interstitial) lung disease. The pathological processes involved depend on the underlying disease with the functional result usually a restrictive defect. On the whole, unlike many patients with COPD, these patients retain the capacity to increase their ventilation at altitude, but impairment of gas transfer is frequently a problem. As a result, oxygen takes longer to diffuse from the alveolar gas into the pulmonary capillary blood. At sea level, provided the blood does not transit the pulmonary capillary too quickly, there may be enough time for equilibration, but arterial haemoglobin desaturation may occur on exertion because of the faster passage of the blood through the lungs. One factor determining how quickly oxygen passes from the alveolar gas to the capillary blood is the driving pressure – the difference between the alveolar Po_2 and the mixed venous Po_2. This partial pressure difference is adversely affected at altitude because of the fall in alveolar Po_2. The mixed venous Po_2 falls only slightly because of the shape of the haemoglobin dissociation curve. Clearly there is the potential for gas exchange in patients with interstitial lung disease to be much worse at altitude – especially on exertion. Much will depend on the severity of the disease and the degree of functional impairment, but since the functional defect differs from that of obstructive lung disease the formulas and nomograms derived for COPD

patients are not appropriate. If there is any doubt about the need for oxygen supplementation during air travel, an hypoxic challenge should be carried out.

ASTHMA

Asthma is a common condition characterized by variable breathlessness associated with inflammation and narrowing of the peripheral airways. Typically the airflow obstruction is reversible, but in some patients the obstruction is relatively fixed and their disease really forms part of the spectrum included under the umbrella term COPD. Patients with asthma should be managed according to current guidelines, which identify five treatment steps (British Thoracic Society 1997b). Treatment should be optimized well in advance of air travel. Patients whose asthma is resistant to treatment, but are stable, may require an hypoxic challenge to determine their need for oxygen on board. All patients must be sure to take on board an adequate supply of tablets and inhalers, including any additional drugs such as oral corticosteroids that may be required in an emergency. Inhalers and spacers may be used in-flight. Nebulizers may need to be battery powered and passengers should check with the airline. If there is a problem, a spacer is likely to suffice. Patients with asthma should be given written instructions describing current treatment and what action to take in an emergency. Some patients with brittle asthma are subject to sudden and severe life-threatening attacks. Air travel is contraindicated. Patients who have recently suffered an attack of acute severe asthma should wait until they have fully recovered before travelling by air.

PLEURAL EFFUSION

The healthy pleural cavity contains a small amount of fluid. Normally water and other small molecules are ultrafiltered from capillaries in the parietal pleura and absorbed into the capillaries of the visceral pleura. However, a number of disease states may interfere with this process and lead to the accumulation of fluid in the pleural space – a pleural effusion. The three main mechanisms are increased capillary pressure, as in cardiac failure, reduced plasma oncotic pressure, as in hypoalbuminaemia, increased capillary permeability, as in pulmonary infection or infarction, and lymphatic obstruction as may occur with carcinoma. Whether or not a patient with a pleural effusion is fit to travel by air will depend to some extent on the underlying disease process. Small pleural effusions may be functionally unimportant but large effusions cause breathlessness and need to be drained well in advance of air travel. A chest radiograph should be taken as close to the time of travel as practicable to check that there has been no significant re-accumulation of fluid, as well as to exclude a pneumothorax.

RESPIRATORY INFECTION

Many passengers on international flights come from developing countries with a high prevalence of tuberculosis. It is estimated that nearly 8 million new cases of tuberculosis occur each year world wide (World Health Organization 1998). Evidence suggesting transmission of tuberculosis from an infectious flight attendant to other aircrew and perhaps also to passengers (Driver et al. 1994) has led to concern that the airliner environment may facilitate droplet spread. The possibility that re-circulation of air may spread airborne disease is unlikely. Provided the ventilation system is operating, air is filtered at a rapid rate and airborne particles and micro-organisms greater than 0.3 microns will be removed. The tubercle bacillus measures about 0.5–1 micron. The observation that transmission of tuberculosis on board aircraft seems to require proximity to the index case (Kenyon et al. 1996) suggests that the ventilation system is effective. A reported outbreak of influenza aboard a commercial airliner had a very high attack rate of 72 per cent, but this was attributed to an inoperative ventilation system during a 3-hour ground delay after an engine failure during an aborted take-off. Measles may also have been transmitted during air travel.

In an investigation of aircraft contacts of six airline passengers with highly infectious tuberculosis, two with multi-drug-resistant organisms, evidence for transmission was found only on one flight lasting more than 8 hours and then only to passengers sitting close to the index case. No case of active tuberculosis occurring as a result of contact while on board a commercial aircraft has yet been reported. A patient with active tuberculosis may be infectious long before the diagnosis is made, and it is during this period that transmission of the disease is most likely. Patients with known infectious tuberculosis should be advised to remain in isolation at home or in hospital, but some are known to ignore this advice and have boarded commercial flights. There is probably little that can be done to prevent this. However, if a person with infectious tuberculosis is known to be planning travel on a commercial airliner, the health authorities should inform the airline concerned. The captain of an aircraft has a legal right to deny boarding to a person who may be a threat to the safety of other passengers or crew.

Healthy patients with open tuberculosis and fully sensitive organisms become non-infectious after 2 weeks of treatment, which includes rifampicin and isoniazid (Joint Tuberculosis Committee of the British Thoracic Society 1994). Patients with drug-resistant and multi-drug-resistant tuberculosis present a special problem as they may remain infectious for a considerable time. Advice on control of infection in these difficult cases, as well as tuberculosis in an HIV setting, can be found in the latest guidance issued by the Interdepartmental Working Group on Tuberculosis (1998). Multi-drug-resistant tuberculosis may be particularly difficult to treat and patients may travel by air without the knowledge of the airline in search of a cure (Centers for Disease Control and Prevention 1995). The latest guidelines on chemotherapy reflect the increasing frequency of multi-drug-resistant organisms (Joint Tuberculosis Committee of the British Thoracic Society 1998).

If a person with potentially infectious tuberculosis is found to have travelled aboard an aircraft, it is necessary to decide whether to inform other passengers and the flight crew. The first step is to find out whether the person was infectious or not. According to the World Health Organization guidelines, individuals should be considered infectious at the time of the flight if all the following conditions are met:

- at diagnosis they have positive acid-fast bacillus (AFB) smears from sputum specimens and positive cultures for *Mycobacterium tuberculosis*; and

- at the time of the flight they were symptomatic with a cough and were not receiving treatment for tuberculosis or treatment had been started, but there was no evidence of a response.

Even if an individual was infectious, action is only deemed necessary if the flight was longer than 8 hours. The recommended procedure is summarized in Figure 11.5.

CYSTIC FIBROSIS

Cystic fibrosis is the most common fatal inherited disease in European populations. With time the underlying abnormalities of ion and water transport affect lung function, leading to airflow obstruction and impaired gas exchange. Improved treatment means that patients are living longer and many are well enough to holiday abroad. Unfortunately, holidays at altitude may provoke severe exacerbations. The mechanism may be increased airway resistance or pulmonary vascular resistance in response to hypoxia. In this group of patients, the best predictor of desaturation during air travel is an hypoxic challenge at sea level. Predictions based on spirometry or sea level saturations may underestimate hypoxia in some individuals (Oades *et al.* 1994).

ADVANCED LUNG DISEASE

Occasionally it is necessary for patients with advanced lung disease to travel by air for an operation that is only available in a specialized centre. Lung transplantation and pulmonary thromboendarterectomy are two examples. Transporting patients with this severity of illness on ordinary commercial flights is not without problems. In a series of 21 patients flying from Israel to various sites in Europe and the USA, one severely ill patient died and three developed severe cyanosis and near syncope when they attempted to go to the lavatory without oxygen (Kramer *et al.* 1995). One of these, a patient with emphysema, had an arterial P_{O_2} on air at sea level above the 50 mmHg (6.5 kPa) cut-off recommended in the Guidelines of the British Thoracic Society (1997a). A further emphysematous patient with a sea level P_{O_2} of 55 mmHg (7.3 kPa) had a fall in saturation after her oxygen had been removed to 80 per cent when the aircraft altitude was 37 000 feet. However, despite the severity of their illness, most of the patients were able to maintain a saturation of above 85 per cent while on oxygen – though some were given as much as 8 l min^{-1}. Two patients ran out of oxygen 30 minutes before landing and had to rely on an emergency supply. Essentially, patients with stable severe lung disease can usually be transported safely by air provided sufficient oxygen is given, but they may be at serious risk if the oxygen supply is interrupted. In planning oxygen use, it is important to allow for unexpected delays. Patients with this severity of disease must be accompanied by a physician with resuscitation facilities.

THORACIC SURGERY AND TRACHEOSTOMY

Patients who have undergone major thoracic surgery should allow ample time for recovery before flying. Ideally 6 weeks should elapse, but some airlines will accept passengers after just 2 weeks. Assessment should focus on the possibility of air remaining in the pleural space and any underlying disease. The low humidity of the aircraft cabin may cause problems to patients with tracheostomies. In one case, a patient with a tracheostomy became distressed and cyanosed and developed intercostal recession during the flight. The cause was a thick mucus plug. Humidification and adequate suction may help such problems.

IN-FLIGHT OXYGEN

It is not usually possible for patients to bring their own oxygen on board a commercial airliner. Most carriers require notification of oxygen requirements from the physician, but this is not always straightforward because the in-flight oxygen is not standardized and airline practices tend to vary. Flow rates available range from a choice of just two and within a range of 1–15 l min^{-1}. Most carriers offer nasal cannulae and for many this is the only device available. A few

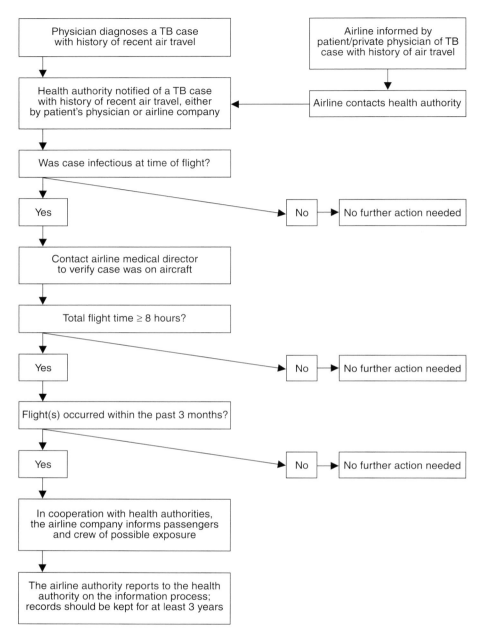

Figure 11.5 *Recommended procedure for action after diagnosis of patient with infectious disease who has travelled recently.*

provide masks. Charges vary enormously. Many patients who meet the criteria for long-term home oxygen are smokers. Despite warnings, a considerable number continue to smoke while on oxygen. This is not without hazard in the home and in an aircraft would be extremely dangerous.

CONCLUSION

The cabin environment is not the only problem facing the respiratory patient wishing to fly. For many patients, the greatest stress may be found on the ground. Modern airports tend to be very large, porters are in short supply and passengers can be expected to walk long distances. Simple measures such as wheelchairs can make all the difference. Best of all is a fit travelling companion. Airports in some resorts can themselves be at high altitude. The physician's advice needs to take all these aspects into account. No patient with a respiratory disorder should smoke, but unfortunately many do. A number of studies have shown that even patients with established COPD may improve their lung function if they stop smoking. Smoking also interferes with the function of haemoglobin. Carboxyhaemoglobin not only decreases the number of haemoglobin sites available for oxygen transport, but also alters the shape of the haemoglobin dissociation curve. Stopping smoking just 48 hours before a flight should significantly improve oxygen delivery.

If it is decided that a patient is fit to fly, it is important to ensure that treatment is optimized, appropriate immunizations given and the patient has an adequate supply of drugs including, if indicated, emergency supplies of antibiotics and corticosteroids. It may not be possible to obtain identical preparations abroad. Drugs needed on board must be readily available in hand luggage. Eight per cent of airline luggage goes astray, so it is wise to take duplicate supplies in both hand and main luggage. Some dry powder devices need to be kept away from damp. Patients need to be reminded of the cost of health care in foreign countries and must ensure they are in a position to meet the costs of emergency treatment. They should carry a list of current treatment. This is particularly important for patients on theophyllines who might otherwise be given excessive doses of aminophylline in an emergency.

When organizing travel, the patient should try and book a direct flight, especially if oxygen is required. The cost of oxygen is variable. The best advice is to shop around. Adequate insurance may prevent the temptation to travel if the patient is not feeling well on the day. An early check-in avoids the need to rush and has the added advantage that luggage is less likely to go astray. There is also a better chance of a suitable seat away from smokers and close to the toilet. During the flight, most patients would be well advised to avoid alcohol and sedatives and drink plenty of clear fluids. Many will have a number of risk factors for venous thromboembolism and should follow the guidelines given in Chapter 15.

Finally, patients on long-term oxygen present a special problem. They can still fly, but they are likely to need an extra $1-3$ l min^{-1} of oxygen during the flight. They may also require an increased flow at their destination if this is at high altitude. Difficulties can arise if they are permanently dependent on oxygen because airlines cannot provide oxygen for boarding or at stopovers and may not take the patient's own supply on board unless it is empty.

REFERENCES

Aerospace Medical Association, Air Transport Committee. Medical guidelines for air travel. *Aviat Space Environ Med* 1996; **67**: B1–15.

Bense L. Spontaneous pneumothorax related to falls in atmospheric pressure. *Eur J Respir Dis* 1984; **65**: 544–6.

British Thoracic Society. BTS guidelines for the management of chronic obstructive pulmonary disease. *Thorax* 1997a; **52** (Suppl 5): S1–28.

British Thoracic Society, The National Asthma Campaign, The Royal College of Physicians of London *et al*. The British guidelines on asthma management. 1995 review and position statement. *Thorax* 1997b; **52** (Suppl 1): S1–21.

Centers for Disease Control and Prevention. Exposure of passengers and flight crew to *Mycobacterium tuberculosis* on commercial aircraft, 1992–1995. *J Am Med Assoc* 1995; **273**: 911–12.

Dillard TA, Berg BW, Rajagopal KR, Dooley JW and Mehm WJ. Hypoxemia during air travel in patients with chronic obstructive pulmonary disease. *Ann Intern Med* 1989; **111**: 362–7.

Driver CR, Valway SE, Morgan WM, Onorato IM and Castro KG. Transmission of *Mycobacterium tuberculosis* associated with air travel. *J Am Med Assoc* 1994; **272**: 1031–5.

Gong H Jr, Tashkin DP, Lee EY, Simmons MS. Hypoxia-altitude simulation test: evaluation of patients with chronic airway obstruction. *Am Rev Respir Dis* 1984; **130**: 980–6.

Interdepartmental Working Group on Tuberculosis. *The Prevention and Control of Tuberculosis in the United Kingdom: UK guidance on the prevention and transmission of 1. HIV-related tuberculosis 2. Drug resistant, including multiple drug-resistant tuberculosis.* London: Department of Health, 1998.

Joint Tuberculosis Committee of the British Thoracic Society. Control and prevention of tuberculosis in the United Kingdom: code of practice 1994. *Thorax* 1994; **49**: 1193–200.

Joint Tuberculosis Committee of the British Thoracic Society. Chemotherapy and management of tuberculosis in the United Kingdom: recommendations 1998. *Thorax* 1998; **53**: 536–48.

Kenyon TA, Valway SE, Ihle WW, Onorato IM and Castro KG. Transmission of multidrug-resistant *Mycobacterium tuberculosis* during a long airplane flight. *N Engl J Med* 1996; **334**: 933–8.

Kramer M, Jakobson DJ, Springer C and Donchin Y. The safety of air transportation of patients with advanced lung disease: experience with 21 patients requiring lung transplantation or pulmonary thromboendarterectomy. *Chest* 1995; **108**: 1292–6.

Lien D and Turner M. Recommendations for patients with chronic respiratory disease considering air travel: a statement from the Canadian Thoracic Society. *Can Respir J* 1998; **5**: 95–100.

Neidhart P and Suter PM. Pulmonary bulla and sudden death in a young aeroplane passenger. *Intens Care Med* 1985; **11**: 45–7.

Oades PJ, Buchdahl RM and Bush A. Prediction of hypoxaemia at high altitude in children with cystic fibrosis. *Br Med J* 1994; **308**: 15–18.

Schwartz JS, Bencowitz HZ and Moser KM. Air travel hypoxaemia with chronic obstructive pulmonary disease. *Ann Intern Med* 1984; **100**: 473–7.

Sinha RK. Travel by air for patients with COPD. *Thorax* 1998; **53**: 625.

Vohra P and Klocke RA. Detection and correction of hypoxaemia associated with air travel. *Am Rev Respir Dis* 1993; **148**: 1215–19.

World Health Organization. *Tuberculosis and Air Travel: Guidelines for Prevention and Control.* Geneva: WHO, 1998.

Coronary artery disease

J SIMON R GIBBS

Although it is safe for most patients with coronary artery disease to undertake a commercial flight (Shesser 1989), just less than one quarter of in-flight medical incidents involve chest pain. In-flight deaths are rare (25.1 per million departures) but heart disease still accounts for more than half the fatalities (Cummins 1988). Since the majority of in-flight medical emergencies are associated with a pre-existing medical condition, pre-flight assessment of patients known to have heart disease is important. Indeed, pre-flight assessment has shown that of patients cleared to fly, none is likely to have significant in-flight medical problems (Gong *et al.* 1993).

HYPOXIA

The cabin pressure of commercial aircraft is reduced compared with sea level and is equivalent to an ascent to moderate altitude. During take-off, cabin pressure decreases at a rate of about 100 m min^{-1}, although the aircraft itself ascends more rapidly. Cabin pressure is maintained between 5000 and 8000 feet. The low cabin pressure causes a reduction in the arterial oxygen tension (Pa_{O_2}) from 94 mmHg (12.5 kPa) at sea level to a range between 60 and 66 mmHg (8 and 8.8 kPa) with an arterial oxygen saturation between 89 and 92 per cent in the aircraft cabin during flight.

This exposure causes few symptoms in healthy subjects. However, at minimum levels of cabin pressure, the fall in blood-oxygen content does have the potential to cause problems. These may be exacerbated in the elderly because they have reduced ventilatory capacity, ventilatory efficiency and hypoxic ventilatory drive. Above about 6500 feet, cigarette smokers over the age of 70 years have an arterial saturation of <90 per cent, and so are at particular risk. As the arterial oxygen tension falls to below 60 mmHg (8 kPa), all subjects will experience the effects of sympathetic activation initiated by hypoxic stimulation of the carotid bodies. This leads to an increase in heart rate, blood pressure, cardiac output and the force of myocardial contraction. Normally, the circulation vasodilates and coronary flow increases to compensate for the hypoxaemia, and this permits maximal exercise at high altitude without anaerobic metabolism.

In myocardial ischaemia, the balance between oxygen supply and demand is disturbed. Hypoxaemia, in the presence of coronary stenoses, would be expected to reduce oxygen supply to the myocardium and worsen ischaemia. Sympathetic activation also worsens myocardial ischaemia as a consequence of increased cardiac work and coronary vasoconstriction in regions of abnormal endothelial vasomotor control. The increased work of breathing probably has a minor effect, but respiratory alkalosis induced by hyperventilation may also cause coronary vasoconstriction. Patients with coronary artery disease may experience an increase in symptoms. Nevertheless, neither acute electrocardiographic (ECG) changes of myocardial ischaemia at rest nor symptomatic deterioration has been reported in patients with coronary artery disease below the age of 65 years who visited altitudes just over 8000 feet for 5 days – an 'altitude' similar to that of civil aircraft.

Exercise studies in patients with coronary artery disease at altitudes above aircraft cabin pressure have shown decreased exercise tolerance and earlier appearance of angina and ST-segment changes on the ECG. Acute exposure to 8200 feet (2500 metres) is associated with a small but significant reduction in the work required to provoke myocardial ischaemia. This is induced at a lower level of myocardial oxygen demand than at sea level. These findings are in contrast with data collected after long-term altitude acclimatization. In this circumstance angina and ST-segment depression occur at the same level of work at sea level and altitude. This would suggest that the acute effects of hypoxia are due mainly to increased cardiac work, and do not appear to be directly related to myocardial hypoxia. Indeed, it has been suggested that if a patient can reach stage 3 of the Bruce treadmill protocol (>6 minutes) without discomfort, then that patient will be able to tolerate an altitude of 14 000 feet without discomfort (Hultgren 1997).

There are anecdotal reports of patients with coronary artery disease developing myocardial infarction or unstable angina on board aircraft and at moderate altitude. In one survey, 19 patients with coronary disease had no events during a 5-day stay at 8200 feet (2500 metres) (Roach et al. 1995), but, in another similar study, 1 of 20 veterans sustained acute myocardial infarction after exercise (Levine et al. 1997). It is not clear whether the latter was due to the environment or would have occurred, in any case, at sea level. As far as arrhythmias are concerned, these may be precipitated by sympathetic activation, and by respiratory alkalosis, which may reduce serum potassium. No change has been detected in arrhythmic substrate in hypoxia using signal-averaged ECGs. Single premature ventricular complexes during exercise do increase modestly with acute exposure to 8200 feet (2500 metres) without an increase in repetitive forms, but it is unlikely that moderate altitude exposure substantially alters the risk of life-threatening arrhythmias in patients with coronary disease (Levine et al. 1997).

CHRONIC STABLE ANGINA

Patients with uncomplicated chronic stable angina are at low risk, but patients with more severe, but stable, angina should be reviewed by their physician (Table 12.1). If they undertake air travel, they should have supplemental oxygen available on the aircraft. In addition, they may require an increase in medication to control their symptoms. Indeed, patients with angina must ensure that their medications are readily accessible and carried in their hand luggage, and they should carry a fresh supply of glyceryl trinitrate and understand how to use it. Medication should be taken on time. Advice may be required about timing and dose of anti-anginal medication when a patient is crossing multiple time zones, east or west. In particular, the correct time intervals for

Table 12.1 *Canadian Cardiovascular Society Functional Classification of Angina*

Class	Description
I	Ordinary physical activity such as walking and climbing stairs does not cause angina. Angina with strenuous or rapid or prolonged exertion at work or recreation.
II	Slight limitation of ordinary activity. Walking or climbing stairs rapidly, walking uphill, walking or stair climbing after meals, in cold, in wind, or when under emotional stress, or only during the few hours after awakening. Walking more than two blocks on the level and climbing more than one flight of ordinary stairs at a normal pace and in normal conditions.
III	Marked limitation or ordinary physical activity. Walking one or two blocks on the level and climbing more than one flight of stairs in normal conditions.
IV	Inability to carry on any physical activity without discomfort. Anginal syndrome may be present at rest.

taking β-blockers should not be missed as this may precipitate myocardial ischaemia. The timing and doses of medication may need to be adjusted, on an individual basis. Patients with angina should be advised to arrive at the airport in good time so that they do not have to rush to the aircraft. Assistance may be required with heavy luggage and a wheelchair may be required. Patients with severe angina may need to limit their exercise before and during the flight. They should always carry a detailed list of their medications and a copy of a recent electrocardiogram in case of an emergency.

UNSTABLE ANGINA

Unstable angina includes angina of recent onset (within the last month), chronic angina which is increasing in severity and frequency within the last month, rest pain or nocturnal pain. Although the resting ECG may be normal, changes such as ST-segment depression or T-wave inversion may occur during episodes of pain (Figure 12.1). These are associated with a high risk of future cardiac events and the patient usually requires further investigation. A recent study revealed that in a long-haul air evacuation of 59 patients with unstable angina there were six in-flight events (Castillo and Lyons 1999). This would suggest that air travel by patients with unstable angina should only be undertaken with a medical escort, and may need in-flight medical treatment. Unstable angina is thus a contraindication to travel as an airline passenger (Cox et al. 1996).

MYOCARDIAL INFARCTION

Traditional advice has been that travel after myocardial infarction should be delayed to between 4 and 24 weeks after the event, but this advice has been challenged. Of 196 adults carried on commercial aircraft between 3 and 53 days after a myocardial infarction, 5 per cent developed symptoms requiring in-flight attention from their escorting physician (Cox et al. 1996). Six of the nine episodes occurred in patients flying within 2 weeks of myocardial infarction, leaving the authors to conclude that air travel between 2 and 3 weeks after a myocardial infarction was safe, but only in the presence of an escorting physician.

Patients with recent myocardial infarction may fly after 3 weeks, providing their recovery has been uncomplicated. They should be able to perform normal daily activities. A treadmill exercise test should demonstrate a low risk of cardiac events, i.e. no symptoms or myocardial ischaemia at maximum exercise, no significant arrhythmias and a normal blood pressure rise. If a treadmill exercise test cannot be undertaken for medical reasons, then an alternative stress test such as myocardial scintigraphy or stress echocardiography should be considered. Patients who are symptomatic or demonstrate signs of myocardial ischaemia on a stress test (Figure 12.1) should undergo appropriate investigation and treatment before flying. There is no role for performing stress tests in hypoxia.

Patients with recent myocardial infarction associated with complications such as heart failure, post-infarction angina, or arrhythmias should undergo appropriate investigation and treatment before air travel is considered. They should normally be stable for at least 3 weeks after treatment, be able to perform normal daily activities and have a negative stress test. Each case requires individual assessment and delay in travel for several weeks or months is preferable (Alexander 1995). An old myocardial infarction (Figure 12.2) is only a problem when there is significant angina, left ventricular dysfunction, or arrhythmias. These patients should undergo medical examination prior to travel. It is essential to ensure that all patients continue their usual medications during the flight.

CORONARY SURGERY AND ANGIOPLASTY

Successful coronary artery surgery from which the patient has fully recovered without complications presents a low risk. Post-operatively, patients should not fly for at least 2 weeks or until any air introduced into the chest cavity at the time of operation has resorbed. Clinical examination prior to travel is required to ensure a successful and stable post-operative outcome with no evidence of heart failure, arrhythmias, or residual ischaemia. Patients who have undergone surgery in the more remote past require a medical examination and a stress test prior to travel. Patients may travel after uncomplicated percutaneous transluminal coronary angioplasty

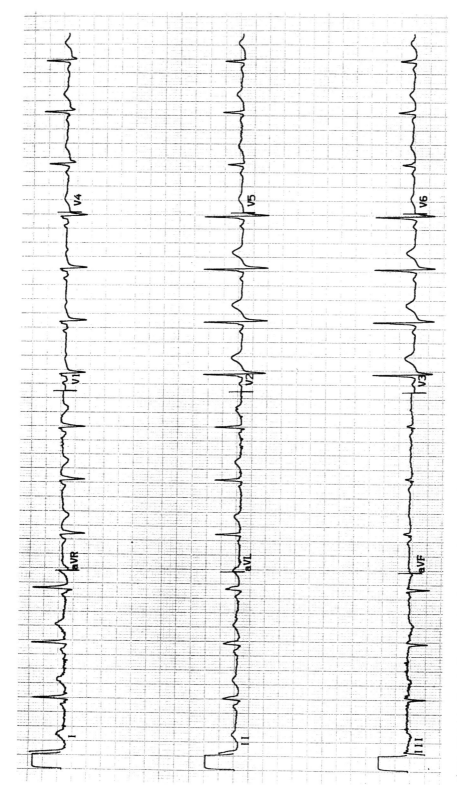

Figure 12.1 (a) *Treadmill exercise test demonstrating myocardial ischaemia. Electrocardiogram recorded at rest.*

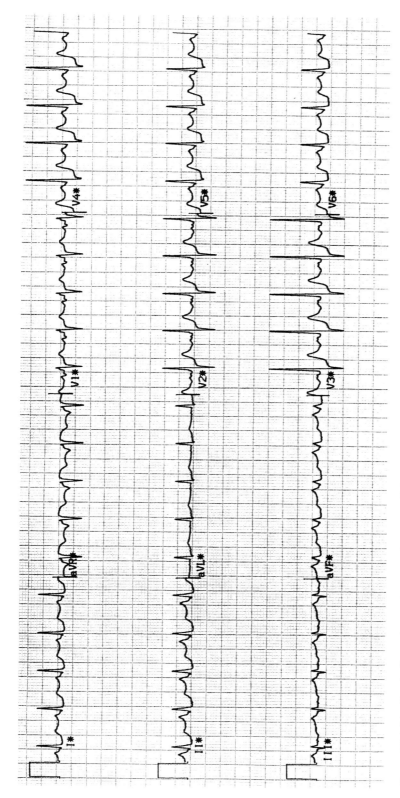

Figure 12.1 (b) *Treadmill exercise test demonstrating myocardial ischaemia. Electrocardiogram recorded at peak exercise. It shows depression of the ST segment in leads V4–V6.*

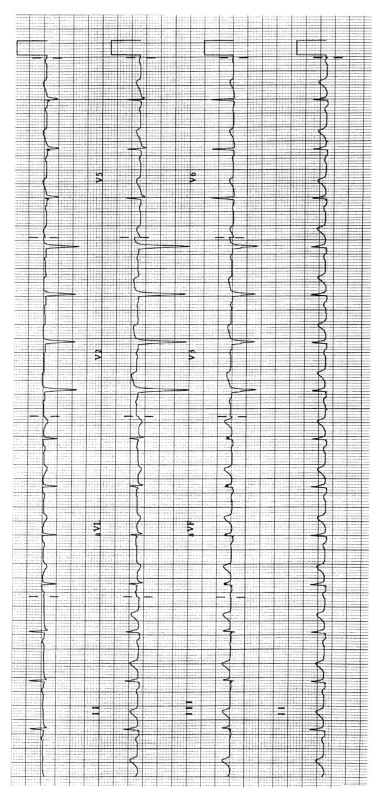

Figure 12.2 An electrocardiogram with evidence of an old anterior myocardial infarction. Such a patient may have significant left ventricular dysfunction. Note the q waves in leads V1–V3.

Table 12.2   *New York Heart Association Functional Classification*

Class	Description
I	Patients with cardiac disease but without resulting limitations of physical activity. Ordinary physical activity does not cause undue fatigue, palpitation, dyspnoea or anginal pain.
II	Patients with cardiac disease resulting in slight limitation of physical activity. They are comfortable at rest. Ordinary physical activity results in fatigue, palpitation, dyspnoea or anginal pain.
III	Patients with cardiac disease resulting in marked limitation of physical activity. They are comfortable at rest. Less than ordinary physical activity results in fatigue, palpitation, dyspnoea or anginal pain.
IV	Patients with cardiac disease resulting in inability to carry on any physical activity without discomfort. Symptoms of heart failure or of the anginal syndrome may be present even at rest. If any physical activity is undertaken discomfort is increased.

when they are asymptomatic, medically stable and can perform normal daily activities. Medical assessment is essential prior to air travel after an angioplasty performed for unstable angina or with an angioplasty associated with complications. In such cases it is advisable to wait 1–2 weeks before travel. Patients who have sustained myocardial infarction perioperatively should be treated in the same way as other patients with myocardial infarction.

CO-MORBIDITY

It should be appreciated that co-morbid conditions, in particular chronic lung disease (see Chapter 10), may affect patients with coronary artery disease by worsening the hypoxaemia. Appropriate measures should be taken in the management of such conditions and account taken of their effect on myocardial ischaemia. Uncontrolled hypertension is a contraindication to flying and may be exacerbated by hypoxia. Hypertension must be controlled prior to air travel, the ideal level being below 140/85 mmHg. Patients with coronary artery disease with mild to moderately impaired left ventricular function, but without residual ischaemia, have good tolerance to exposure to an altitude of 8000 feet.

Heart failure is a clinical syndrome caused by ventricular dysfunction and associated with symptoms of breathlessness and fatigue and typical physical signs. Most patients will, at least, be on diuretics and angiotensin-converting enzyme (ACE) inhibitors. Acute or decompensated heart failure is a contraindication to air travel. Patients in classes I and II of the New York Heart Association Functional Classification (Table 12.2) may travel provided they are medically stable and their baseline arterial oxygen is above 70 mmHg (9.3 kPa). Supplemental oxygen is required if the Pao_2 is <70 mmHg (Mohr 1997). Patients in classes III or IV must be medically stable. They require supplemental oxygen and advice about exercise on the aircraft.

Patients with uncontrolled ventricular or supraventricular arrhythmias are not permitted to fly. Frequent or high-grade ventricular ectopy is also a contraindication to air travel (Alexander 1995). Permanent pacemakers and internal cardioverter defibrillators present a low risk for air travel providing the patient is medically stable. The increasing sophistication of these devices is a consequence of more complex software, which renders them more prone to interference with airport security devices and aircraft electronics. However, problems are unlikely and advice may be obtained from pacemaker clinics and companies. Patients should carry a pacemaker card.

CONCLUSION

Medical screening before air travel is highly likely to determine which patients can fly safely. The doctor must assess the physical fitness of the patient, estimate the risk, recommend precautions and prescribe appropriate medication. When reviewing patients with coronary artery disease, advice must be tailored to the circumstances of the individual. Prior to air travel, special attention should be given to the stability of symptoms and the known severity of heart disease, and patients with unstable symptoms should be advised not to fly. An adequate supply of medication (including fresh glyceryl trinitrate) should be ensured and medication must be readily accessible and carried in hand luggage. The patient should carry a list of their medications and the timing and doses may need to be reviewed, especially where time-zone changes occur. The need for in-flight oxygen and for special assistance at the airport, such as a wheelchair, should be anticipated. The patient should be given a copy of a recent electrocardiogram. It is important to ascertain the altitude of the destination airport and whether problems were encountered on previous flights.

Where there is any doubt about the safety of flying, then an opinion should be sought from the airline medical advisers and from a cardiologist. In considering air travel in high-risk patients, it is the patients who must make their own decision, but this should be based on advice provided by their advisers.

REFERENCES

Alexander JK. Coronary problems associated with altitude and air travel. *Cardiol Clin* 1995; **13**: 271–8.

Castillo CY and Lyons TJ. The transoceanic air evacuation of unstable angina patients. *Aviat Space Environ Med* 1999; **70**: 103–6.

Cox GR, Peterson J, Bouchel L and Delmas JJ. Safety of commercial air travel following myocardial infarction. *Aviat Space Environ Med* 1996; **67**: 976–82.

Cummins RO. High-altitude flights and risk of cardiac stress. *J Am Med Assoc* 1988; **260**: 3668–9.

Gong H, Mark JA and Cowan MN. Preflight medical screenings of patients. Analysis of health and flight characteristics (see comments). *Chest* 1993; **104**: 788–94.

Hultgren H. *High Altitude Medicine*. Stanford, CA: Hultgren Publications, 1997.

Levine BD, Zuckerman JH and deFilippi CR. Effect of high-altitude exposure in the elderly: the Tenth Mountain Division study. *Circulation* 1997; **96**: 1224–32.

Mohr LC. Hypoxia and air travel. In Houston CS and Coates G (eds), *Hypoxia, Women and Altitude*. Berlington, VT: Queen City Printers Inc., 1997; 222–41.

Roach RC, Houston CS, Honigman B *et al*. How well do older persons tolerate moderate altitude? *West J Med* 1995; **162**: 32–6.

Shesser R. Medical aspects of commercial air travel. *Am J Emerg Med* 1989; **7**: 216–26.

13

Defibrillation

DOUGLAS A CHAMBERLAIN

HISTORICAL INTRODUCTION

Although the first definite human defibrillation was recorded only a little over 50 years ago, the ability of electricity to both stop and start the heart had aroused interest over a century earlier. Prescient advice was offered, for example, by one Richard Reece in the Medical Guide of 1820. Among the articles that were to be available for resuscitation was an electrifying machine to be attached to a metal tube placed in the oesophagus and to a wire for touching successively 'the regions of the heart, the diaphragm, and the stomach...' with the very topical comment: '... in cases of suspended animation what is necessary to be done should be done quickly...' (Eisenberg 1996). Electricity was known to stimulate muscular contraction, but true resuscitation as opposed to simple movement from the use of this (and other similar devices of the time) would have been unlikely.

The strictly scientific trail began in Leipzig in 1850 when Ludwig and Hoffa (1850) showed that the application of constant or faradic current could create in the dog heart a state of irregular arrhythmic contraction. McWilliam (1889) later developed these observations in experiments at University College London and in Aberdeen. He recognized that 'arhythmic [sic] fibrillar contraction' represented uncoordinated ventricular activity, and in 1889 suggested that this rhythm abnormality was probably a frequent cause of sudden death in man. Until McWilliam's experiments, it had been assumed that the heart became incapable of pumping blood only because of cessation of all activity, with no concept that disordered activity could be an alternative cause. Prevost and Battelli (1899) noted, but only as an incidental finding, that a strong electrical shock could reverse fibrillation that had been caused previously by a weaker current. But the possibility of therapeutic implications had to wait many years until an electricity company funded the research into 'countershock' ably conducted by Kouwenhoven and Hooker (Hooker et al. 1933) who showed in dogs that the heart could be defibrillated through the intact chest. Progress was interrupted by the war, but experiments were resumed afterwards.

Based on the progress that had been made in laboratory studies, the first successful human defibrillation in 1947 was achieved by Claude Beck who had worked for several years towards that goal (Beck et al. 1947). The cardiac arrest had occurred during surgery for a chest deformity and was achieved at the second attempt by paddles placed directly on the heart. External defibrillation through the intact chest wall followed in 1955. Zoll was able to report several successes after three earlier disappointments and thus introduced the modern era of cardiac resuscitation (Zoll et al. 1956). Rapid progress was made because two other crucial advances followed soon after the introduction of external defibrillation. First, expired air ventilation was shown to be far more effective than the previous methods of first aid for apnoea (Safar *et al.* 1958). Second, the window of opportunity for resuscitation from cardiac arrest was widened by the demonstration that external chest compression could maintain some forward flow of oxygenated blood (Kouwenhoven *et al.* 1960). Thus, the three key components of resuscitation were all available and widely practised by the early 1960s: chest compression and ventilation as first aid measures, and defibrillation as definitive treatment.

At first, defibrillation was necessarily a hospital technique. The alternating current defibrillators that became available commercially were large and heavy, suitable to be moved only on sizeable trolleys. They also had unnecessarily complex controls with panels that demanded a considerable degree of familiarity for confident and successful operation. Some of these controls were used to adapt defibrillators for giving shocks to terminate non-cardiac arrest arrhythmias including commonplace conditions such as paroxysmal tachycardias and atrial fibrillation – a procedure that is distinguished by the term cardioversion. This has remained one of the most important strategies for rhythm control, but will not be discussed further here.

The next breakthrough came with the development of units using direct current that did not require a heavy inductor and could be battery operated (Lown *et al.* 1962). The way was open to take defibrillation with portable machines into the community where the great majority of sudden cardiac death occurs. Pantridge and colleagues in Belfast demonstrated that this strategy was feasible and rewarding, although it was aimed specifically at the pre-hospital care of victims of myocardial infarction that had the primary objective of preventing cardiac arrest (Partridge and Geddes 1967). By 1970, a number of cities had developed systems of pre-hospital defibrillation for attempting to rescue victims who had already suffered sudden death. The sites were predominantly in the USA. New York and Charlottesville employed physicians after the Belfast model. Later Seattle, Columbus, Miami, Portland, Los Angeles and Boston used non-medical personnel who later came to be known as paramedics. Alongside these early initiatives, Brighton in the UK had its first paramedic ambulance operative by mid-1971 (White *et al.* 1973).

Defibrillation was still basically a medical procedure and the extension of the skill to paramedics was considered by some to be bold. It was also perceived as requiring extensive training, which would inevitably constrain any wide application in the community. But again, technology came to the rescue. The introduction of the automated external defibrillator (AED) depended on the development of software that could distinguish the waveform of ventricular fibrillation from other rhythms for which electrical treatment was not needed or not appropriate (Diack *et al.* 1979). Even the earliest commercial models could achieve reasonable sensitivity and specificity – accurate enough for successful clinical use (Jaggarao *et al.* 1982; Stults *et al.* 1986). They are now sufficiently developed for the European Resuscitation Council to commend their widespread use by first responders from organized trained groups, not necessarily medical (Bossaert *et al.* 1998) and for the American Heart Association to take an even broader view in promoting so-called public access defibrillation with an aim to make training available to the general public (Weisfeldt *et al.* 1995).

RHYTHMS OF SUDDEN CARDIAC DEATH

Sudden cardiac death (cardiac arrest) occurs as a result of any of four abnormalities of heart rhythm that may or may not occur in the context of myocardial infarction or unstable angina. Two are amenable to defibrillation and two are not. The arrhythmia that is most commonly found if an electrocardiogram can be recorded within minutes of death is **ventricular fibrillation**, representing the total breakdown of the electrical organization of the heartbeat. Whilst all the fibres may be contracting, they do so with little or no coordination so that the heart only quivers and pumps no blood. The coarse, undulating and apparently random electrical activity seen on the electrocardiogram gradually loses amplitude as metabolic stores become exhausted until – after many minutes – only a straight line is seen.

Even coordinated activity may be fast enough to prevent any detectable forward flow of blood. So-called **pulseless ventricular tachycardia** represents the response to abnormal electrical signals within the pumping chambers driving the heart at rates that may reach 300–400 beats per minute –

leaving little time for blood to enter the ventricles even if contractions were strong enough to pump effectively. This rhythm may be fundamentally similar to other types of ventricular tachycardia at rates that do permit forward flow – so that a spectrum of possibilities exists, from almost normal flow to no detectable flow. But even in this latter case, some circulation may exist that is not apparent as a peripheral pulse. Minimal but undetectable flow may, however, be capable of useful oxygen delivery and thus widen the window of opportunity for treatment before irreversible changes occur in the brain or heart. Collapse and loss of consciousness from a malignant arrhythmia is, therefore, not always synonymous with cardiac arrest. Pulseless ventricular tachycardia cannot be sustained because the progressive loss of unreplenished metabolic substrate soon makes coordinated activity impossible. Ventricular fibrillation supervenes and this in turn slowly progresses to a total absence of electrical activity as described above.

A coordinated electrical rhythm even at a satisfactory rate may fail to generate any effective flow of blood if the heart muscle has been deprived of metabolic substrate and thus cannot contract effectively, or if venous return is impeded or if forward flow is blocked. Whilst in most cases electrical and mechanical activity degenerate together, satisfactory electrical signals may be preserved for several minutes in a motionless or ineffective heart. This phenomenon is usually called **electromechanical dissociation** in Europe and **pulseless electrical activity** in North America. The latter may be a better term in that the observer cannot know whether or not some pumping action is preserved, but only that it is insufficient to generate a palpable pulse. One common form of pulseless electrical activity occurs if the heart should rupture hours or a few days after a myocardial infarction. This complication is relatively common after undiagnosed heart attacks and is, therefore, well known to pathologists. Blood escapes into the pericardial cavity and quickly compresses the heart chambers, thus preventing venous return and further forward flow. In such cases the heart rhythm as seen electrocardiographically can appear to be normal or near normal initially, but inevitably it degenerates within a few minutes. A similar phenomenon occurs in the presence of a massive pulmonary embolus when forward blood flow is obstructed by clot within the pulmonary arteries. Cardiac arrests with initial preservation of a relatively normal electrocardiogram seen on an aircraft may more often be due to a pulmonary embolus than to myocardial rupture.

Whilst all of the rhythm abnormalities described above will eventually degenerate to show only a straight line on an electrocardiogram, this total absence of electrical activity can occur as the initial abnormality. It is known as **asystole**, which can, therefore, be either a primary event or – more commonly – the end result of another form of cardiac arrest after progressive decay of the amplitude of any electrical signal. Primary asystole typically occurs if the total blood supply to the heart is cut off by the formation of a clot at the origin of the main coronary artery – an irrecoverable situation.

PATHOPHYSIOLOGY: IMPLICATIONS FOR RESUSCITATION

Cardiac arrest in the major developed countries is usually a complication of coronary heart disease, which is the most common or second most common cause of premature death, rivalled only by cancer (taking all types together). Most events occur without prolonged warning and are classified as 'sudden cardiac death', which is usually defined as death within one hour of the onset of any symptoms. Until relatively recently, it was believed that sudden cardiac death with an ischaemic aetiology occurred only as an early complication of myocardial infarction with manifestations, such as pain, that might or might not have been reported by the victim. Only when pre-hospital resuscitation became feasible was this view challenged. Cobb and his associates (1975) reported that over half of those resuscitated in Seattle had no clinical, electrocardiographic, or enzymatic evidence of infarction when assessed later in hospital. Some victims have been resuscitated so promptly that they have little or no retrograde amnesia. They have been able to report that receding consciousness was the first and only symptom of their cardiac arrest. This is consistent with the frequency with which victims may die during sleep without apparent disturbance; others collapse whilst performing some task seemingly without distraction. Thus, sudden ischaemic cardiac death may be unheralded following subtle distur-bances within the coronary circulation that cause no premonitory symptoms. We still do not know the proportion of ischaemic cardiac arrests that occur without warning. Data such as that from Seattle are restricted to victims who have been resuscitated suc-cessfully. Having no recent myocardial damage would be a prognostically favourable feature – thus biasing the sample. But it is clearly common and presents an additional challenge for rescue services. In the absence of warning symptoms, the need for a defibrillator becomes apparent only after the col-lapse has occurred, so the delay is usually too long for a successful outcome to be likely. Moreover, in an aircraft cabin, a painless arrhythmic death of a seated or sleeping passenger will sometimes go unnoticed for a lengthy period.

Approximately 60 per cent of community cases of 'natural' sudden death in the UK are due to coronary disease with or without warning symptoms, but 40 per cent have other protean causes (Thomas et al. 1988), some of which are also cardiovascular in the broadest sense, including conditions such as pul-monary embolus or aortic dissection and rupture. The distribution will be a little different in airline pas-sengers – with less respiratory illness for example – and more will be a result of coronary disease or pul-monary embolism. Some fatalities due to heart dis-ease will have been diagnosed previously whilst others can be detected at post-mortem examination, including congenital abnormalities such as aortic stenosis, hypertrophic cardiomyopathy, myocarditis, dilated cardiomyopathy, complex cyanotic defects, and structural abnormalities of the right ventricle. Yet others are purely electrical and can defy the best efforts of careful pathologists at post-mortem exami-nation, and may or may not be manifest electrocar-diographically during life – the long QT syndromes (Camm et al. 2000) and Brugada syndrome (Brugada et al. 1998) being the best known in this group. Whilst coronary death occurs more frequently in the mid-dle-aged and elderly – and at a younger age in men than in women, reflecting the epidemiology of vascu-lar disease – the non-coronary deaths may occur at any age.

The proportion of cases of sudden cardiac death that occur with ventricular fibrillation or pulseless ventricular tachycardia as the primary arrhythmia and thus potentially amenable to defibrillation is not known with certainty because these rhythms may give way – abruptly or more slowly from pro-gressive amplitude attenuation – to asystole. Observational studies have confirmed what might be expected. The sooner an electrocardiogram can be taken after collapse the more likely it is to show one of the two 'shockable' rhythms. Yet we know from hospital practice and monitored out-patients that some cases do have electromechanical dissoci-ation or asystole from the onset and are, therefore, not amenable to defibrillation. Calculations from the best evidence available show that approxi-mately 70 per cent of cases of out-of-hospital cardiac arrest have a potentially shockable arrhyth-mia initially (Holmberg et al. 2000), but this does not imply that all can be resuscitated because success also depends on reasonable residual myocardial function and the absence of determin-ing co-morbidity.

DEFIBRILLATION

Of the sudden cardiac death rhythms described above, only the first two are readily amenable to treatment. An appropriate electrical discharge from a defibrillator usually terminates the abnormal activity of ventricular fibrillation or pulseless ven-tricular tachycardia. All electrical activity stops at least for a few seconds after a successful shock. But, provided the original abnormal rhythm had been present for no more than a very few minutes and any underlying damage is not severe, a natural pace-maker will soon take over to provide coordinated electrical activity, often at a very slow rate at first but progressively speeding up. This 'rescue rhythm' (technically called an escape rhythm) rarely arises from the normal pacemaker in the first instance. It is more likely to be generated from a subsidiary pace-maker in one of the ventricles, a feature of the remarkable fail-safe system that can protect the heart from all but the most major catastrophes. In favourable cases, sinus rhythm from the dominant pacemaker in the right atrium takes over and restores a normally generated heartbeat within a minute or so. Not infrequently, ventricular fibrilla-tion will recur – especially whilst the heartbeat is still slow or generating little blood flow despite an adequate rate because of damage or electrical 'stun-ning' of the heart muscle. This recurrence is not an indication of an untreatable situation. Many victims of cardiac arrest recover after multiple shocks, but in general the fewer that are required the better the eventual outlook.

Success of defibrillation

The success of defibrillation depends on several factors. By far the most important is the interval from collapse to the first defibrillation shock. Particularly in the pre-hospital setting, this may not be the same as the interval from true cardiac arrest to shock. Other poorly perfusing, but organized, rhythms are a common prelude to ventricular fibrillation (Hays *et al.* 1989) or even asystole, and may have rates fast enough to impair consciousness whilst retaining some useful blood flow. This may explain the relatively long intervals that sometimes occur in cases for whom resuscitation is eventually successful. Nevertheless, every minute that passes after collapse before a shock can be given costs many percentage

points of lost opportunity for eventual recovery: 10 per cent per minute is close to what is usually observed. The use of bystander cardiopulmonary resuscitation (CPR) increases the window of opportunity for success, but should not be allowed to delay defibrillation. Whilst there is controversy as to whether initial CPR may be helpful before shock delivery in cases where delay has been relatively long (Cobb *et al.* 1999), all agree that within the first 4 minutes of collapse the most successful strategy is shock delivery as quickly as it can be achieved. Figure 13.1 shows how the prospects of a successful outcome diminishes with the delay to first shock, but also how the success rate is enhanced if bystander CPR is given whilst awaiting the possibility of defibrillation (Holmberg *et al.* 2000).

The second major factor that determines success rate is the pathology that caused the arrest. Primary ventricular fibrillation or pulseless ventricular tachycardia occurring without a recent coronary occlusion or infarction has a better short-term prognosis in response to resuscitation attempts than would a situation where a critical

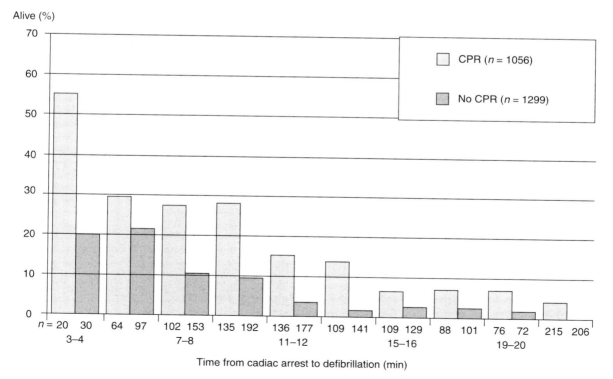

Figure 13.1 *The decreasing prospects for survival to one month in relation to time from collapse to defibrillation. Note the improved survival in those who had received bystander CPR. (Reproduced with permission from Holmberg M et al. 2000).*

area of the myocardium has been deprived of its blood supply by a recent occlusion. The presence of pre-existing heart disease will also have an adverse effect. Less important factors are the patient's physical characteristics that determine the proportion of electrical energy crossing the heart during an external shock and the characteristics of the shock itself.

Defibrillating waveforms and available energy levels can vary, and although practice has been largely standardized, interesting developments have occurred in recent years. After the general adoption of direct current devices for the treatment of cardiac arrest, it became clear that success could be achieved at a range of energy levels, with the prospects of success increasing, within limits, as the number of joules increased. Two considerations led all reputable guidelines to set a sequence of 200 J, 200 J and 360 J (or in some countries 200 J, 360 J, 360 J) for the first three shocks, with continuing use of 360 J thereafter. The first consideration was to avoid wasting time with low energy levels that were unlikely to be successful, the second was to avoid myocardial damage or prolonged electrical 'stunning' from unnecessarily high levels. The conventional doses seemed satisfactory and appropriate – using a variety of waveforms favoured by different manufacturers. The most frequently used in Western countries have been the monophasic truncated and truncated-exponential waveforms, and the monophasic damped sine waveform. In Eastern Europe, however, a biphasic discharge was adopted from the outset. In this case, the flow of electricity is reversed – first travelling in one direction and then in the other. The shapes of the common waveforms, including a recent biphasic truncated exponential type, are shown in Figure 13.2. Little comparative clinical research was undertaken to compare the efficacy of the different types of monophasic discharge in general use, and assumptions were made that they were approximately equivalent.

The need to miniaturize defibrillators to be implantable for the protection of individuals expected to have recurrent ventricular fibrillation proved a stimulus for new research. It was discovered that biphasic shocks tended to be successful at appreciably lower energies than those required by monophasic ones, allowing capacitor size to be greatly reduced. Whilst this was readily accepted at the low energy levels needed for internal defibrillation, the adoption of the biphasic waveform for external defibrillation by Western countries took somewhat longer, perhaps due in part to conservatism of both manufacturers and physicians, and indeed, most units that are in operation at the start of the new millennium still use the older waveforms. Studies in electrophysiological laboratories with facilities for the investigation of patients with serious electrical disorders of the heart showed that 150 J was usually adequate for external biphasic defibrillation (Bardy et al. 1996), and a subsequent randomized trial (Schneider et al. 2000) during out-of-hospital resuscitation has confirmed the superiority in everyday use of the same waveform over the standard 200 J discharge used in monophasic shocks. Most new units now provide biphasic waveforms, including many of the automated external defibrillators that are likely to be used in aircraft. Some have fixed energy levels and others permit escalation of energy for refractory fibrillation – but the need for this strategy has not been proved by clinical trials.

Automated external defibrillators

Automated external defibrillators (AEDs) are designed for use by minimally trained personnel. When the devices are opened, operation should be totally intuitive, aided by simple written instructions and/or audible prompts. The number of control buttons to be pressed is restricted to one or two – including a 'press to shock' command. The AED analyses one or more segments of the electrocardiogram over a few seconds and determines whether a shockable rhythm is present or not. If such a rhythm (ventricular fibrillation or pulseless ventricular tachycardia) is detected, then the operator is invited to deliver the shock but need not do so. Thus both the machine and the operator must make independent decisions that a shock is indicated before any discharge can occur, the former on the basis of an electrical waveform and the latter on the evident lifeless state of the patient. This dual check makes for near total safety – the operator cannot shock an individual who has an effective heartbeat. Poor electrode contact or movement does not cause spurious instructions as their detection by the algorithm is followed by an appropriate prompt to correct the

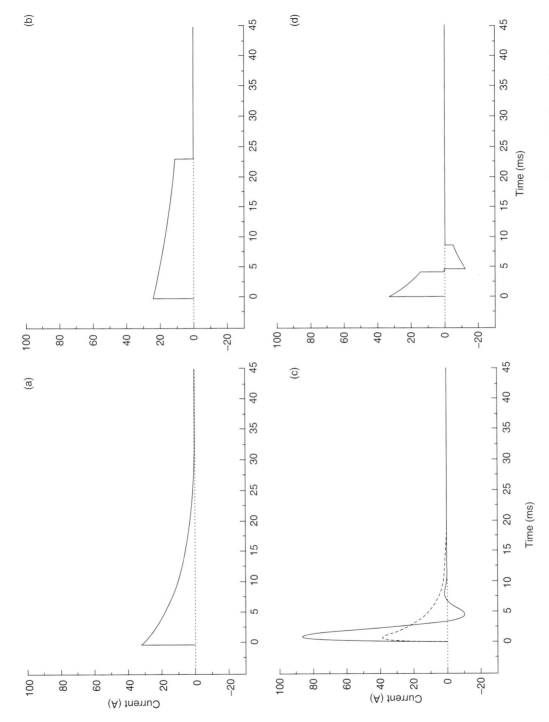

Figure 13.2 *Common defibrillation waveforms: (a) monophasic exponential; (b) monophasic exponential truncated; (c) monophasic and biphasic damped sine; (d) a recent biphasic truncated exponential. (Reproduced with permission from Achleitner et al. 1999, p. 195)*

cause of artefact. The claim is realistic that AEDs are easier to use than a domestic television set – and accordingly in a different league of simplicity from a video recorder! Such statements can reassure those who may be required to undergo the simple training that is provided for their use. Within the environment of an aircraft the algorithms are not influenced by nearby avionics, and defibrillating discharges cause no significant disturbance of flight control systems.

Successful defibrillation in flight

At the time of the first deployment of defibrillators on British Caledonian aircraft in 1987, a calculation was made of the prospects of successful resuscitation if the equipment can be used promptly and correctly. The calculation remains valid today, at least for populations that have a relatively high incidence of coronary disease. It can be made first by considering the likely number of cardiac deaths on aircraft, then by assessing what proportion of these might be resuscitated successfully. Countries such as the UK that have high rates of death from coronary disease can expect about 1500 cases of sudden death per million population per year – sudden being defined in the usual epidemiological sense of within one hour of the onset of any symptoms. Coronary death rate is heavily dependent on age, but aircraft passengers will be reasonably representative – with smaller than average numbers being very young or very old. It equates to four sudden deaths per million per day, suggesting one death per million passengers if one considers flights of 6 hours' duration. This is reasonably consistent with the incomplete figures that are available for air travel. Recent British Airways experience, for example, shows an in-flight mortality rate of 1.2–1.8 passengers per million carried. In 1988, however, a report based on a survey by the International Air Transport Association (Cummins *et al.* 1988) gave a figure of 3.1 deaths per million passengers, although at that time the average flight lasted little more than 2 hours.

The figure of one passenger per million suffering on-board sudden death is a reasonable approximation, and most will be due directly or indirectly to myocardial ischaemia. At most, 70 per cent of these deaths will occur with ventricular fibrillation as the initial rhythm (Holmberg *et al.* 2000), but on the evidence mentioned earlier only about half of them may have had warning symptoms that have drawn the attention of cabin staff. Thus 35 per cent should have a reasonable chance of receiving an appropriate shock within 3 or 4 minutes – the period during which success rates are high. The instances that occur without premonitory symptoms will usually pass unnoticed – collapse is not apparent in those who are sitting and often asleep. An initial success rate of 70 per cent in this group would be high by hospital standards, but might be achieved in an aircraft with a defibrillator and trained staff since prompt treatment should be available. With this assumption, the 35 per cent receiving a prompt shock might be reduced to 25 per cent initial survivors. Data from the largest series of in-hospital resuscitations (Turnstall-Pedoe *et al.* 1992) suggest that of those with a cardiac aetiology, about half of the initial survivors will be discharged alive from hospital. This equates to 12.5 per cent of the (approximately) one per million passengers with in-flight sudden death. The provision of on-board defibrillation facilities and staff trained to use the equipment competently might, therefore, save the lives of at best *one passenger for every 8 million carried on an average (6-hour) international flight, but correspondingly less for short-haul operations.* Whilst this is a relatively small number, the considerations that might lead an airline to provide such facilities are more complex.

SHOULD AIRLINES CARRY AEDs?

This question can have no scientific answer, but may now have a pragmatic one. More lives could be saved if defibrillators put on all the world's large aircraft were deployed instead in some of the many acute hospital wards that do not at present have one. But the aviation industry is justifiably proud of its safety record, and is prepared to spend large amounts of money to preserve and enhance it. The expense incurred for the purchase of AEDs and for the necessary staff training is not excessive when compared with other safety costs. Other considerations will sway opinion. The isolation of passengers from usual medical facilities does carry some obligation for the airlines to provide reasonable first aid equipment that can mitigate problems until an aircraft can land – and for cardiac arrest no first aid will be successful unless the provision includes a defibrillator. Marketing pressures play some role, particularly when one or more airlines are known to be already carrying defibrillators: many opportunities exist for making this known without the need for overt advertising. Medico-legal considerations have come to the fore after several claims for damages in the USA for alleged failure to deal appropriately with a cardiac arrest (Crewdson 1996). The media pressure that has been brought to bear was highly effective, although it took a somewhat simplistic approach to the problem. Finally, and most persuasively, the former President of the United States lent his support with the proposition that all US commercial airlines should carry a defibrillator (Crewdson 2000), with the result that the American Department of Transportation has ruled that all large passenger aircraft must be equipped by May 2004 (Department of Transportation 2001). Although dissenting voices have been heard in the recent past (Wolbrink and Borrillo 1999), the pressures on major world airlines is becoming irresistible, whatever the cost-benefit equation in comparison with other health issues. At least 43 airlines had adopted the policy by early 2001, and most others are likely to follow.

British Caledonian was the first airline to carry defibrillators on all its wide body aircraft in 1987, though they were removed shortly afterwards following the merger with British Airways. Qantas followed suit with a more successful programme. At the time of a report in 1997 (O'Rourke *et al.* 1997), 27 cardiac arrests had occurred amongst 30 million passengers with two successful defibrillations – a close approximation to predictions made on *a priori* grounds. But in addition, four successes were achieved in airports using equipment carried on the aircraft – a bonus that had not previously been widely considered. American Airlines currently have the greatest experience (Page *et al.* 2000), with shocks administered to 13 passengers with documented ventricular fibrillation from July 1997 to July 1999, with first shock defibrillation in all – resulting in six long-term survivors. During this time, approximately 71 million passengers were carried, again with a success rate consistent with theoretical predictions. All 28 000 cabin staff have been trained, a policy also adopted by British

Airways. Other successes have been achieved by Virgin Atlantic, British Airways, and by Delta – whose first defibrillation was of a member of the airline cabin staff only one week after the devices had been put on board.

TRAINING OF CABIN STAFF

As for all First Responder schemes, those who undertake to provide defibrillation with AEDs must be able to show proficiency in basic life support – and in many situations training to achieve this is the principal requirement in terms of instruction. The training of cabin crew routinely ensures that staff are competent in basic life support so that instruction in the use of AEDs may be seen as an additional module. The European Resuscitation Council (Bossaert *et al.* 1998) considers that all aspects of training should take about 8 hours, but that this might be 'considerably shorter' depending on previous training and experience. Instruction directed solely to AEDs can generally be accomplished in 2 hours, and many appropriate courses are now available that can be used or adapted by airlines. The frequency of refresher training or practice drills has not been standardized, but is recommended to be at least every 6 months (Bossaert *et al.* 1998). Ideally, this should be continued indefinitely, but the logistics of this policy may pose major problems for airlines that have adopted the policy of training all cabin staff. Methods of computer-assisted self-instruction may offer a solution. Modern AEDs need little or no maintenance and are designed for regular self-checks, usually on a daily basis with alerts programmed in the event of any potential ¡malfunction. Whilst this is convenient, the previous requirement for operator checks did have value as a reminder of defibrillation procedures. Some form of regular familiarization with the equipment should be required of cabin staff as part of routine duties.

Resuscitation in aircraft has unique problems that must be addressed in training. Moving an unconscious passenger from a seat, removal of clothing, finding space for adequate basic life support and for safe defibrillation all present difficulties not met in most other situations. Careful simulations under realistic conditions are important. Another problem may be more difficult to overcome. During a life-threatening medical emergency, the assistance of physicians (or nurses) who are on board as passengers is likely to be requested and is potentially helpful. Cabin staff must realize, however, that they themselves may have received more training in dealing with a cardiac arrest and in defibrillation procedures than many who are medically qualified. Thus, a crew member should remain 'in charge', willing to accept appropriate advice but mindful that physicians may feel an inappropriate obligation to give instructions that may reduce the chances of a successful outcome. Such difficulties can usually be avoided by firm statements of protocols that are laid down by the airline medical advisors and that are expected to be followed. Those not familiar with the science of resuscitation may also express anxieties that few drugs are available as adjuvant therapy. Cabin staff will be reassured to know that no drugs used in resuscitation from cardiac arrest have been shown to improve outcome and it is at least possible that none does so. Only CPR and defibrillation are of proven value.

Cabin staff have limited experience dealing with medical emergencies and so the use of defibrillators may be daunting. But the ease of use and safety of equipment will rapidly become apparent. An AED will report 'no shock advised' unless the rhythm analysis detects ventricular fibrillation or rapid ventricular tachycardia. This does NOT mean that basic life support should also be withheld. A prompt to check for an effective circulation will follow. Training for on-board defibrillation must also instil zeal for good CPR given with as few and as brief interruptions as possible. During cardiac arrest, every second without chest compression reduces the prospects of recovery, and efforts must not slacken because a shock has been given. Effective basic life support should be restarted without delay after defibrillation if evidence of a satisfactory circulation is not immediately apparent. This might be the result of a non-perfusing rhythm, poor heart muscle contraction, or a very slow heart rate. A satisfactory circulation can be recognized if the patient's colour improves, if there is normal breathing, coughing, or evidence of returning consciousness. Current international resuscitation guidelines accept that non-health professionals must not be called upon to make decisions based on the perceived absence or presence of a palpable pulse. 'If in doubt, compress' is a sound policy: chest compression is unlikely to cause damage, but lack of compressions in the absence of an effective spontaneous circulation may eliminate any prospect of a successful outcome.

Most airlines will provide training for cabin staff in-house. Any other policy would be impractical if large numbers are to receive instruction integrated with the first aid component of regular courses. Ideally, senior trainers should have had first-hand experience of resuscitation procedures and also hold a recognized Advanced Life Support Instructor certification. The European Resuscitation Council states that all first-responder defibrillation programmes must operate under strict medical control by physicians qualified and experienced in emergency programme management (Bossaert et al. 1998). Their responsibility should include appropriate audit. In relation to airline defibrillation, any external advisor must work in close collaboration with airline medical departments – or, if no such department exists, with the appropriate supervisory staff.

REFERENCES

Achleitner U, Amann A, Stoffaneller M and Baubin M. Waveforms of external defibrillators: analysis and energy contribution. *Resuscitation* 1999; **41**: 193–200.

Bardy GH, Marchlinski FE *et al.* for the transthoracic investigators. Multicenter comparison of truncated biphasic shocks and standard damped sine wave monophasic shocks for transthoracic ventricular defibrillation. *Circulation* 1996; **94**: 2507–14.

Beck CS, Pritchard WH and Feil HS. Ventricular fibrillation of long duration abolished by electric shock. *J Am Med Assoc* 1947; **135**: 985–6.

Bossaert L, Handley A, Marsden A *et al.* European Resuscitation Council guidelines for the use of automated external defibrillators by EMS providers and first responders. A statement from the Early Defibrillation Task Force, with contributions from the Working Groups on Basic and Advanced Life Support, and approved by the Executive Committee of the European Resuscitation Council. *Resuscitation* 1998; **37**: 91–4.

Brugada J, Brugada R and Brugada P. Right bundle-branch block and ST-segment elevation in leads V1 through V3. *Circulation* 1998; **97**: 457–60.

Camm AJ, Janse MJ, Roden DM, Rosen MR, Cinca J and Cobbe SM. Congenital and acquired long QT syndrome. *Eur Heart* 2000; **21**: 1232–7.

Cobb LA, Baum RS, Alvarez H and Schaffer WA. Resuscitation from out-of-hospital ventricular fibrillation; 4 years follow-up. *Circulation* 1975; **51–52** (Suppl III): 223–8.

Cobb LA, Fahrenbruch CE, Walsh TR *et al*. Influence of cardiopulmonary resuscitation prior to defibrillation in patients with out-of-hospital ventricular fibrillation. *J Am Med Assoc* 1999; **281**: 1182–8.

Crewdson J. Ill in the air? Don't count on fast landing. *Chicago Tribune* August 4, 1996.

Crewdson J. Clinton calls for defibrillators on all US Airliners. Federal sites could get heart-savers. *Chicago Tribune* May 21, 2000.

Cummins RO, Chapman PJC, Chamberlain DA, Schubach JA and Litwin PE. In-flight deaths during commercial air travel. How big is the problem? *J Am Med Assoc* 1988; **259**: 1983–8.

Department of Transportation. 14 CFR Parts 121 and 135 (Docket No FAA-2000–7119; Amendment No. 121–280 and 135–78) RIN 2120-AG89 Emergency Medical Equipment Agency: Federation Aviation Administration (FAA) DOT. April 13, 2001.

Diack AW, Welborn WS, Rullman RG, Walter CW and Wayne MA. An automatic cardiac resuscitator for emergency treatment of cardiac arrest. *Med Instrum* 1979; **13**: 78–83.

Eisenberg MS. Quoted in Paradis NA, Halperin HR and Nowak RM (eds), *Cardiac Arrest. The Science and Practice of Resuscitation Medicine*. Baltimore: Williams & Wilkins, 1996, 15. [Reece R. Electroresuscitation. In *The Medical Guide*. London, 1920.]

Hays LJ, Lerman BB and DiMarco JP. Nonventricular arrhythmias as precursors of ventricular fibrillation in patients with out-of-hospital cardiac arrest. *Am Heart J* 1989; **118**: 53–7.

Holmberg M, Holmberg S and Herlitz J. Effective bystander cardiopulmonary resuscitation in out-of-hospital cardiac arrest patients in Sweden. *Resuscitation* 2000; **47**: 59–70.

Hooker DR, Kouwenhoven WB and Langworthy OR. The effect of alternating electrical currents on the heart. *Am J Physiol* 1933; **103**: 444–54.

Jaggarao NSV, Heber M, Grainger R, Vincent R, Chamberlain DA and Aronson AL. Use of an automated external defibrillator-pacemaker by ambulance staff. *Lancet* 1982; **2**: 73–5.

Kouwenhoven WB, Jude JR and Knickerbocker GG. Closed-chest cardiac massage. *J Am Med Assoc* 1960; **173**: 1064–7.

Lown B, Amarasingham R and Neuman J. New method for terminating cardiac arrhythmias. Use of synchronized capacitor discharge. *J Am Med Assoc* 1962; **182**: 548–54.

Ludwig CFW and Hoffa A. Einige neue Veruche üher Herzbewegung. *Z rat Med* 1850; **ix**: 107–44.

McWillian JA. Cardiac failure and sudden death. *Br Med J* 1889; **1**: 6–8.

O'Rourke MR, Donaldson E and Geddes JS. An airline cardiac arrest program. *Circulation* 1997; **96**: 2849–53.

Page RL, Joglar KA, Kowal RC *et al*. Use of automated external defibrillators by a US airline. *N Engl J Med* 2000; **343**: 1210–16.

Partridge JF and Geddes JS. A mobile intensive-care unit in the management of myocardial infarction. *Lancet* 1967; **ii**: 271–3.

Prevost J-L, Battelli F. La mort par les courants électriques – courants alternatifs à haute tension. *J Physiol Pathol Gen* 1899; **ii**: 427–42.

Safar P, Escarraga LA and Elam JO. A comparison of the mouth-to-mouth and mouth-to-airway methods of artificial respiration with the chest-pressure arm-lift methods. *N Engl J Med* 1958; **258**: 671–7.

Schneider T, Martens PR, Paschen H *et al*. for the ORCA Investigators. Multicenter, randomized, controlled trial comparing 150-J biphasic shocks and 200- to 360-J monophasic shocks in the resuscitation of out-of-hospital cardiac arrest victims. *Circulation* 2000; **102**: 1780–7.

Stults KR, Brown DD and Kerber RE. Efficacy of an auto-mated external defibrillator in the management of out-of-hospital cardiac arrest: validation of the diag-nostic algorithm and initial clinical experience in a rural environment. *Circulation* 1986; **73**: 701–9.

Thomas AC, Knapman PA, Krikler DM and Davies MJ. Community study of the causes of 'natural' sudden death. *Br Med J* 1988; **297**: 1453–6.

Tunstall-Pedoe J, Bailey L, Chamberlain DA, Marsden AK, Ward ME and Zideman DA. Survey of 3765 cardiopul-monary resuscitations in British hospitals (the BRESUS study): methods and overall results. *Br Med J* 1992; **304**: 1347–51.

Weisfeldt ML, Kerber RE and McGoldrick P *et al*. Public access defibrillation. A statement for healthcare professionals. From the American Heart Association Task Force on auto-matic external defibrillation. *Circulation* 1995; **92**: 2763.

White NM, Parker WS, Binning RA, Kimber ER, Ead HW and Chamberlain DA. Mobile coronary care provided by ambulance personnel. *Br Med J* 1973; **3**: 618–22.

Wolbrink A and Borrillo D. Airline use of automatic external defibrillators: shocking developments. *Aviat Space Environ Med* 1999; **70**: 87–8.

Zoll PM, Linenthal AJ, Gibson W, Paul MH and Normal LR. Termination of ventricular fibrillation in man by externally applied electric countershock. *N Engl J Med* 1956; **254**: 727–32.

FURTHER READING

The American Heart Association in collaboration with the International Liaison Committee on Resuscitation (ILCOR). Guidelines 2000 for cardiopulmonary resuscitation and emergency cardiovascular care – an international consensus on science. Part 3 Adult basic life support. *Resuscitation* 2000; **46**: 47–8.

14

Haematological disorders and transfusion

PAUL LF GIANGRANDE

Several blood disorders can affect fitness to fly and, at the same time, flight itself may lead to various problems. An example of the former is anaemia and an important example of the latter is thrombo-embolism. The problem of thrombosis is covered in the next chapter.

ANAEMIA

Haemoglobin in red blood cells (erythrocytes) is necessary for the uptake of oxygen in the lungs, and its transport and transfer to peripheral tissues. The normal haemoglobin level is 13.5–17.5 g dl^{-1} for males and 11.5–15.5 g dl^{-1} for females. Anaemia may be the consequence of a wide variety of disorders, and it is important to determine the cause. Whatever the aetiology, cardiovascular reserve could be impaired and this could pose a problem in an aircraft with a cabin altitude up to 8000 feet. As a general rule, patients with a haemoglobin level of 7.5 g dl^{-1} or more are not likely to experience problems with commercial air travel. However, the haemoglobin level alone cannot be relied upon to decide whether a patient is fit to travel.

A distinction must be made between chronic and acute anaemia. Patients with long-standing anaemia, such as that associated with renal failure, often have good cardiovascular compensation and experience

few problems with travel. By contrast, patients with anaemia of recent onset, such as after surgery, are more likely to experience problems. It is also important to bear in mind that examination whilst at rest may prove misleading and exercise tolerance should be assessed. As a general guideline, those who are able to walk about 50 metres and climb 10–12 stairs without symptoms should be able to fly without incident (Peters 1978). Signs of haemodynamic instability precipitated by exertion include tachycardia or other arrhythmias, hypotension, chest pain and changes in the ST segment of the electrocardiogram. In addition to possible difficulties associated with the journey, travellers with anaemia should be advised of the possible hazards of blood transfusion in developing countries. This is particularly important for patients with chronic haematological conditions where periodic transfusion is required.

Iron deficiency

Iron deficiency is the commonest cause of anaemia, but it is important to establish the underlying cause. It may reflect poor intake (vegetarians) or poor absorption (coeliac disease), but the commonest cause is chronic blood loss (menorrhagia, peptic ulcers or other gastrointestinal pathology). The typical picture associated with iron deficiency is a low haemoglobin associated with hypochromia (mean corpuscular haemoglobin <27 pg) and microcytosis (mean corpuscular volume <80 fl) of the red cells. The diagnosis can be confirmed by the finding of a low serum ferritin level (Gaul 1999).

Folate and B$_{12}$ deficiency

Deficiency of folic acid or vitamin B$_{12}$ may also cause anaemia. In this case, the red cells are unusually large (macrocytosis) with a mean corpuscular volume of 100 fl or more. Serum levels should be checked. Severe vitamin B$_{12}$ deficiency may be associated with both peripheral neuropathy and spinal cord demyelination, but this does not occur in association with folic acid deficiency. Isolated macrocytosis associated with a normal haemoglobin also merits documentation, as it may be an indicator of several conditions including chronic liver disease, sustained high alcohol intake, and hypothyroidism, although it is a normal finding in pregnancy and neonates. Anaemia in association with thrombocytopenia and/or an abnormal leucocyte count deserves investigation, and referral to a haematologist should be considered.

Sickle cell disease

Sickle cell disease is a congenital haemolytic anaemia in which the mutation renders the molecule unstable. The gene is encountered predominantly in people of Afro-Caribbean origin, among whom the gene frequency may be as high as 5 per cent. The gene is found with a lower frequency amongst people of the Mediterranean, Middle East and Indian subcontinent. Carriers of this condition have no clinical problems, but homozygotes are prone to recurrent episodes of painful 'crises'. Often there is no obvious precipitating cause, but it is recognized that infections, dehydration and exposure to cold or low levels of oxygen can provoke crises. These painful crises are due to necrosis in the bone marrow, secondary to occlusion of small vessels. The most frequently involved areas are the knee, lumbosacral spine, elbow and femur. Less often the ribs, sternum, clavicles, calcaneus and facial bones are affected.

The course of sickle cell disease is variable and many patients lead essentially normal lives punctuated by only occasional painful crises. Crises in bones and joints should be treated conservatively with bed rest, maintenance of fluid balance and correction of hypoxia if the lungs are affected. Crises can be extremely painful, and opiate analgesics are usually needed. Extensive sickling within the lungs can be life-threatening ('chest crisis'). This can initially present with cough, fever and pleuritic chest pain, and a chest radiograph shows extensive infiltration of either one or both lung fields. Typically, adults with sickle cell anaemia have a chronic haemolytic anaemia, with a haemoglobin level in the range of 7–10 g dl^{-1}. The blood film is characteristic, with numerous hyperchromatic and irreversibly sickled cells (which are evident even in the absence of clinical sickling) and target cells. The chronic haemolytic process results in consumption of folic acid, and oral supplementation is often required.

Fetal haemoglobin is composed of paired α- and γ-chains, but by approximately 6 months of age production of β-chains replaces that of fetal γ-chains and this is when the first symptoms of the condition appear. Dactylitis ('hand–foot syndrome') is often the first manifestation of the condition. The digits of the hand or feet become painful, swollen, hot and tender due to sickling within the bone. Avascular necrosis of the hip is a not infrequent complication in adolescents as well as adults, and may be bilateral. Repeated episodes of splenic infarction may lead to loss of immune function with particular susceptibility to capsulated bacteria. There is a risk of vaso-occlusive stroke in patients with sickle cell anaemia, which may present as sudden onset of seizures, coma, visual disturbances or hemiplegia. Gallstones of aggregates of bilirubin often form in sickle cell anaemia. Repeated infarction within the hypertonic environment of the renal medulla often results in recurrent episodes of painless haematuria. Eventually, the ability to concentrate urine is impaired, and patients are thus prone to dehydration. It is vital that attention be paid to fluid balance.

In the past, flight at altitude in unpressurized aircraft has been a cause of sickling. Even now, some physicians dissuade patients with sickle cell disease from travelling, or insist on administration of in-flight oxygen during the flight. However, recent data suggest that, perhaps contrary to expectations, sickling crises and related problems in patients with sickle cell disease (Hb SS) flying in pressurized commercial aircraft are extremely rare (Ware et al. 1998).

There are reassuring data available now which permit a more relaxed attitude. People with sickle cell disease should certainly be encouraged to drink plenty of water during the journey, as they are particularly prone to dehydration due to the impaired ability of the kidneys to concentrate urine. The risk of sickling with other variants, including haemoglobin S/C disease and haemoglobin S/β-thalassaemia is higher. In such cases, it would be sensible to have oxygen available on board, although it is not necessary to use it in flight on a prophylactic basis.

By contrast, sickle cell trait is a benign condition in which 20–40 per cent of the circulating haemoglobin is Hb S and the rest is normal Hb A. The haemoglobin level is normal. *In vitro* tests show that sickling does not occur in sickle cell trait until the P_{O_2} falls to about 10 mmHg (1.33 kPa) and thus clinical problems will only occur in conditions of extreme hypoxia. Flight in pressurized commercial aircraft certainly poses no problems whatsoever, and in this context it should be noted that the sickle cell trait is not a bar to the granting of a licence for a commercial pilot (Bendrick 1997).

The thalassaemias

The thalassaemias are a group of haematological disorders in which a defect in the synthesis of one or more of the globin polypeptide chains is present and erythrocyte precursors are destroyed prematurely. A classification of the thalassaemias is beyond the scope of this chapter, but the principal division is that between disorders involving the α-chain and the β-chain of the haemoglobin molecule. The prevalence of the genes for thalassaemia is high in Mediterranean countries, particularly Greece, Italy, Cyprus and North Africa, the Middle East, the Indian subcontinent and South East Asia. Carriers of β-thalassaemia ('thalassaemia trait'), the commonest form in European countries, have no clinical problems, apart from a mild and persistent microcytic anaemia with a haemoglobin typically in the range from 10–12 g dl^{-1}. This should present no problems for flying.

The homozygous form, β-thalassaemia major, runs an entirely different course. The condition is characterized by severe anaemia and is accompanied by massive enlargement of the liver and spleen. Examination of the blood film shows severe hypochromic, microcytic anaemia with reticulocytosis. Normoblasts, target cells and basophilic stippling of erythrocytes are also seen. Haemoglobin electrophoresis is required for definitive diagnosis, and the hallmark of β-thalassaemia major is the absence of normal haemoglobin A, which is replaced by fetal haemoglobin (Hb F) and some Hb A2. Somewhat paradoxically, many of the serious medical complications seen in thalassaemia result from treatment of the condition.

These patients are dependent upon regular blood transfusions but this eventually results in iron overload with deposition of iron in various organs, causing fibrosis. Iron overload may result in serious medical complications such as diabetes mellitus and cirrhosis and cardiac complications such as arrhythmias or congestive cardiac failure. Subcutaneous infusions of the chelating agent desferrioxamine may postpone the onset of iron overload.

MALIGNANCY

Advances in recent years offer the prospect of a cure for many haematological malignancies, including acute leukaemias and lymphomas. A description of acute leukaemias is outside the scope of this chapter, but it should be borne in mind that treatment of haematological malignancies often involves prolonged courses of chemotherapy and/or radiotherapy. Some conditions require treatment with steroids. Immunosuppression with cyclosporin or other agents will be required after bone marrow transplantation, as with other solid organ transplants. Live vaccines should not be given to patients who are immunocompromised by steroid treatment, chemotherapy or radiotherapy. Such vaccines include yellow fever, BCG (bacille Calmette-Guérin), poliomyelitis and typhoid. Vaccination should be postponed until at least 3 months after stopping corticosteroids and 6 months after stopping chemotherapy.

Chronic lymphocytic leukaemia

Chronic lymphocytic leukaemia (CLL) is a malignant proliferation of B-lymphocytes and occurs chiefly in the elderly. It typically runs an indolent course and is often picked up as an incidental finding, e.g. when a routine full blood count is taken prior to elective surgery. Many patients die of a completely unrelated condition. In advanced stages, there may be evidence of bone marrow failure, with anaemia and thrombocytopenia, diffuse lymphadenopathy and splenomegaly. Most patients will not require treatment initially. Treatment with steroids and alkylating agents may ultimately be needed as the disease progresses over a period of some years to control bone marrow failure or significant lymphadenopathy. Autoimmune haemolytic anaemia is also a recognized complication, which responds well to steroid therapy. Patients with chronic leukaemia are prone to bacterial, fungal and herpes zoster infections because of hypogammaglobulinaemia, neutropenia and disturbances of cellular immunity.

Chronic myeloid leukaemia

Chronic myeloid leukaemia (CML) occurs most frequently in the age range of 40–60 years, although it can rarely affect children. The course of the disease is characterized by two distinct phases. The initial chronic phase lasts 3–4 years. There are often signs of hypermetabolism, including weight loss, fever and night sweats. The condition is associated with high white cell counts, and often marked splenomegaly. The patient will suffer anaemia due to bone marrow infiltration, as well as thrombocytopenia, which can result in haemorrhagic complications. Gout due to hyperuricaemia from excessive purine breakdown may be a problem. Other rare complications are priapism and visual disturbances, due to the high blood viscosity associated with high white cell counts. Eventually, transformation into an acute 'blast' phase occurs. This can develop quickly, over a period of days or weeks. The white cell count rises rapidly and is less responsive to chemotherapy and the spleen enlarges. Chemotherapy with busulphan or hydroxyurea is effective in controlling the condition in the chronic phase and interferon-α is also effective. Steroids are not used in the treatment of this condition. Bone marrow transplantation offers a good prospect of cure in younger patients with compatible donors, and this is best carried out during the chronic phase.

Multiple myeloma

Multiple myeloma is another malignancy affecting lymphoid precursor cells. Like CLL, it affects mainly elderly subjects and often runs an indolent course for several years. However, progressive marrow infiltration occurs, causing bone pain and progressive pancytopenia. Accumulation of plasma cells in the marrow results in the development of discrete osteolytic areas, which are a diagnostic feature on radiography, and can result in pathological fractures. Extensive bone disease is often associated with hypercalcaemia, which can present with polyuria and psychiatric symptoms, e.g. acute confusional state. The malignant cells secrete large amounts of non-functional immunoglobulin into plasma. This can result in plasma hyperviscosity, leading to neurological disturbances (including ataxia, neuropathies, psychiatric and visual disturbances) and even coma, as well as haemorrhagic problems due to interaction with the coagulation proteins.

The abnormal monoclonal protein also accumulates in the kidney, frequently resulting in progressive renal failure. Standard treatment consists of a combination of oral melphalan, often in combination with prednisolone. This will only control the disease, leading to a 'plateau phase' with a stable paraprotein level, and does not cure the disease. More radical treatment, including bone marrow transplantation, may be offered to younger patients. There are thus a number of potentially serious complications that can arise in myeloma, which would require urgent intervention. These include pathological fractures, spinal cord compression, hypercalcaemia, recurrent bacterial infections and renal failure.

Diagnosis

The diagnosis of malignant haematological disease does not necessarily constitute a bar to travel. No problems would be anticipated with air travel if well controlled on appropriate therapy, but each case merits consideration on an individual basis. Live vaccines, for example yellow fever, should not be given to subjects with leukaemia or lymphomas, particularly if they have had treatment with immunosuppressive agents such as steroids and alkylating agents. A low white cell count (neutropenia) can also render a patient unusually susceptible to infections, and so the count should be checked before travel, although it should be borne in mind that the nadir may only be achieved a week or so after the treatment has been completed. As a rough guide, the white cell count should be $1.0 \times 10^9 \, l^{-1}$ or more for travel. Similarly, the platelet count should be at least $50 \times 10^9 \, l^{-1}$.

THROMBOCYTOPENIA

The normal range for the platelet count is 150–400 $\times 10^9 \, \text{l}^{-1}$. Many conditions result in thrombocytopenia, including autoimmune thrombocytopenia and various malignant diseases. The nature of the underlying disease will need to be considered when assessing a patient for travel as will the trend in the count. When assessing the risk of the bleeding tendency, it should be borne in mind that far more platelets are produced than are actually required to control bleeding. Easy bruising and persistent bleeding from cuts and scratches only develop when the platelet count falls below approximately $80 \times 10^9 \, \text{l}^{-1}$. Serious internal bleeding, such as intracranial haemorrhage, may occur if the platelet count falls below $20 \times 10^9 \, \text{l}^{-1}$, although the trigger for prophylactic transfusion of platelets in most haematology units is now even lower at $10 \times 10^9 \, \text{l}^{-1}$.

However, the risk of bleeding is not just related to the absolute platelet count. In autoimmune thrombocytopenia there is a rapid turnover of young platelets and serious bleeding is rarely a problem, even with very low counts. Indeed, commercial pilots may only be disqualified from flying when the platelet count falls below $75 \times 10^9 \, \text{l}^{-1}$. For passengers in civil aircraft, it would be reasonable to permit a patient to fly with a much lower threshold of $\leq 40 \times 10^9 \, \text{l}^{-1}$. Patients with thrombocytopenia should not be given aspirin or similar non-steroidal drugs, as these will exacerbate the bleeding tendency through their inhibitory effect on platelet function. Paracetamol (acetaminophen) is a safe alternative analgesic. Patients who have undergone splenectomy for autoimmune thrombocytopenia will be permanently vulnerable to certain infections.

HAEMOPHILIA

Haemophilia A is a congenital disorder of coagulation, characterized by hereditary deficiency of factor VIII. Deficiency of factor IX results in an identical clinical condition known as haemophilia B (Christmas disease). These are both sex-linked recessive disorders that only affect males. Very occasionally, acquired haemophilia may be encountered in which the deficiency of the coagulation factor is a result of autoantibody formation, and this can affect both males and females. The hallmark of haemophilia is recurrent and spontaneous bleeding into joints, principally the knees, elbows and ankles. Repeated bleeding into joints can, in the absence of treatment, result in disabling arthritis at an early age. Bleeding into muscles and soft tissues is also seen frequently. Although the diagnosis of haemophilia is not compatible with the granting of a commercial pilot's licence, travel as a passenger in a commercial aircraft should present no problems. However, it should be borne in mind when assessing a patient for fitness to fly, that a significant number of haemophiliacs have been exposed to hepatitis and human immunodeficiency virus (HIV) through their treatment. Some countries (e.g. USA) insist on a special entry visa for people with these communicable diseases. HIV-positive patients should not receive yellow fever, BCG or oral typhoid vaccines. People with haemophilia should also carry an adequate quantity of coagulation factor concentrate for their stay abroad. The World Federation of Haemophilia maintains a database of the addresses and other contact details for specialist haemophilia centres around the world.

In summary, passengers with haemophilia should take adequate stocks of coagulation factor with a letter from their doctor for Customs as bottles of white powder may invite suspicion. Travel insurance should be arranged with haemophilia and other conditions declared, and special visas are required for some countries (including USA) for those patients with infectious diseases such as HIV and hepatitis C. It is also important to identify treatment centres *en route* and the contact details.

SPLENECTOMY

Some discussion of the hazards of splenectomy is relevant to the well-being of the airline passenger. The commonest reason for splenectomy, nowadays, is traumatic rupture following abdominal injury, but it is also performed for the treatment of several haematological conditions, including certain haemolytic anaemias, autoimmune thrombocytopenia and hairy cell leukaemia. The operation used to be carried out routinely in Hodgkin's lymphoma as part of the staging process before starting treatment. Patients with sickle cell disease are effectively asplenic due to repeated infarction within the organ. Whilst splenectomy may control the underlying haematological condition, the patient will be left permanently vulnerable to certain infectious diseases (Conlon 1993, Mileno and Bia 1998). Asplenic individuals are particularly susceptible to encapsulated organisms such as *Streptococcus pneumoniae*, *Haemophilus influenzae* and *Neisseria meningitidis*. Vaccination should be offered where possible, although the immunological response is better when the vaccine is given before elective splenectomy. Bacteraemia in asplenic individuals often has a fulminating course, leading rapidly to shock and coma accompanied by disseminated intravascular coagulation. The diagnosis may not be immediately obvious in a patient who has collapsed, although the presence of a surgical scar in the left hypochondrium is an important clue. Patients should be treated with an antibiotic at the first sign of fever or respiratory illness, however trivial. Amoxicillin is preferred to penicillin V because of better absorption following oral administration, and also because it has a broader antibacterial spectrum which includes *H. influenzae*. Malaria in asplenic subjects is often fatal, and it is vital that asplenic subjects take appropriate prophylaxis where indicated.

TRANSFUSION

Blood transfusion in many parts of the world still poses very real risks with regard to transmission of viral and other infections. Systematic screening of blood donations is not yet feasible in many developing countries and needles may not even be sterilized before re-use. Infections which may be transmitted by transfusion of blood or plasma include HIV, hepatitis B and C, malaria, babesiosis, *Trypanosoma cruzi* (Chagas' disease), brucellosis, syphilis, cytomegalovirus (CMV) and human T-cell lymphoma virus (HTLV-I). Whilst it is difficult to generalize, the risks are particularly high in sub-Saharan Africa where there is a particularly high prevalence of HIV and malaria. Patients with chronic disorders must be counselled about the possible risks in certain parts of the world if transfusion might be required.

Patients sometimes enquire about the possibility of taking blood from their home country with them abroad. This raises a number of technical as well as logistical problems (blood has to be stored at 4°C and has a limited shelf-life of up to 6 weeks), which are not easy to resolve. The international shipment of blood for transfusion is only practical when handled by agreement between two responsible organizations, such as national blood transfusion services. This mechanism is not feasible for the emergency needs of individual patients and should not be attempted by private individuals. In fact, emergency blood transfusion is rarely required and is likely to be needed only in the setting of massive haemorrhage after trauma, gastrointestinal bleeding or obstetric emergencies. In developed countries, a decision to transfuse is far too often based solely on the haemoglobin level. In fact, the decision should be based on the clinical state and haemodynamic stability (pulse, blood pressure, respiratory rate) of the patient. It is by no means essential, for example, to transfuse someone just because the haemoglobin has fallen to 8 g dl^{-1}. Even in the case of massive haemorrhage, resuscitation can often be achieved through the use of colloid (e.g. 'Haemaccel', derived from partially degraded gelatin) or crystalloid plasma expanders instead of blood. Whilst it is not feasible to transport packs of blood abroad, plasma expanders may be transported much more readily as they have a much longer shelf-life and do not require storage at room temperature. It is also advisable in some cases to take sterile needles and other disposable equipment such as giving sets.

REFERENCES

Bendrick GA. You're the flight surgeon: sickle cell trait and beta-thalassemia. *Aviat Space Environ Med* 1997; **68**: 244–5.

Conlon CP. The immunocompromised traveller. *Br Med Bull* 1993; **49**: 412–22.

Gaul MP. You're the flight surgeon. Borderline anemia. *Aviat Space Environ Med* 1999; **70**: 826.

Mileno MD and Bia FJ. The compromised traveler. *Infect Dis Clin North Am* 1998; **12**: 369–412.

Peters ASR. Carriage of invalids by air. *J R Coll Physicians Lond* 1978; **12**: 136–42.

Ware M, Tyghter D, Staniforth S and Serjeant G. Airline travel in sickle-cell disease. *Lancet* 1998; **352**: 652.

APPENDIX: NORMAL HAEMATOLOGICAL VALUES

Haemoglobin
  Males: 13.5–17.5 g dl^{-1}
  Females: 11.5–15.5 g dl^{-1}
MCV (mean corpuscular volume): 80–95 fl
MCH (mean content haemoglobin): 27–34 pg
WBC (white blood count): 4.0–11.0 $\times$ 10^9 l^{-1}
  Neutrophils: 2.5–7.5 $\times$ 10^9 l^{-1}
  Lymphocytes: 1.5–3.5 $\times$ 10^9 l^{-1}
  Monocytes: 0.2–0.8 $\times$ 10^9 l^{-1}

Eosinophils: 0.04–0.44 $\times$ 10^9 l^{-1}
Platelets: 150–400 $\times$ 10^9 l^{-1}
Serum ferritin
  Males: 40–340 μg l^{-1}
  Females: 14–150 μ g l^{-1}
Serum folate: 3.0–15 μg l^{-1}
Red cell folate: 160–640 μg l^{-1}
Serum vitamin B$_{12}$: 160–925 ng l^{-1}

Normal ranges for coagulation tests cannot be stated, as these vary according to the method and reagents used. The normal range for the laboratory that carried out the tests must, therefore, be consulted.

15

Venous thrombosis

PAUL LF GIANGRANDE

It is now generally accepted that long-distance air travel is associated with a risk of deep vein thrombosis and pulmonary embolism, which may be fatal. The consensus at a meeting convened by the World Health Organization (2001) to review the evidence was that there probably is a link, but that the incidence is low and involves mainly passengers with additional risk factors. The exact incidence of thromboembolism in relation to air travel is uncertain, though it has been estimated that at least 5 per cent of all cases of deep vein thrombosis may be linked to air travel. The term 'economy class syndrome' has been coined to describe the phenomenon and this emphasizes the role of impairment of venous circulation due to prolonged immobility in a cramped position. However, venous thrombosis is not exclusively associated with air travel, and it has been documented following long car, bus or even train journeys. Furthermore, thrombosis is by no means restricted to those in the relatively confined conditions of economy class, and thus the alternative term of 'travellers' thrombosis' has been suggested.

Most reports involve venous thrombosis in the lower limbs, but there are also reports of cerebral venous thrombosis and arterial thrombosis associated with long flights. Venous thrombosis in the lower limbs may be confined to the superficial leg veins, but may involve the deep veins of the calf or the more proximal such as the superficial femoral, common femoral or iliac veins. The risk of pulmonary embolism is much higher when proximal veins are involved. In addition to the potential for embolism, organization of the venous thrombus in the leg can ultimately cause long-term problems including chronic ulceration and the post-phlebitic syndrome. Thrombosis is more common in the left leg, possibly due to the fact that the femoral artery on that side passes anterior to the vein and so may compress it.

It is possible to derive some general conclusions from a survey of published cases (Giangrande 2000). Thromboembolism is rarely observed after flights of less than 5 hours' duration and, typically, the flights are of 12 hours' duration or more. The risk rises with age and subjects over the age of 50 are more at risk whilst those under the age of 40 years are less vulnerable. Symptoms of thromboembolism do not usually develop during or immediately after the flight, but tend to appear within 3 days of arrival when the patient may be far away from the airport and thus the causal link not be immediately apparent. Symptoms of thrombosis or pulmonary embolism have been reported up to 2 weeks after a long flight. Pulmonary embolism may be the first manifestation, without any symptoms in the lower limbs (Lapostolle et al. 2001).

RISK FACTORS

A number of risk factors has been recognized, primarily through clinical experience in the setting of surgery, which predispose to venous thromboembolism (Table 15.1). There are also risk factors specific to air travel, including relative immobility for a prolonged period in a cramped position. Most airline seats have fairly rigid metal frames designed for safety in the event of an accident, but the bar at the front edge of the seat may compress the popliteal vein. It has been suggested that exposure to the mild hypobaric hypoxia of a pressurized aircraft may result in activation of the coagulation cascade (Bendz *et al.* 2000, 2001). Although cabin air is of low humidity, the net loss of body water associated with a long-haul flight is low, and has been estimated to be only 100 ml (Nicholson 1998). However, excessive consumption of alcohol or gastrointestinal infections associated with vomiting and diarrhoea may lead to the development of dehydration. Ingestion of alcohol will also encourage immobility and the use of sedatives may be associated with an increased risk of thrombosis (Zornberg and Jick 2000).

In some patients, a haematological abnormality may exist which predisposes to the development of thromboembolism. Such disorders include the relatively rare congenital, inherited deficiencies of natural anticoagulants, such as antithrombin, protein C or protein S. By far the commonest genetic abnormality which predisposes to thrombosis is the factor V Leiden genotype which is associated with resistance to activated protein C. The defect involves a single mutation in the factor V molecule which renders the molecule resistant to cleavage by protein C. This mutation is encountered in approximately 4 per cent of the white population, although it is very rare or even absent in other racial groups. It is associated with an approximately eight-fold increased risk of venous thrombosis, but with a considerably higher risk in women taking oestrogen-containing oral contraceptives.

Elevation of the plasma prothrombin level in association with a point mutation in the prothrombin gene is another newly identified genetic risk factor for venous thrombosis. It is encountered in approximately 2 per cent of the European population and is associated with an approximately three-fold risk of thromboembolism. In addition to these inherited defects, the development of a lupus anticoagulant is associated with an increased risk of venous thromboembolism. Although first identified in subjects with systemic lupus erythematosus, the antibody is found typically in otherwise healthy individuals, and is paradoxically associated with a thrombotic tendency. Other haematological disorders associated with an increased risk of thrombosis include myeloproliferative disorders such as polycythaemia and thrombocythaemia. Screening for thrombophilic defects prior to long-haul flights is often raised, but offers no tangible benefits in passengers without a personal history of thrombosis. Screening may be of value in subjects who have had an episode of venous thromboembolism, or where there is a strong family history, but these tests should be done through a haematologist once the subject has been off anticoagulants for at least one month.

DIAGNOSIS

Typical symptoms of venous thrombosis include pain, swelling and tenderness in the calf, which is

Table 15.1 *Risk factors for venous thromboembolism*

Age: greater than 40 years (but especially the elderly)
Previous thrombotic episode (especially pulmonary embolism)
Documented thrombophilic abnormality (e.g. antithrombin deficiency)
Other haematological disorders (polycythaemia and thrombocythaemia)
Pregnancy and puerperium
Malignancy
Congestive heart failure or recent myocardial infarction
Recent surgery (especially lower limb)
Chronic venous insufficiency
Oestrogen therapy (e.g. oral contraceptive pill, HRT)
Obesity
Prolonged recent immobility (e.g. after recent stroke)
Dehydration (diarrhoea)

often warm to touch with distended superficial veins. However, it must be emphasized that it is not possible to rely on clinical examination alone to exclude the diagnosis of venous thrombosis in the lower limbs. There may be no abnormality, even when extensive thrombosis is present, so objective tests are required for proper evaluation. Furthermore, other diagnoses such as local infection or a muscle strain may mimic the condition. In the author's experience, only 15–20 per cent of patients referred with symptoms suggestive of deep venous thrombosis actually turn out to have positive test results. The first symptoms of venous thrombosis in the legs may actually be due to pulmonary embolism, without any problem in the legs. Typical symptoms of pulmonary embolism include pleuritic chest pain (sharp, stabbing pains in the side of the chest, which are exacerbated by breathing in), dyspnoea (breathlessness) at rest or on only mild exertion and haemoptysis (coughing up blood).

The principal tools used for objective diagnosis are contrast venography and ultrasonography. Contrast venography is regarded by many as the definitive method, and will identify thrombosis confined to veins of the calf as well as the larger proximal vessels. However, it may be difficult to arrange at short notice. Compression ultrasonography is, therefore, increasingly preferred for initial screening. In this technique the proximal veins are compressed gently using the ultrasound transducer. Inability to occlude the vein indicates the presence of a venous thrombosis. This method is of more limited sensitivity in identifying the presence of thrombosis confined to the distal calf, but these probably require no treatment anyway.

More recently, measurement of the level of D-dimers in the blood has been developed as a complementary initial screening test to detect deep vein thrombosis. D-dimers are degradation fragments of fibrin of which a thrombus is composed, and sensitive tests have been developed which may be used as an initial screening procedure for thromboembolism. The test has a negative predictive value, and thromboembolism can be excluded with a high degree of confidence if the level of D-dimers in the blood is in the normal range. The result can be available within as little as 40 minutes after venepuncture, so it is a test of practical value. The result of the D-dimer test is used alongside clinical evaluation of other risk factors in selecting patients for further radiological examinations.

TREATMENT

The conventional approach to the treatment of venous thromboembolism involves immediate anticoagulation with heparin followed by a more prolonged period of oral anticoagulation with warfarin or with other similar coumarin, such as nicoumalone. Low molecular weight heparins (dalteparin, tinzaparin, enoxaparin, reviparin) are increasingly adopted in preference to conventional, unfractionated heparin. These have the advantage of a single daily subcutaneous injection, and treatment can be monitored on an out-patient basis so that admission to hospital is no longer necessary in uncomplicated cases. One regimen uses dalteparin 200 iu kg^{-1} daily by subcutaneous injection into the lower abdomen or thigh, and warfarin (10 mg) at the same time. Heparin is stopped after 5 days, or when the International Normalized Ratio (INR) reaches 2, whichever is shorter. Anticoagulation should not automatically be embarked upon in all patients as some are at risk of bleeding, and may not be suitable for anticoagulation in the first place.

Recent haemorrhagic stroke should be regarded as a contraindication. Elderly or confused patients may not cope with the demands of anticoagulation, particularly if they are taking several other drugs. Patients with peptic ulceration, pre-existing haemorrhagic diathesis, hepatic cirrhosis, disseminated malignancy, uncontrolled hypertension, or proliferative retinopathy may not be suitable. Pregnancy is not a contraindication, but does pose special problems. The usual duration of treatment with warfarin after an uncomplicated deep vein thrombosis in the lower limb is 3 months. If pulmonary embolism has occurred, it is advisable to extend treatment for a total of 6 months. Warfarin treatment can be stopped abruptly. If thrombosis is confined to the distal calf, it is not absolutely necessary to initiate anticoagulation as the risk of pulmonary embolism or the postphlebitic syndrome is low. However, if this strategy is adopted, it will be necessary to repeat imaging a week later to rule out the possibility of proximal extension.

PROPHYLAXIS

A number of general measures may be taken to minimize the risk of thrombosis associated with long flights. The most important step is to consider whether the patient is fit to fly. For example, since major orthopaedic surgery is a well-recognized risk factor for thrombosis, patients who have had total hip or knee replacement are advised to postpone non-essential journeys for 3 months. The single most important measure during the flight is to carry out leg exercises from time to time whilst seated. In-flight magazines often give illustrated examples, but simple stretching exercises such as flexion, extension and rotation of the ankles will help to promote circulation in the lower limbs. Periodic deep breaths assist the venous return and the pulmonary circulation.

It is not actually necessary to get up and walk around the cabin from time to time. Many airlines, quite reasonably, discourage this as there is always the possibility of encountering unexpected clear air turbulence. An aisle seat or one next to an exit offers more space and some airlines allow seats to be reserved at the time of booking. Hand luggage stowed under seats will also restrict movement. Passengers should also take advantage of refueling stops on long-haul flights to get off the plane and walk around for a while. Adequate hydration should be ensured during the flight. It is not necessary to abstain from alcohol, but excessive consumption should be avoided as this will both promote diuresis and discourage mobility. Similarly, the use of sedatives is best avoided. Although oestrogen-containing oral contraceptives, as well as hormone replacement therapy (HRT), are recognized risk factors for venous thrombosis, it is not advocated that such hormonal medication should be interrupted for the period of travel.

In the absence of randomized controlled studies, it is not possible to give evidence-based recommendations regarding prophylactic treatment. Nevertheless, some conclusions may be drawn from experience in the setting of surgery. For people at risk of thrombosis the wearing of below-knee elasticated stockings on both legs may be helpful. In a recent study, passengers who did not wear stockings developed asymptomatic thrombosis in the calf, whilst none who wore stockings developed a deep venous thrombosis (Scurr et al. 2001). Stockings have the advantages of being readily available without prescription and are washable. They apply graduated pressure to the leg, which is maximal at the ankle (20–30 mmHg), thus encouraging venous return.

It is important to note that the usual full-length stockings used in hospital for prophylaxis of thrombeoembolism in patients undergoing surgery are not suitable for use in flight. They provide a lower pressure at the ankle as they are designed for recumbent patients. It is also important that the patient is provided with the correct size of compression stocking and that they are worn correctly and do not cause constriction in the popliteal area. Quite apart from reducing the risk of thrombosis, elasticated stockings help to prevent oedema of the legs and feet, which can itself cause discomfort after a long flight. Stockings are contraindicated in cases of peripheral vascular disease as the additional compression could provoke ischaemia. The wearing of stockings may precipitate superficial thrombophlebitis in subjects with varicose veins (Scurr et al. 2001).

Aspirin has been advocated in the prophylaxis of thrombosis associated with travel, although this is not based on compelling clinical data. The ability of aspirin to inhibit thrombosis in the arterial tree is well documented, but there is controversy over whether aspirin confers any degree of protection against venous thrombosis. A meta-analysis of several surgical studies concluded that aspirin does offer some protection (Antiplatelet Trialists' Collaboration 1994). This has been supported in a recent prospective study which demonstrated that aspirin reduced the risk of both venous thrombosis and pulmonary embolism by at least one-third in the setting of hip fracture or major orthopaedic surgery [The Pulmonary Embolism Prevention (PEP) Collaborative Group 2000]. The consensus at the meeting of the World Health Organization was that indiscriminate use of a pharmacological agent, such as aspirin, should not be encouraged in view of the potential side effects such as allergic reactions or gastrointestinal bleeding. A single aspirin tablet taken a few hours prior to a long flight may thus be of some prophylactic value but is primarily intended for individuals with no documented high-risk factors for thrombosis or contraindications to aspirin such as allergy or symptoms suggestive of peptic ulceration.

The use of heparin may be considered in the relatively few passengers at high risk of thrombosis, i.e. with a history of more than one thrombotic episode and an identified thrombophilia, although many are already likely to be on long-term anticoagulation. A single subcutaneous injection (into the lower abdomen or thigh) of low molecular weight heparin 2 or 3 hours before the outward and return flights will suffice. The precise dose will vary according to the particular product used. Care should be taken to avoid inadvertent intramuscular injection, as this is likely to result in the formation of a haematoma. Heparin should not be used when there is a pre-existing haemorrhagic condition, e.g. thrombocytopenia, or other medical condition where there is a potential for bleeding, e.g. peptic ulceration. In the unlikely event of significant bleeding after such a low dose of heparin (or after inadvertent overdosage), protamine sulphate may be given as an intravenous bolus injection to neutralize the effect of the circulating heparin.

ANTICOAGULATION

Oral anticoagulants are used widely in the management of common conditions such as deep venous thrombosis, pulmonary embolism, atrial fibrillation and peripheral arterial disease. Physicians may be asked to advise on fitness to travel whilst on such drugs, or to deal with bleeding complications. Warfarin and other similar oral anticoagulants, such as nicoumalone, are competitive antagonists of vitamin K and reduce the synthesis of coagulation factors II (prothrombin), VII, IX and X, resulting in prolongation of the prothrombin time. Warfarin is well absorbed from the gastrointestinal effect, but its effect on coagulation is delayed for up to 24 hours. The prothrombin time is the laboratory test used to monitor warfarin therapy. To promote uniformity in results from laboratories, reagents used for monitoring warfarin treatment are calibrated against an international standard. The results of the prothrombin time are expressed as the International Normalized Ratio (INR). The therapeutic range of the INR for a patient on warfarin is between 2.0 and 4.5, but target values for specific conditions have been recommended (Haemostasis and Thrombosis Task Force 1998). A target INR of 2.5 is appropriate for venous thromboembolism, atrial fibrillation, cardiac mural thrombosis, cardiomyopathy and prior to cardioversion. A higher target INR of 3.5 is suitable for subjects with a mechanical heart valve although long-term anticoagulation is not required with a biological valve, patients who have experienced recurrent venous thromboembolism, and those with the antiphospholipid syndrome ('lupus anticoagulant').

The INR should be monitored periodically. Testing will need to be carried out initially at weekly or fortnightly intervals, although the interval can be extended to a maximum of 12 weeks in the case of patients who are stable on long-term warfarin. Many drugs interact with warfarin and it is prudent to check the INR 1 week after starting a new drug. Patients receiving anticoagulants should never receive intramuscular injections, as this is likely to result in a large haematoma at the site of injection. Patients on warfarin should avoid aspirin or similar non-steroidal inflammatory agents such as ibuprofen, diclofenac and indomethacin. These will exacerbate the potential for bleeding through their inhibitory effect on platelets as well as by their potential to cause mucosal ulceration in the gastrointestinal tract. Paracetamol is a perfectly safe alternative medication for people on warfarin.

Anticoagulation is not a contraindication to travel *per se*, even though anticoagulation is not compatible with the duties of a commercial pilot. Travellers should be advised to ensure that they have an adequate supply to cover the whole of their stay abroad. They must carry their medication with them rather than pack the tablets in a case that will be carried in the aircraft hold. It is vital to arrange the usual INR blood test to monitor treatment. Indeed, changes in diet, alcohol intake and climate may well result in significant changes to the INR, even in subjects who have been stable previously. Illnesses such as diarrhoea or vomiting may impair absorption of warfarin. All patients should carry their treatment booklets, which should contain clear clinical details and the results of previous blood tests. Finally, medical insurance for overseas trips is strongly recommended and medical conditions should be declared when the policy is taken out.

Haemorrhage is the most important complication of warfarin therapy and the risk is proportional to the degree of anticoagulation. The risk of bleeding whilst on oral anticoagulants rises significantly when the INR is greater than 5. The elderly are particularly prone to serious bleeding complications with oral anticoagulation. The treatment of bleeding problems due to over-anticoagulation depends upon the clinical circumstances and the INR. Temporary suspension of warfarin is often all that is required for minor bleeding problems such as bleeding from gums, epistaxis or haematuria. Diversion of an aircraft does not need to be considered if such a problem arises in flight. Vitamin K may be given to partially reverse the effect of warfarin and reduce the INR. Tablets will have only a limited effect, as absorption is delayed and the INR will not be reversed for a minimum of at least 8 hours, but is better than nothing. If the patient is not carrying any vitamin K, it is quite possible that another passenger will be carrying multivitamin pills of some sort. If available, a slow intravenous injection of 0.5–2.0 mg vitamin K is usually enough for a faster partial correction of the INR within 2–4 hours.

In the case of a major bleeding episode, such as intracranial haemorrhage or gastrointestinal bleeding, rapid and complete reversal is required and even intravenous vitamin K will be of little use. If such a problem occurs during flight, diversion of the aircraft will be required so that fresh-frozen plasma or other blood products (prothrombin-complex concentrates, which contain coagulation factors II, VII, IX and X) can be infused. In due course, the reason for the bleeding problem and/or prolonged INR should be identified, e.g. interaction with a new medication or confusion over intake of warfarin tablets. Haemorrhagic problems associated with an INR in the therapeutic range also deserve investigation, particularly in the elderly, to exclude latent pathology. For example, haematuria may be associated with a tumour of the bladder and melaena may be the first manifestation of a peptic ulcer.

REFERENCES

Antiplatelet Trialists' Collaboration. Collaborative overview of randomised trials of antiplatelet therapy III. Reduction in venous thrombosis and pulmonary embolism by antiplatelet prophylaxis against surgical and medical patients. *Br Med J* 1994; **308**: 235–46.

Bendz B, Rostrup M, Sevre K, Andersen TO and Sandset PM. Association between hypobaric hypoxia and activation of coagulation in human beings. *Lancet* 2000; **356**: 1657–8.

Bendz B, Sevre K, Andersen TO and Sandset PM. Low molecular weight heparin prevents activation of coagulation in a hypobaric environment. *Blood Coag Fibrinol* 2001; **12**: 371–4.

Giangrande PLF. Thrombosis and air travel. *J Travel Med* 2000; **7**: 149–54.

Haemostasis and Thrombosis Task Force for the British Committee for Standards in Haematology. Guidelines of oral anticoagulation (third edition). *Br J Haematol* 1998; **101**: 374–87.

Lapostolle F, Surget V, Borron SW *et al*. Severe pulmonary embolism associated with air travel. *N Engl J Med* 2001; **345**: 779–83.

Nicholson AN. Dehydration and long haul flights. *Travel Med Int* 1998; **16**: 177–81.

Scurr JH, Machin SJ, Bailey-King S, Mackie IJ, McDonald S and Smith PD. Frequency and prevention of symptomless deep-vein thrombosis in long-haul flights: a randomized trial. *Lancet* 2001; **357**: 1485–9.

The Pulmonary Embolism Prevention (PEP) Trial Collaborative Group. Prevention of pulmonary embolism and deep vein thrombosis with low dose aspirin: the Pulmonary Embolism Prevention (PEP) trial. *Lancet* 2000; **355**: 1295–302.

World Health Organization. World Health Organization consultation on air travel and thromboembolism: Geneva 12–13th March, 2001: http://www.who.int/ncd/cvd/dvt.htm.

Zornberg GL and Jick H. Antipsychotic drug use and risk of first-time idiopathic venous thromboembolism: a case-control study. *Lancet* 2000; **356**: 1219–23.

Otolaryngology

DAVID A JONATHAN

The upper aerodigestive tract is particularly at risk due to pressure changes encountered during flight. As Boyle stated in 1662, the volume of gas within any enclosed cavity will vary inversely with the pressure to which it is subjected, at a constant temperature, and so the air-containing cavities of the middle ear cleft and paranasal sinuses are potentially vulnerable to pressure changes. In certain circumstances, such changes may give rise to acute symptoms and, possibly, on-going problems after completion of the journey. With appropriate advice, most of these problems can be avoided. This chapter deals with conditions affecting the ears, nose and throat. Each topic is addressed in terms of advice that should be given prior to flying, steps that should be taken if problems occur during flight and finally, the management of disorders that might persist after the flight. The demands of modern life mean that susceptible patients will frequently find that advice not to fly is simply unacceptable, and so the risk has to be assessed carefully and advice not to fly given only when this is realistic.

THE EAR

The middle ear or tympanic cavity is an air-containing space within the petrous temporal bone and is in continuity with the nasopharynx via the Eustachian tube. The tympanic membrane forms the lateral boundary of the middle ear, separating it from the external auditory canal. Medial to the middle ear cavity lie the structures of the bony labyrinth (inner ear) – the cochlea and the vestibular apparatus. Superiorly lies the middle fossa and posteriorly the mastoid air cells. In front of the middle ear lies the carotid artery and just below that, the opening to the Eustachian tube. The middle ear cleft is a continuation of the upper respiratory tract and is lined with a modified respiratory epithelium (Figure 16.1).

The volume of air within the middle ear and mastoid system varies between 2.5 and 13 cm^3 (Moser 1990). Under normal circumstances the pressure within the middle ear cleft is equal to the ambient air pressure as a result of brief and regular openings of the Eustachian tube, prompted by swallowing or yawning. This tube is 3.5 cm long and runs downwards, forwards and medially from the middle ear to open into the lateral wall of the nasopharynx. The lateral third of the tube is bony, the medial two-thirds is cartilaginous. The cartilaginous portion, whilst normally remaining closed, opens briefly on swallowing, yawning or jaw manipulations as a result of the action of several muscles, most notably the tensor and levator palati.

Otitic barotrauma

The volume of air within the middle ear cleft varies considerably in response to pressure changes: 5 cm^3 at sea level will occupy nearly 7 cm^3 at a cabin altitude of 8000 feet (Moser 1990). Otitic barotrauma

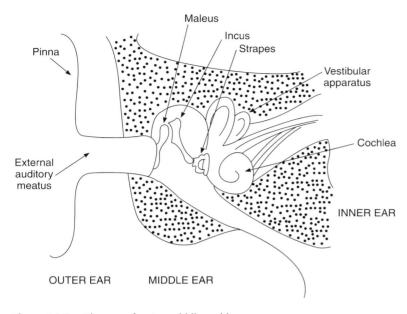

Figure 16.1 *Diagram of outer, middle and inner ear.*

occurs when the Eustachian tube is unable to equalize middle ear pressure with ambient pressure during aircraft flight. It is difficult to estimate its true incidence, but in its mild form it is very common. Otoscopic signs of barotitis have been demonstrated in 10 per cent of adults and 22 per cent of children (Strangerup *et al.* 1998). It is uncommon for the sufferer to have symptoms during ascent of the aircraft because the gradual reduction in cabin pressure results in a relative positive middle ear pressure. Under these circumstances there is a passive opening of the Eustachian tube and equilibration. However, during descent the reverse is true. The gradual increase in cabin pressure results in a relatively negative middle ear pressure and opening of the Eustachian tube requires active muscular function (Figure 16.2). With impaired tubular function, equalization of pressure will not happen, with resultant symptoms. Therefore, otitic barotrauma is almost universally felt on descent rather than ascent of the aircraft.

The symptoms may vary in severity from mild popping of the ears to increasing pain, often described as sharp and stabbing. Hearing acuity may also be affected. Submucosal oedema may develop within the middle ear, leading to haemorrhage and, in extreme cases, perforation of the tympanic membrane may occur (King 1979). Often a slight pressure differential will resolve within minutes or hours of landing, but in some circumstances symptoms may persist, in which case medical advice is frequently sought.

The most common predisposing factor is a simple upper respiratory infection where oedema of the Eustachian tube mucosa results in narrowing of the lumen and tubal dysfunction. There are some specific circumstances where tubal function may be impaired, such as nasal obstruction secondary to a grossly deviated nasal septum, nasal polyps and acute or chronic rhinosinusitis. Nasopharyngeal masses and any palatal defect may also impair tubal function. Middle ear pathologies are themselves sometimes caused by dysfunction of the Eustachian tube, and recent middle ear surgery (see below) may also have some impact. There are, however, some individuals without a past history of any ear disorder who, under normal circumstances, have no symptoms referable to the ears, but, nevertheless, experience severe otitic barotrauma. They must be presumed to have borderline function of the Eustachian tube which only becomes apparent when there is the requirement to overcome a greater than normal pressure differential.

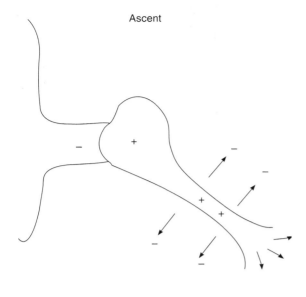

Ascent

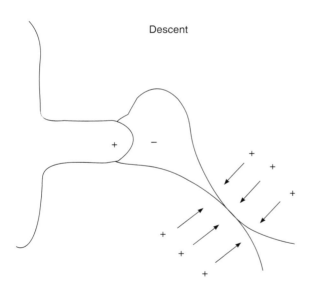

Descent

Figure 16.2 *Middle ear pressure changes during ascent and descent.*

PRE-FLIGHT ASSESSMENT

To advise travellers as to the likelihood of developing otitic barotrauma, it is important to gain some idea as to whether they suffer from impaired function of the Eustachian tube. Reliable testing of tubal function is difficult. Some tests assess function directly, whereas others use indirect methods and make inferences from the observations. Some direct

tests are confined to the laboratory and involve sophisticated pressure chamber equipment. There are also acoustic techniques (Jonathan *et al.* 1986). A simple direct test is observation of tympanic membrane during the Toynbee manoeuvre. The Toynbee manoeuvre (King 1979) is carried out by swallowing whilst the nose and mouth are occluded, thus creating a negative pressure within the pharynx. Under normal circumstances swallowing will also provoke opening of the Eustachian tube. Movement of the tympanic membrane confirms normal tubal function. A positive Toynbee test is an excellent predictor of normal function, but, unfortunately, a negative Toynbee does not necessarily imply dysfunction. It is sometimes easier to observe tympanic membrane movement after a Valsalva manoeuvre (forced expiration with mouth and nose closed), but this is simply a test of patency rather than actual function. Nevertheless, a positive Valsalva is useful.

Simple indirect tests rely upon the premise that a well-ventilated middle ear with normal pressure is indicative of normal function. Therefore, the presence of a normal-looking tympanic membrane, which is mobile on pneumatic otoscopy, suggests there is unlikely to be any significant dysfunction. Similarly, observation of a good peak on tympanometry with normal middle ear pressure would suggest the same. These tests, whilst contributing to the clinical picture, do not necessarily represent how the Eustachian tube will behave once subjected to the need to overcome a significant pressure difference between the middle ear and its surroundings as might be encountered during descent of the aircraft. Unfortunately, therefore, they cannot be regarded as infallible – one study has indicated that tympanometry (see above) is a poor predictor of otitic barotrauma (Ashton and Watson 1990).

PREVENTION AND TREATMENT

As a general rule, flying whilst suffering from a heavy head cold should be avoided. If unavoidable, then decongestants should be used. Oral pseudoephedrine has been shown to be more effective than topical oxymetazoline (Jones *et al.* 1998). Topical medications have the advantage of not inducing drowsiness, which can occur when oral pseudoephedrine is combined with an antihistamine. Sympathomimetics should be avoided in travellers with hypertension, hyperthyroidism, coronary heart disease, diabetes and in patients taking monoamine-oxidase inhibitors. General advice should be given to encourage swallowing; sucking boiled sweets may help, and advice not to sleep during descent of the aircraft may prove to be helpful. Performing the Valsalva manoeuvre (see above) may be effective.

An alternative manoeuvre described by Frenzell (King 1979), should, in theory, be more effective than the Valsalva, although as it is a technique that requires some instruction it is less widely used. It consists of closing the glottis, mouth and nose, whilst simultaneously contracting the muscles of the floor of the mouth and the superior pharyngeal constrictors. This technique can be performed in any phase of respiration and is independent of intrathoracic pressure. The Otovent® device may be a suitable alternative, especially for children. This is an auto-inflation device that consists of a simple balloon with nozzle. The nozzle is placed against one nostril, the other nostril being occluded, and the subject is asked to blow through the nose, thereby inflating the balloon to a predetermined size. In so doing, a gentle pressure is placed on the nasal cavity, nasopharynx and, therefore, also the Eustachian tube. This has been demonstrated, both in adults and children, to be more successful than the Valsalva manoeuvre in normalizing middle ear pressure during aircraft flight (Strangerup et al. 1998).

On completion of the journey, symptoms of otitic barotrauma may persist. Depending upon the severity, medical advice may be necessary and further treatment will be along the lines of decongestants, inhalations and antibiotics. If a tympanic membrane rupture were to occur, this will probably heal spontaneously although, in the meantime, the individual should keep the ear dry. Swimming should not be resumed until it is confirmed that the tympanic membrane is healthy. Individuals with a history of otitic barotrauma, for whom flying is a frequent necessity, might benefit from middle ear ventilation. Insertion of a ventilating tube into the tympanic membrane will ensure that no pressure differential exists across the tympanic membrane and should, therefore, guarantee pain-free flying. Ordinary grommets or long-term ventilating tubes might be considered, but individuals have to be aware that all these tubes will extrude at some point (Hern and Jonathan 1999). There is also a low risk of associated morbidity, such as otorrhoea, acute otitis media, or persistent tympanic membrane perforation (von Schoenberg et al. 1989).

CHILDREN

The function of the Eustachian tube in childhood is frequently suboptimal, and so a significant factor in the high incidence of childhood middle ear problems. Not surprisingly, therefore, otitic barotrauma is common in children, and it is not uncommon for the first few days of a family summer holiday to be marred by the onset of acute otitis media provoked by an episode of barotrauma. Methods of prevention and treatment have already been outlined. Mothers of babies would be well advised to breast- or bottle-feed their child during descent. Dysfunction of the Eustachian tube is probably a key factor in the aetiology of otitis media with effusion (glue ear). Ironically, the presence of thick tenacious fluid within the middle ear with immobility of the tympanic membrane may 'protect' the middle ear against the adverse effects of pressure change, which depend on the presence of gas.

Middle ear surgery

Patients who have recently undergone middle ear surgery are more likely to suffer the effects of barotrauma. Among this group are individuals whose Eustachian tube is in any case suboptimal. In addition, for a period of time after surgery, the middle ear cleft may contain blood, which can occlude the Eustachian tube and increase the likelihood of barotrauma. Apart from the pain and suffering which result from barotrauma, the pressure changes encountered during an aircraft flight may, in some circumstances, threaten the outcome of surgery. Appropriate advice must be given to all patients who have undergone ear surgery as to when it is safe to resume flying.

MIDDLE EAR VENTILATING TUBES

Middle ear ventilating tubes (grommets) for the treatment of established childhood otitis media with effusion is a recognized and effective form of treatment. When repeat grommet insertion is necessary, a different-shaped tube ('long-term tube') may be used. Similarly, these tubes may be inserted in adults who have also developed persistent middle ear effusions. The surgical treatment of glue ear with grommet insertion will, at the very least, ensure that there is no otitic barotrauma because the grommet acts as a conduit for air, preventing any pressure differential across the tympanic membrane. Parents of children with grommets can, therefore, be reassured that flight should not cause any problems.

MYRINGOPLASTY

Myringoplasty, which is an operation to close a long-standing perforation of the tympanic membrane to reduce the likelihood of further infection, is commonplace. Usually temporalis fascia is used and, placed under the existing tympanic membrane as a 'graft', it acts as a scaffold and allows healing of the membrane. Whilst myringoplasty surgery has a high success rate, the tympanic membrane is not as robust as usual for a period afterwards and so flying should be avoided until a satisfactory appearance is evident. Usually after about a month the tympanic membrane can be well visualized and, if intact, simple Eustachian tube function tests (see above) can be used to confirm an air-filled middle ear with normal tube function. Flying is then permissible. An untreated simple perforation of the tympanic membrane would, in itself, not be a contraindication to flying.

MASTOID SURGERY

Mastoid surgery to eradicate cholesteatoma (open or closed cavity mastoidectomy) may result in a significant disruption of the normal architecture of the middle ear cleft. These individuals are quite likely to have had long-standing Eustachian tube dysfunction and may already have experienced otitic barotrauma. The likelihood of further barotrauma after surgery is difficult to predict. Nevertheless, flying should be avoided until the operative changes have settled – perhaps for 4–6 weeks. Predicting the likelihood of further otitic barotrauma is also difficult, but if the ear is dry and the middle ear well ventilated, there is every possibility of pain-free flying. In extreme circumstances, middle ear ventilation is worth considering.

STAPEDECTOMY SURGERY

Otosclerosis is an hereditary condition which, by virtue of gradual fixation of the stapes footplate, results in a conductive hearing loss. A stapedectomy (or, more correctly, a stapedotomy) is a surgical

option for the treatment of this condition. It involves the removal of the stapes superstructure and the creation of a small opening through the stapes footplate. A prosthesis is placed into this fenestrum, with the other end fixed to the long process of the incus, thus reconstituting a mobile ossicular chain. This is an effective procedure in the vast majority of cases, although there is a definable, but small, risk of sensorineural hearing loss. If this does occur, it is probably secondary to leaking of perilymph through the stapedotomy.

The pressure changes that may be encountered during aircraft flight could result in excessive movement of a newly placed prosthesis and could result in such a perilymph leak. The likelihood of this happening may be reduced with the interposition of a vein graft between the footplate and the prosthesis, thereby creating an effective seal. Indeed, this technique is regarded by many as standard though opinions vary. It is the author's belief that flying after stapedectomy surgery should be avoided until the post-operative changes have settled, usually about 4 weeks. A normal tympanic membrane should be observed with mobility and normal middle ear pressure on tympanometry testing. In addition, tests as outlined above should be carried out to ensure normal function of the Eustachian tube.

OSSICULAR RECONSTRUCTION

Ossicular reconstruction can dramatically improve hearing after gradual destruction of the ossicular chain due to chronic ear disease (ossiculoplasty). This may be carried out in conjunction with a myringoplasty. As with myringoplasty surgery, flying is inadvisable until the operative changes have settled, usually for about a month. Depending upon the exact nature of the reconstruction, there is the possibility that otitic barotrauma will result in excessive force being applied to the stapes footplate, with a resultant perilymph leak and a risk of sensorineural hearing loss and vertigo. It is, therefore, advisable, especially in the early stages after surgery, for the specialist to indicate when flying can safely be undertaken.

Hearing loss

Sensorineural hearing loss is extremely common in the population at large (Davis 1987), and of itself is not a contraindication to flying. Nevertheless, whilst with modern aircraft the ambient noise level for passengers is relatively low, in old commercial aircraft and some light aircraft, the noise encountered may reach a level where prolonged exposure may be injurious to the cochlea and induce a noise-induced hearing loss. Most individuals with a sensorineural hearing loss, in particular the predominantly high-frequency loss that is typically seen in presbyacusis (age-related hearing loss), frequently find their auditory discrimination is impaired in the presence of background noise. These individuals, therefore, may well find that whilst travelling in an aircraft, their auditory abilities may be impaired.

Vertigo

Normal equilibrium relies upon the coordination of sensory input from a variety of areas – vestibular, visual and proprioceptive. Malfunction of any of these areas may result in the false perception of movement and may be perceived by the individual in a variety of different ways. Rotatory vertigo may be experienced; alternatively, the sensation may be one of more generalized imbalance. The causes of vertigo are many and varied and often complex. Aircraft flight itself is unlikely to influence any of these underlying causes, although vertigo sufferers may experience stress at the prospect of being confined to a seat for perhaps a long period of time without any prospect of help, and this may aggravate their symptoms. The pressure changes occurring in the middle ear as a result of otitic barotrauma can have an impact on the fluid within the inner ear and it is occasionally reported that Ménière's sufferers may experience vertiginous symptoms whilst flying.

Whilst a perilymph fistula may well be iatrogenic (as with stapedectomy surgery), rupture of the oval or round window membrane can occur as a result of barotrauma (King 1979). This is more likely to happen in those travelling in military aircraft where pressure changes are more extreme than those encountered during commercial flights. Nevertheless, if a passenger were to develop sudden-onset rotatory vertigo, together with a perceived reduction in hearing in one ear, then a perilymph fistula should be suspected and on completion of the flight, a specialist opinion should be sought urgently.

Alternobaric vertigo is an unusual cause of vertigo during flight. The mechanism by which this occurs is not understood, but it is likely to be due to the effect of positive pressure within the middle ear on the inner ear via the oval and round windows. Any further increase in pressure caused by the Valsalva manoeuvre may aggravate the situation (Lundgren and Malm 1966, Tjernstrom 1974, Wicks 1989). The individual will experience a transient vertigo during either ascent or descent.

NOSE AND SINUSES

The nose and paranasal sinuses act together as an efficient air conditioner for the rest of the respiratory tract. Under normal circumstances, air inhaled through the nose will, by the time it reaches the larynx, have been humidified and warmed to within a remarkably constant level irrespective of the external humidity and temperature (Drake-Lee 1987). However, prolonged exposure to excessively dry air, as encountered during a long-haul aircraft flight, may lead to excessive drying and even crusting within the nasal cavity. Whilst this in itself is unlikely to create an acute problem, it may be a contributing factor if other conditions are present.

The paranasal sinuses are air-containing cavities within the facial skeleton – maxillary, ethmoid, frontal and sphenoid (Figure 16.3). The lining of these sinuses is an extension of the nasal mucosa, being a mucus producing ciliated respiratory epithelium. Close inspection of the anatomy of the lateral nasal wall will reveal the various ostia through which, under normal circumstances, air can travel between the nose and the paranasal sinuses, and through which the mucociliary clearance mechanism can clear mucus and any debris from within the sinuses (Figure 16.4).

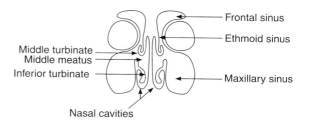

Figure 16.3 *Schematic drawing of paranasal sinuses.*

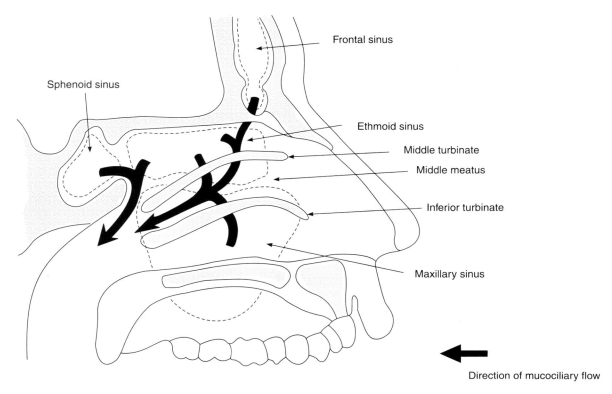

Frontal sinus

Sphenoid sinus

Ethmoid sinus

Middle turbinate

Middle meatus

Inferior turbinate

Maxillary sinus

Direction of mucociliary flow

Figure 16.4 *Lateral nasal wall with direction of mucociliary clearance.*

Sinus barotrauma

Sinus barotrauma, like otitic barotrauma, is due to an inability to equalize the pressure within some or all of the paranasal sinuses with the ambient air pressure. Again, like its otitic counterpart, the problems are encountered typically during descent of the aircraft. The frontal sinus is most commonly affected (O'Reilly 1999) and usually the individual will quickly become aware of discomfort with, at times, an excruciating sharp pain over the affected sinus. Epistaxis is a recognized accompaniment. During sinus barotrauma the sudden onset of negative pressure within the affected sinus results in submucosal haemorrhage, with shearing of the sinus mucosa from the bony wall (Weissmann *et al.* 1972). Often an upper respiratory infection predisposes to this condition and may affect individuals who hitherto have not had any sinus problems whilst flying. However, other factors may predispose on a more predictable basis to repeated episodes of sinus barotrauma, namely anatomical variations (deviated

nasal septum, enlarged middle turbinate), nasal polyps and chronic rhinosinusitis. The mechanism by which these factors cause sinus barotrauma is occlusion of the all-important middle meatus, which is the anatomical area under the middle turbinate into which the majority of the sinus ostia open.

It is difficult to predict those who may suffer from sinus barotrauma. A past history of nasal or sinus symptoms is, of course, relevant. More specifically, a history of nasal allergy, recurrent acute or chronic sinusitis, or nasal polyposis are all important. Examination of the nose may reveal an obvious problem such as a displaced nasal septum or nasal polyps. Close inspection of the nasal passage with a rigid endoscope may reveal more subtle evidence of sinus disease, such as small middle meatal polyps, infection or abnormal mucus streaming. Sinus x-rays are of little benefit in assessing the paranasal sinuses, but computed tomography (CT) scanning provides excellent images and can reveal variations of bony anatomy. It can also give an indication of the health of the nasal and sinus mucosa and so is an essential prerequisite to surgery. However, it is not a predictor of the likelihood of developing sinus barotrauma. More sophisticated investigations of nasal function such as mucociliary clearance tests and rhinomanometry, are unlikely to provide any further information.

Ideally, individuals with an upper respiratory infection should avoid flying to prevent barotrauma. If flying is unavoidable, then systemic or topical nasal decongestants may help to reduce nasal mucosal oedema and so prevent barotrauma. Individuals with the aforementioned nasal conditions, which might predispose to sinus barotrauma, are at a greater risk and consideration of surgical correction should be given. There is evidence that the surgical clearance of the middle meatus and the enlargement of the natural sinus ostia result in a reduced likelihood of subsequent sinus barotrauma (Parsons *et al.* 1987, O'Reilly *et al.* 1996). Similarly, correction of a deviated nasal septum and removal of nasal polyps are likely to be of benefit. Once sinus barotrauma is established, the immediate use of decongestants may be beneficial and, if symptoms persist after landing, their use should continue for up to 7 days together with antibiotics if there is evidence of an infection. Individuals in whom there is no obvious predisposition, but who, nevertheless, suffer from frequent sinus barotrauma, may be candidates for endoscopic sinus surgery if frequent flying is a necessity.

Nasal and sinus surgery

As with ear surgery, patients who have recently undergone nasal or sinus surgery are potentially at greater risk of barotrauma. Mucosal oedema, inevitable as a consequence of surgery, together with blood clots and crusting that may settle in the nose for some days after surgery, can result in the occlusion of the sinus ostia with resultant inability for pressure equalization. After nasal or sinus surgery, all patients should be reviewed by their specialist before undertaking a flight.

Epistaxis

Epistaxis is a common problem and, fortunately, usually mild. It can affect all ages but is seen more frequently in children and the elderly. Typically in children the bleeding arises from the anterior nasal septum (Little's area), where there is an arterial anastomosis. The trigger for bleeding may be a superficial infection or mild trauma caused by rubbing or picking. Often the bleeding, whilst frequent, is short lived. In the elderly, the bleeding may come from the anterior part of the nose, but it arises commonly further back and can occasionally be very heavy, even life threatening. Somebody with a history of repeated epistaxis, especially frequently, should seek advice prior to any flight. Simple nasal cautery is likely to be effective in many cases, but in children a topical antiseptic cream is often effective.

First aid measures may be necessary if an epistaxis occurs during flight. Fortunately, in the majority of occasions, the bleeding is likely to be from the anterior part of the nose and direct pressure can be applied by squeezing the soft cartilaginous portion firmly between finger and thumb. Whilst doing this the individual should be encouraged to sit upright, mouth open, with a bowl or receptacle under their chin (Trotter's manoeuvre). They should be instructed not to swallow any blood, but to spit it out into the bowl. This allows for the assessment of blood loss, and will reduce the likelihood of blood entering the stomach with irritation and vomiting. Ice packs applied to the forehead and bridge of the nose are still used frequently. Whilst their efficacy is as yet unproved, they may lead to reflex vasoconstriction, and, at the very least, soothe and calm a possibly distressed individual. The nose can, of course, be compressed for as long as is necessary, although if bleeding continues advice will have to be sought once the aircraft has landed.

THE THROAT

The relatively hostile atmosphere of the cabin during flight may give rise to minor symptoms referable to the larynx, although these are unlikely to cause any significant problems. However, there are certain circumstances where this may be relevant. Whilst early laryngeal cancer can be treated very effectively with radiotherapy, or even limited surgery, for more advanced tumours total laryngectomy may be performed. This has the immediate effect of disconnecting the lower from the upper respiratory tract and the individual will have an end stoma sited in the midline of the neck just above the sternal notch. Once the humidifying and warming functions of the nasal passages are removed, there is, in the early days after surgery, a tendency for quite significant crusting within the upper trachea. If this is left undisturbed, it can cause distressing and even life-threatening obstruction to the trachea and so requires careful monitoring. Good stoma care is vital, especially in the early days after surgery, and it is usual to wear a sponge bib applied loosely over the stoma. This can be moistened to provide for adequate humidification of inhaled air.

Under normal circumstances, an individual in this situation should seek advice from a department of laryngology where equipment is available for 'decrusting'. It is for this reason that flying when medical help may be unavailable is probably unwise in the early days after surgery. Fortunately, in most cases, after a matter of weeks, the tracheal mucosa has, to some extent, acclimatized to the new situation and there is little, if any, crusting. Nevertheless, a patient with a laryngectomy who is to undertake a prolonged flight should wear a humidifying bib to prevent excessive drying and crusting. Patient associations advise passengers to seek the advice of their consultant with respect to the first flight and, ideally, advise a short-haul flight first. The patient should wear a laryngectomy bib and keep it moist, and carry all medical supplies including spare bibs in hand luggage. In the unlikely event of cabin depressurization, the standard face masks supplied would be inappropriate for a laryngetomee. Some airlines carry stoma masks, so individuals should enquire before flying whether these are available.

Increasingly after total laryngectomy, vocal rehabilitation is achieved with the use of a variety of prostheses. These involve the surgical creation of a small communication between the upper trachea and the pharyngeal remnant, into which the prosthesis (a type of valve) is inserted. When a finger or a fixed one-way valve is placed over the prosthesis, air is forced from the trachea up into the pharyngeal remnant and thence into the mouth and excellent speech can be achieved. These prostheses may become dislodged, even inhaled, although if the latter occurs it is possible for it to be expelled with a sharp cough. Such is their size, they are unlikely to cause complete airway obstruction. Nevertheless, the event may induce considerable alarm and panic. An increased incidence of dysfunction of the Eustachian tube is seen after laryngectomy. Individuals must be made aware of this, bearing in mind that after surgery, manoeuvres such as Valsalva or Frenzell's are not possible.

CONCLUSION

The ears, nose and throat are potentially at risk during a flight, but fortunately the majority of symptoms are mild, and, with forethought and some simple precautions, these can often be avoided. In certain circumstances, particularly after any form of surgery, it is sensible for the potential passenger to seek advice from their specialist before undertaking a flight.

REFERENCES

Ashton DH and Watson LA. The use of tympanometry in predicting otitic barotrauma. *Aviat Space Environ Med* 1990; **61**: 56–61.

Davis AC. Epidemiology of hearing disorders. In Stephens D (ed.), *Scott-Brown's Otolaryngology*, 5th edn. London: Butterworths, 1987; **2**: 90–126.

Drake-Lee AB. Physiology of the nose and paranasal sinuses. In Wright D (ed.), *Scott-Brown's Otolaryngology*, 5th edn. London: Butterworths, 1987; **1**: 162–82.

Hern JD and Jonathan DA. Insertion of ventilating tubes – does the site matter? *Clin Otolaryngol* 1999; **24**: 424–5.

Jonathan DA, Chalmers P and Wong K. Comparison of sonotubometry with typanometry to assess eustachian tube function in adults. *Br J Audiol* 1986; **20**: 231–5.

Jones JS, Sheffield W, White LJ and Bloom MA. A double-blind comparison between oral pseudoephedrine and topical oxymetazoline in the prevention of barotrauma during air travel. *Am J Emerg Med* 1998; **16**: 262–4.

King PF. The Eustachian tube and its significance in flight. *J Laryngol Otol* 1979; **93**: 659–78.

Lundgren CEG and Malm LU. Alternobaric vertigo among pilots. *Aerosp Med* 1966; **37**: 178–80.

Moser M. Fitness of civil aviation passengers to fly after ear surgery. *Aviat Space Environ Med* 1990; **61**: 735–7.

O'Reilly BJ. Otorhinolaryngology. In Ernsting J, Nicholson AN and Rainford DJ (eds), *Aviation Medicine*. Oxford: Butterworth-Heinemann, 1999; 319–36.

O'Reilly BJ, Lupa H and McRae A. The application of endoscopic sinus surgery to the treatment of recurrent sinus barotrauma. *Clin Otolaryngol* 1996; **21**: 528–32.

Parsons DS, Chambers DW and Boyd EM. Long term follow up of aviators after functional endoscopic sinus surgery for sinus barotrauma. *Aviat Space Environ Med* 1987; **58**: 1029–34.

Stangerup SE, Tjernstrom O, Klokker M, Harcourt J and Stockholm J. Point prevalence of barotitis in children and adults after flight and effect of autoinflation. *Aviat Space Environ Med* 1998; **69**: 45–9.

Tjernstrom O. Further studies on alternobaric vertigo. Posture and passive equilibration of middle ear pressure. *Acta Otolaryngol* 1974; **78**: 221–31.

von Schoenberg M, Wengraf CL and Glesson M. Results of middle ear ventilation with Goode's tubes. *Clin Otolaryngol* 1989; **14**: 503–8.

Weissman B, Green RS and Roberts PT. Frontal sinus barotrauma. *Laryngoscope* 1972; **82**: 2160–8.

Wicks RE. Alternobaric vertigo: an aeromedical review. *Aviat Space Environ Med* 1989; **60**: 67–72.

17

Aviation dentistry

ANDREW J GIBBONS

High-altitude flying affects the orofacial system in a variety of ways due to changes in ambient pressure, oxygen inhalation and temperature. This can lead to in-flight dental problems, and the most painful of these is barodontalgia. Flying may also precipitate dysfunction of the temporomandibular joint, complications with the sockets of extracted teeth and difficulties with dentures. Even cases of vertigo have been reported at altitude due to dental pathology. However, for the airline passenger, most conditions can be prevented by good oral health and prompt treatment when problems arise, although the aeromedical transport of passengers with facial trauma poses a particular problem.

BARODONTALGIA

Barodontalgia is dental pain due to a change in barometric pressure and includes the pain felt in the teeth, but referred from elsewhere. The pain often comes on suddenly, though the intensity is unpredictable. When severe, it can lead to total incapacitation, and for pilots barodontalgia can be especially serious, leading to distraction from the task. The onset of pain occurs typically between altitudes of 5000 feet and 15 000 feet (Hodges 1978). In civil aircraft with the cabin altitude limited to 8000 feet, the incidence of barodontalgia is low. Nevertheless, with the variable standard of dental health in airline passengers, and with the large number of travellers,

many elderly, barodontalgia represents an important problem.

It was dental pain in military aircrew operating at high altitudes in unpressurized aircraft that stimulated research into barodontalgia. Lipson and Weiss (1942) speculated that aeroembolism, accelerations of flying manoeuvres and prolonged vasoconstriction due to extreme cold could all play a role in the genesis of the condition. It is true that aeroembolism could occur if the cabin pressure was suddenly lost. This could lead to air emboli in the capillaries of the pulpal or periodontal tissues, but aeromedical cases of dental aeroembolism have not been proven (Bengel 1980). Decreased temperature at high altitude was later found to be a negligible factor (Harvey 1943). Further, when air spaces are left deliberately under a restoration to ascertain whether air trapped beneath would expand and cause barodontalgia, no correlation was established on altitude testing (Rauch 1985). Nevertheless, the latter study, which concluded that pain was related to the proximity of the caries to pulpal tissue in restored teeth, supported the long established view that protective linings should be used more frequently under large restorations (Mitchell 1944).

Pathophysiology

The precise pathophysiology of barodontalgia remains unclear. The possibility that pulpal vessels dilating during decreases in pressure could be a cause of pain was put forward by Harvey (1947). The dilated vessel would exert an abnormal pressure on pulpal nerve tissue. It was also suggested that rotary instruments used for cutting cavities could cause pulpal hyperaemia. This results in teeth being susceptible to barodontalgia for a few days. The histological examination of teeth extracted from patients who have experienced pain under hypobaric conditions has shown a high incidence of extravascular vacuoles, indicating an impaired microcirculation and, therefore, pre-existing pathology (Orban and Ritchey 1945, Orban et al. 1946). From this it was hypothesized that the pathological basis of dental pain during decompression is a circulatory disturbance in the pulp which prevents the equalization of pulpal pressure. An expansion of vacuole gas and an increase in intrapulpal pressure cannot be dissipated by the unyielding surrounding dentine, but must be accommodated by the pulp itself, causing pain. Normal pulps without circulatory disturbance do not have vacuoles and can accommodate changes in pressure.

However, this theory has recently been called into question with the suggestion that the vacuoles were fixation artefacts (Kollmann 1993). An alternative hypothesis was proposed that reduced blood flow in inflamed pulps at altitude result in the discharge of impulses in the nerves, as occurs in other ischaemic tissues. In a survey of over 11 000 personnel exposed to an altitude of 43 000 feet, it was found that most cases of barodontalgia were actually due to an inflamed pulp (Kollmann 1993). This was also found in another series (Holowatyj 1996) and confirms that the majority of barodontalgia is due to pulpitis.

Much less frequently non-vital pulpal tissue, tooth abscesses and inadequate root fillings may cause barodontalgia. An investigation of dental pain during decompression found that a number of cases involved teeth with necrotic, gangrenous pulps (Joseph et al. 1943). Expansion and contraction of gases within the abscess or necrotic tissues may cause pressure on adjacent nerve endings. Air trapped in root fillings near to vital tissues may have similar effects (Levy 1943). Further, chronic periapical infection may become acute and painful on decompression (Coons 1943). Rarely, a periodontal abscess may be the cause of sudden acute pain on descent from altitude (Hodges 1978).

Maxillary sinusitis should always be included in the differential diagnosis of barodontalgia. Indeed, investigation of toothache under conditions simulating high-altitude flight have found approximately 10 per cent of symptoms are due to maxillary sinusitis (Orban and Ritchey 1945). Similarly, studies on barodontalgia in submariners have found that most had either congestion of the maxillary sinus or a dental problem, with pain associated with sinus trauma referred to the posterior maxillary teeth (Shiller 1965). The differential diagnosis of dental and sinus pain may prove difficult and the diagnosis may only be reached after treatment has proved successful (Senia et al. 1985). In general, barodontalgia on ascent is most likely due to pulpitis whereas on descent it is more likely to be due to maxillary sinusitis. Pain referred to the posterior mandibular teeth may arise when the pressure between the middle ear and the nasopharynx has not equalized due to closure of the Eustachian tube. Aero-otitis media may ensue.

Aetiology

From this literature review, there are three main causes of barodontalgia: first, pulpitis; second, periapical and periodontal pathology due to necrotic pulps, abscesses or cysts; and finally, maxillary sinusitis. Pulpitis is the most common form and occurs on ascent to cabin altitudes to over 5000 feet. The pain may be severe and is usually relieved by descent. The teeth have often been filled recently, with sound restorations that conceal an old exposure of the pulp. Histologically, the pulps show inflammatory changes, though these may be minimal. On the other hand, the pain from a necrotic pulp occurs mainly during descent and is dull and throbbing in nature. Periapical abscesses may cause persistent pain after ascent or descent, and pain may develop a few hours or days post-flight with an acute abscess. Expansion of air bubbles in the necrotic pulp or periapical/periodontal abscess and cysts is thought to cause pressure effects on adjacent nerve endings, generating pain. Otherwise, a quiescent infection within a necrotic pulp abscess may be stimulated by gaseous expansion during flying, leading to an acute infection. Finally, barodontalgia can be due to maxillary sinusitis and is a referred pain that affects the posterior maxillary teeth. The mucosa of the sinus swells on ascent and closes the ostium. On descent, pressures across the ostium do not equalize, leading to stimulation of nociceptors in the sinus mucosa. The pain is usually sudden in onset, dull, poorly localized and usually affects more than one tooth. Symptoms occur mostly on descent and postural changes, together with coughing and bending, exacerbate the pain. Paraesthesia related to the infra-orbital nerve may occur.

Most forms of subclinical dental pathology can become symptomatic at altitude (Kollmann 1993) and it may be the degree of change in pressure rather than the ambient pressure itself that precipitates the pain (Rauch 1985). Nevertheless, as the incidence of in-flight dental pain is low, it has to be concluded that, despite the many potential causes of barodontalgia, few passengers experience the condition. A diagnostic classification based on symptom aetiology, clinical examination and radiography was prepared by Ferjentsik and Aker (1982). Maxillary sinusitis with referred pain in the teeth was not included in this classification as it was ruled out by prior examination. Table 17.1 is a modified version which includes maxillary sinusitis.

Treatment

One of the first recorded treatments of acute barodontalgia was in 1937 when the pain which occurred at altitudes above 6000 feet was alleviated by a diagnostic pulpectomy (Dreyfus 1937). Nowadays, a careful history of the type, site, onset, duration and aggravating and relieving factors of the pain is taken. It must always be borne in mind that the majority of cases will be due to pulpitis and that this occurs most frequently on ascent, whilst, by contrast, sinus barotrauma occurs most frequently on descent. Pain from the pulp is poorly localized and the patient may only be able to indicate the side of the mouth affected rather than specify the tooth or even the jaw. All teeth on the affected side should be carefully inspected for evidence of caries or infection, and the vitality of each tooth tested, if possible, with an electric pulp tester. Detailed bite wing and periapical radiographs should also be taken. If no obvious dental cause for the pain is found, then replacement of the deep fillings with sedative, zinc oxide and eugenol dressings is required. If this does not alleviate the symptoms, or if a pulpal exposure is found in a suspected tooth, root canal treatment should be undertaken. Periapical pathology is treated by an initial root canal followed by apicectomy. If symptoms persist, extraction of symptomatic teeth is the final option. Direct pulp capping of exposed nerves with calcium hydroxide is not a satisfactory treatment for patients with barodontalgia. If barodontalgia persists despite treatment of suspected lesions, then a careful recording of the pain symptoms during simulated flight in a decompression chamber can help to localize the source of the pain.

PROBLEMS IN-FLIGHT

Astronauts do not take part in space missions for 90 days after dental restorative treatment. This is to prevent the risk of barodontalgia due to any hyperaemia or pulpal problems caused by the preparation of cavities within the teeth, but for the airline passenger recommendations are less restrictive. They should not fly on the same day after restorative procedures with a local anaesthetic. Air forced into extraction sockets after tooth removal has been suggested as a potential problem of cabin pressurization. In addition, changes in barometric pressure may precipitate secondary haemorrhage at the extraction site. Hence, passengers should not fly the same day of an extraction. However, recommendations concerning flying after a restorative procedure with a local anaesthetic or after an extraction are relative rather than absolute. Flying after intravenous sedation or general anaesthetic should be delayed for at least a couple of days.

Aeromedical evacuation of patients with maxillofacial trauma fixed with mini-plates is not uncommon. In this technique, the fracture is plated directly and the teeth are not wired together in intermaxillary fixation, allowing the airway to be free. However, when intermaxillary fixation has been carried out, it is important that the patient carries a pair of wire cutters and that the cabin crew are aware when to cut and where to cut the wires in the event of an emergency. Some airlines will not allow passengers to fly with intermaxillary fixation. The most serious life-threatening emergency is vomiting with inhalation of food debris occluding the airway. In this event, the patient should be sat upright and encouraged to lean forward. Most liquid foods taken in through wired teeth can be easily expelled, but releasing the fixation allows the airway to be cleared.

Table 17.1 *Modified classification of barodontalgia based on Ferjentsik and Aker (1982)*

Chief complaint	Clinical findings	Diagnosis	Treatment
Class I Sharp sometimes severe pain during ascent (decompression), being asymptomatic on descent (compression) and afterwards	Caries or restoration with inadequate lining in tooth. Tooth is vital. Radiograph shows no periapical pathosis	Acute pulpitis	Zinc oxide-eugenol temporary dressing followed in 2 weeks by a well-lined permanent restoration. Root canal therapy if pulp exposed or pain persists
Class II Dull throbbing pain during ascent (decompression), being asymptomatic on descent (compression) and afterwards	Deep caries or restoration in tooth. Tooth is vital/non-vital. Radiograph shows no periapical pathosis	Chronic pulpitis	Root canal therapy or extraction of unrestorable tooth
Class III Dull throbbing pain during descent (compression), being asymptomatic on ascent (decompression) and afterwards	Caries or restoration in tooth. Tooth is non-vital. Radiograph shows periapical pathosis	Necrotic pulp	Root canal therapy or extraction of unrestorable tooth
Class IV Severe persistent pain after ascent (decompression) or descent (compression)	Caries or restoration in tooth. Tooth is non-vital. Radiograph shows definite periapical pathosis	Periapical abscess or cyst	Root canal therapy with or without periapical surgery. Extraction of unrestorable tooth
Class V Dull pain in more than one maxillary posterior tooth on descent (compression), poorly localized and sudden onset	Teeth vital, no tooth pathology. Symptoms made worse by postural changes, coughing and bending. Pathology of antrum on occipitomental radiograph	Maxillary sinusitis	Referral to ENT surgeon for treatment of the cause of sinusitis

Fixation can be applied again after the flight. Some pain may be experienced during the descent due to the blockage of facial sinus openings with blood, but this is rare.

Temporomandibular joint dysfunction as a manifestation of decompression sickness has been reported in a military aviator (Fabian 1998), but this condition is unlikely to be encountered in an airline passenger because of the limited cabin altitude. It is due to microvascular thrombi causing pain and more commonly affects the large rather than the small joints. Treatment with oxygen can be useful. However, temporomandibular pain in-flight due to anxiety is a much more common problem. Increased masticatory muscle activity with clenching and teeth grinding can be a response to stress and may cause pain within the masticatory muscles or the joint itself. Other symptoms include trismus and joint clicking. Immediate treatment is to take a non-steroidal anti-inflammatory drug and apply heat to the tender muscles while resting the jaw. A soft diet should be taken for several days after an acute episode. If the pain is severe, a muscle relaxant, such as diazepam, in low doses may be useful. Long-term treatment involves physiotherapy, occlusal adjustment and bite-raising appliances, but rarely is surgery indicated.

Vertigo has also been associated with dental pathology. Small, locally asymptomatic lesions involving the sensitive tissues of the oral cavity may, on compression, produce barrages of impulses to the central nervous system. These impulses, via the extensive central ramifications of the trigeminal nerve, may lead to referred symptoms such as vertigo. The finding that treatment of the oral lesion in a particular case relieved the symptoms gives support to this conclusion (Eidelman 1981). However, vertigo due to oral pathology is extremely rare.

Rapid decompression has been found to cause trauma in teeth with restorations of inferior quality (Calder and Ramsey 1983), but the pressure changes necessary to cause such an effect are larger than those that would be encountered by an airline passenger. The differences in expansion between filling materials and the natural tooth with changes in barometric pressure are not a problem in teeth restored with fillings to a satisfactory standard. However, the cement strength of cast metal crowns can be compromised by repeated pressure variations, as in diving (Musajio *et al.* 1992). Whether such an effect could influence the teeth of an airline passenger is unlikely. Shattering of teeth during flying is most likely to be due to clenching or sudden biting with excessive pressure on teeth already weakened by large restorations. Finally, retention of complete upper dentures can be dependent on the atmospheric pressure, though the atmospheric pressure plays little part in the retention of lower dentures. Well-fitting dentures are unlikely to be affected by reduced atmospheric pressure, but poor fitting dentures may become loose.

CONCLUSION

Most in-flight dental problems are prevented by good oral health. The frequent airline passenger should undergo annual dental inspections and have bite-wing radiographs to assess interdental caries at least every 5 years. Sound restorations, well-fitting dentures and the adherence to not flying on the same day as a tooth extraction or a restorative procedure requiring local anaesthetic will prevent the majority, if not all, of in-flight dental problems.

REFERENCES

Bengel W. Aerodontalgia. *Quintessence Int* 1980; **10**: 93–7.

Calder IM and Ramsey JD. Ondontecrexis – the effects of rapid decompression on restored teeth. *J Dent* 1983; **11**: 318–23.

Coons DS. Aeronautical dentistry. *J Can Dent Assoc* 1943; **9**: 320–3.

Dreyfus H. Les dentes des aviateurs. *Odontologie* 1937; **7**: 612–13.

Eidelman D. Vertigo of dental origin: case reports. *Aviat Space Environ Med* 1981; **52**: 122–4.

Fabian BG. Case report: inflight decompression sickness affecting the temporomandibular joint. *Aviat Space Environ Med* 1998; **69**: 517–18.

Ferjentsik E and Aker F. Barodontalgia; a system of classification. *Milit Med* 1982; **147**: 302–4.

Harvey W. Tooth temperature with reference to dental pain while flying. *Br Dent J* 1943; **75**: 221–6.

Harvey W. Dental pain while flying during decompression tests. *Br Dent J* 1947; **82**: 113–18.

Hodges FR. Barodontalgia at 12,000 feet. *J Am Dent Assoc* 1978; **97**: 66–8.

Holowatyj RE. Barodontalgia among flyers: a review of seven cases. *J Can Dent Assoc* 1996; **62**: 578–84.

Joseph TV, Gill CF and Carr RM. Toothache and the aviator. *US Navy Med Bull* 1943; **41**: 643–5.

Kollmann W. Incidents and possible causes of dental pain during simulated high altitude flights. *J Endodont* 1993; **19**: 154–9.

Levy BM. Aviation dentistry. *Am J Orthodont* 1943; **29**: 92.

Lipson HJ and Weiss SG. Biological approach to problems in aviation dentistry. *J Am Dent Assoc* 1942; **29**: 1660.

Mitchell DI. Aerodontalgia. *US Army Med Bull* 1944; **73**: 63–7.

Musajio F, Passi P, Girardello BG and Rusca F. The influence of environmental pressure on retentiveness of prosthetic crowns: an experimental study. *Quintessence Int* 1992; **23**: 367–9.

Orban B and Ritchey BT. Toothache under conditions simulating high altitude flight. *J Am Dent Assoc* 1945; **32**: 145–7.

Orban B, Ritchey BT and Zander HA. Experimental study of pulp changes produced in a decompression chamber. *J Dent Res* 1946; **25**: 299–302.

Rauch JW. Barodontalgia – dental pain related to ambient pressure change. *Gen Dent* 1985; **33**: 313–15.

Senia ES, Cunningham KW and Marx RE. The diagnostic dilemma of barodontalgia. *Oral Surg Oral Med Oral Pathol* 1985; **60**: 212–17.

Shiller WR. Aerodontalgia under hyperbaric conditions – an analysis of forty-five case histories. *Oral Surg Oral Med Oral Pathol* 1965; **20**: 694–7.

18

Gastroenterology

DEVINDER S BANSI, BOB GROVER AND ANDREW V THILLAINAYAGAM

Gastrointestinal diseases are a major cause of ill health throughout the world. Acute and chronic disorders are extremely prevalent in developing and developed nations. For example, in excess of one billion people are infested with hookworms and roundworms, and such infestations represent the commonest cause of iron deficiency anaemia. One in ten of the world's population is afflicted by amoebiasis. More than 10 per cent of all consultations in primary care may be for gastrointestinal complaints. Furthermore, the burden of such disorders in the population is set to increase. Some diseases, such as peptic ulcer, are in decline, whereas others, such as gastro-oesophageal reflux, are rising in frequency. Diseases of the gastrointestinal tract afflict all age groups, and so, with ever-increasing international air travel, problems are likely to be of growing relevance to airline passengers.

IN-FLIGHT EMERGENCIES

Clearly, the possibility exists for an acute in-flight emergency to affect any airline passenger and it will require immediate management, but it should be borne in mind that there are numerous chronic diseases which, provided they remain stable, should not preclude safe airline travel. Obviously, those with severe and rapidly progressive disease, or those with conditions at high risk of acute relapse, should be discouraged from flying. This chapter deals with in-flight emergencies, acute gastrointestinal problems and their implications for air travel, and air travel after gastrointestinal surgery. The transfer of the acutely ill patient by air ambulance is dealt with elsewhere.

Ingestion of a foreign body

The ingestion of a foreign body should be suspected, particularly in toddlers and in the mentally impaired, when the passenger presents with choking, pain and distress. It is important to try to ascertain the nature of the foreign body. Sharp objects, such as broken glass, fish or chicken bones, are likely to cause oesophageal trauma or even a perforation. The passage of blunt objects, for example, small plastic toys, may be assisted by drinking fluids or small pieces of soaked bread. If the episode settles with conservative management, location of the foreign body by radiographic studies on arrival at the flight destination is useful. Ingested batteries that may be within the oesophagus or stomach should be considered for endoscopic removal as soon as possible. They carry the risk of caustic damage. Complete inability to swallow may occur after either ingestion of a foreign body or a large food bolus (e.g. large piece of meat). It is important to establish whether this has happened on a previous occasion, as a passenger with known oesophageal disease, such as strictures or cancer, may suffer from this intermittently. If the bolus does not pass with conservative measures, endoscopic removal with or without dilatation will be necessary on arrival. Until then, the passenger should be given nothing by mouth.

Oesophageal rupture

An oesophageal rupture should be suspected with a sudden onset of severe chest pain, especially after recurrent vomiting or ingestion of a sharp foreign body. Clinical signs include tachycardia, tachypnoea, cyanosis and surgical emphysema. This is a life-threatening condition and requires urgent specialist hospital assessment, preferably at a hospital with a cardiothoracic unit. The initial in-flight management includes strong analgesia (e.g. morphine) and intravenous fluids, but nothing should be given by mouth. The differential diagnosis includes acute myocardial infarction, unstable angina, dissecting thoracic aortic aneurysm, pneumothorax and perforated peptic ulcer. These are all emergencies requiring urgent hospital management and are dealt with elsewhere in the text.

Chest pain

The differential diagnosis of chest pain is wide and proves challenging to the hospital physician even with the benefit of an armoury of diagnostic tools. The cardiac and respiratory causes are discussed in other chapters. Once these have been excluded, or if the history is more suggestive of pain of oesophageal origin (oesophageal reflux), a therapeutic trial of antacid is worthwhile. Alternatively, the chest pain may be due to oesophageal spasm precipitated by anxiety or stress. In this scenario, sublingual glyceryl trinitrate may be beneficial, although cardiac chest pain will also respond favourably. If, however, there is any disturbance in cardiorespiratory status, evidence of vomiting blood or coffee grounds, passage of blood or black stool, or, indeed, if the pain is severe and not relieved with conservative measures, an alternative diagnosis should be sought.

ACUTE GASTROINTESTINAL BLEEDING

Upper gastrointestinal bleeding is the reason for many hospital admissions, and despite sophisticated therapeutic equipment and drug therapy, the mortality remains at 5–15 per cent for those under 60 and over 20 per cent for those over 80 years old (Rockall *et al.* 1996). It is defined as bleeding from above the ligament of Treitz, which is the junction between the third and fourth part of the duodenum. Bleeding from the upper gastrointestinal tract is manifest classically by vomiting of fresh blood or 'coffee-ground vomitus', which may or may not be associated with abdominal pain or passage of a black, tarry stool (melaena). A history of peptic ulcers, use of aspirin (or other non-steroidal anti-inflammatory drugs), oesophageal varices or chronic liver disease may suggest the diagnosis, but is not conclusive. Upper gastrointestinal bleeding is caused by chronic gastric or duodenal ulcers in 50 per cent, acute gastric ulcers in 20 per cent, Mallory–Weiss tear in 5–10 per cent (a mucosal tear at the gastro-oesophageal junction due to forceful vomiting, not uncommonly secondary to alcohol intoxication), oesophageal varices 5–10 per cent (dilated veins at the lower end of the oesophagus, most commonly in patients with chronic liver disease) and reflux oesophagitis in 5–10 per cent (Laine and Peterson 1994, Longstreth 1995).

The passage of either fresh red or altered blood *per rectum*, which may be associated with abdominal pain, is diagnostic of bleeding from the colon. Massive bleeding from the lower gastrointestinal tract causing significant haemodynamic disturbance is uncommon. Careful attention to the patient's symptoms and past medical history will often suggest the most likely source of bleeding. Torrential bleeding is usually secondary to diverticular disease/diverticulitis, ischaemic colitis or colorectal carcinoma. However, people with known inflammatory bowel disease may also suffer from rectal bleeding often associated with loose stools in the context of a flare-up of their disease. Haemorrhoids are a very common cause of fresh rectal bleeding and often the patient will be well aware of their presence. Colorectal polyps rarely cause overt bleeding sufficient to compromise the cardiovascular system. Rare conditions such as angiodysplasia may cause significant blood loss, but are not routinely encountered.

Major bleeding from the gastrointestinal tract requires intravenous fluid resuscitation with colloid, if available, together with regular monitoring of pulse, blood pressure and temperature. Nothing should be given by mouth, and urgent hospital investigation is necessary. The patient should be laid flat in the recovery position to minimize the risk of aspiration and to optimize cardiovascular performance. Serious consideration should be given to the diversion of an aircraft if a suitable medical facility can be ensured.

TRAVELLERS' DIARRHOEA

Travellers' diarrhoea is a significant cause of morbidity and may debilitate the airline passenger either pre- or post-flight (Thillainayagam 1998, von Sonnenburg *et al.* 2000). It may affect up to two-thirds of visitors to high-risk tourist destinations. *Escherichia coli* is a common cause of travellers' diarrhoea. There is usually a history over the preceding 12–48 hours of ingestion of beef or unpasteurized milk, giving rise to acute watery diarrhoea, which rarely may be bloody. Treatment is supportive, as the infection is usually self-limiting, although this may take 10–14 days. For severe infections, ciprofloxacin may be given orally. *Shigella* infections (bacillary dysentery) are transmitted by the faeco-oral route with an incubation period of 2–7 days. They may be contracted from any food, but are classically found in areas with poor sanitation and overcrowding. Victims suffer acute watery diarrhoea, fever and cramping abdominal pain.

Salmonella infections associated with acute diarrhoeal illnesses are transmitted via contaminated meat, eggs and poultry. They have an incubation period of 12–48 hours and are prevalent world wide. These strains of salmonella may present with vomiting, fever, headache and malaise. The clinical course is often limited to 5 days. Treatment is supportive and rarely requires antimicrobial therapy. *Rotavirus* is an important cause of diarrhoea in children. The incidence rises during the winter and the virus is prevalent in both developed and developing countries. Rotavirus rarely causes significant symptoms in adults. Treatment is supportive. *Campylobacter* is a well-recognized cause of bloody diarrhoea both in the returning traveller and in patients with no recent history of foreign travel. There is usually a preceding 2–5-day history of chicken or milk ingestion. The bloody diarrhoea is associated with fever, malaise, headache and abdominal cramping. The illness has usually resolved within 7 days, but severe infections may be treated with ciprofloxacin or erythromycin.

Giardiasis is an important cause of diarrhoea in the traveller returning from Russia and certain parts of Europe. The flagellated organism is water-borne and has an incubation period of 1–4 weeks. After laboratory isolation of the organism in stool, treatment is with high dose oral metronidazole. *Amoebiasis* is a protozoal infection of the bowel that is most common in the tropics. The incubation period is highly variable from days to several months. The clinical syndrome varies from asymptomatic to severe acute dysentery or haemorrhagic colitis. The usual mode of transmission is by consumption of contaminated water or food or, less commonly, by direct person-to-person contact. Atypical organisms are more prevalent in the immunocompromised such as those with HIV or patients on immunosuppressive drug therapy. Causes of bloody diarrhoea include rectal gonorrhoea, primary anorectal syphilis and herpes simplex infection. Parasites such as *Cryptosporidium* and *Strongyloides stercoralis*, and mycobacterial organisms such as *Mycobacterium avium-intracellulare* and *Mycobacterium tuberculosis* need to be considered in non-bloody diarrhoea.

Diarrhoeal symptoms may be present either in isolation or combination with other abdominal symptoms, and, indeed, may be associated with any cause of an acute abdomen. However, in the context of probable food poisoning (gastroenteritis), this can usually be managed with either oral or, if not tolerated, intravenous fluid rehydration. It is important to make an assessment of the degree of dehydration. Dry skin and mucous membranes suggest mild (<5 per cent) dehydration which represents a 2 litre fluid deficit. Moderate dehydration (5–8 per cent) with a 4-litre deficit is suggested by cool peripheries, decreased skin turgor and tachycardia. Sunken eyes, postural hypotension and a urine output of less than 400 ml per 24 hours are compatible with severe dehydration of over 6 litres.

Absorption of sodium and water by the gut is enhanced by carbohydrates such as glucose. The World Health Organization oral rehydration solution to replace fluid and electrolyte loss due to diarrhoea contains 3.5 g sodium chloride, 1.5 g potassium citrate, 2.9 g sodium citrate and 20 g anhydrous glucose, to be dissolved in 1 litre of water. However, there is a wide variety of oral rehydration formulations available. The general recommendation for adults is to drink 200–400 ml after each loose motion. Rehydration should be started as soon as possible after the onset of diarrhoea to prevent symptomatic dehydration. Antiemetics and antidiarrhoeal agents are also useful.

ACUTE ABDOMINAL PAIN

The causes of acute abdominal pain are legion and it usually requires specialist assessment with blood tests and diagnostic imaging. The history and physical signs will usually give clues as to the possible aetiology. Pain in the right upper quadrant is often hepatobiliary in origin. Clues in the history would include previous gallstone disease. Episodic cramping or constant pain, which may be associated with fevers, could be secondary to biliary colic or acute cholecystitis. If these symptoms are associated with jaundice, the diagnosis of ascending cholangitis (bile duct infection) must be entertained. This condition carries a significant morbidity and mortality, requiring prompt diagnosis, intravenous fluids and antibiotics.

Epigastric or central abdominal pain that is burning or sharp in nature may be due to a perforated peptic ulcer. This should be suspected in patients with a history of peptic ulcer disease or use of aspirin (or other non-steroidal anti-inflammatory drugs). If the pain 'bores through' to the back, then acute pancreatitis is a likely diagnosis. This is more likely with a history of chronic pancreatitis, particularly after an alcohol binge. Episodic pain in either flank or pain radiating to the groin may be secondary to renal colic. This is an exquisitely painful condition, and should be considered in patients with known renal stone disease. This condition may be associated with the passing of blood *per urethra*.

Left-sided lower abdominal pain associated with fevers and often the passage of blood *per rectum* is usually due to diverticulitis. Diverticulosis is the presence of outpouchings of the wall of the gut. This is a very common condition in the developed world, and one-third of those over the age of 60 has diverticulosis. This condition can be treated with bed rest, nothing by mouth, intravenous fluids and antibiotics when the aircraft lands at its intended destination. Central abdominal pain moving to the right lower quadrant associated with fevers, is usually due to appendicitis. This is more common in the younger age group. Lower abdominal pain below or lateral to the umbilicus, often associated with a history of vaginal discharge or previous gynaecological problems or instrumentation suggests pelvic inflammatory disease, salpingitis, or ectopic pregnancy. These conditions are discussed elsewhere in this text. Diffuse abdominal pain with a rigid abdomen and fever is due to peritonitis until proven otherwise. This is usually due to a perforated abdominal viscus, such as peptic ulcer, gall bladder, bowel or appendix, and requires prompt assessment.

Abdominal pain that radiates to the back should raise suspicion of an aortic aneurysm. This is an abnormal dilatation of the major artery of the body. Leakage and subsequent rupture is usually catastrophic. There may be an expansile mass in the abdomen and if there is associated bruising in the flanks or cardiovascular compromise, the situation is dire, requiring urgent fluid resuscitation and surgical intervention. All these conditions are difficult to distinguish whilst air-borne without specialist expertise and diagnostic equipment. The initial management consists of strong analgesia and intravenous fluids with regular monitoring of cardiovascular status. The patient should not be allowed to take anything by mouth. Urgent specialist assessment and treatment are necessary and diversion of the aircraft to a suitable facility must be considered.

IMPLICATIONS FOR AIR TRAVEL

Many gastrointestinal disorders, if treated and stable, should not preclude air travel. Gastro-oesophageal reflux disease or a history of peptic ulcer disease where the patient is symptomatically stable, on or off appropriate treatment, is of no consequence to air travel. Oesophageal cancer, provided the patient is clinically stable, should cause no added concern. However, it is wise for the patient to be fully informed regarding the position, length and severity of any stricture should they run into problems whilst away from their home. Coeliac disease is also of no concern, though it is necessary to ensure the availability of gluten-free products at an overseas destination. As far as gastrointestinal lymphoma is concerned, there should be no contraindication to travel provided that the traveller is clinically stable without obstructive symptoms. Gallstones have a prevalence of 9 per cent in those over 60 years old. Their presence *per se* is not a preclusion to air travel. Stable chronic pancreatitis is unlikely to be exacerbated by air travel, though the traveller should remember that excessive alcohol consumption may trigger an acute episode.

Hepatobiliary carcinomatous conditions such as pancreatic cancer, cholangiocarcinoma and hepatocellular carcinoma are not in themselves contraindications to travel. The decision to fly is dependent upon the general condition of the patient and the stage of the cancer. The degree of jaundice and cachexia will influence the decision, which should be made by discussion between the patient and the physician. Patients with chronic autoimmune liver disease should be safe to fly, but like any other patient they may decompensate and this could occur in-flight. If these patients have an upper gastrointestinal bleed, this may be secondary to a combination of variceal haemorrhage and clotting abnormality. A recent gastrointestinal haemorrhage should pose no particular problem provided there was an endoscopic assessment and treatment at the time of the bleed, and that the 5-day post-rebleeding window has been passed and they are stable from a cardiovascular point of view.

Recent acute cholecystitis, cholangitis or acute pancreatitis are not absolute contraindications to travel once the patient is over the acute episode. However, if the event was related to gallstones, the patient should ideally have a cholecystectomy pre-flight to prevent a recurrence. Recent relapse of inflammatory bowel disease, attack of infectious gastroenteritis, recent acute hepatitis or acute liver failure have no particular in-flight restrictions once over the acute episode. However, patients should be encouraged to carry their medicines and details of their current treatment.

SAFE AIR TRAVEL AFTER GASTROINTESTINAL SURGERY

Concerns may be expressed by patients, or, indeed, relatives of those hoping to embark upon overseas airplane travel, who have recently undergone gastrointestinal surgery. A number of areas are worthy of mention. Patients who have undergone either a major colonic or gastric resection should not travel for 10–14 days post-operatively or until they are able to travel comfortably with a significant wound. Those who have undergone either an oesophageal resection or antireflux surgery could travel after 10–14 days, but a thoracotomy with the possibility of air remaining in the pleural cavity requires special consideration and guidance should be sought from a respiratory physician. Patients who have had an oversew of a perforated peptic ulcer should not travel before 10 days, due to the risk of rebleeding. Minor surgery such as an appendicectomy or laparoscopic cholecystectomy should pose no travel problems after one week. The more common complications that occur after an endoscopic retrograde cholangiopancreatogram usually occur within the first 72 hours. Only in exceptional cases should there be a problem with air travel.

As far as hepato-pancreatico-biliary surgery is concerned advice should be sought from the surgical team involved. Liver transplantation may raise questions with respect to suitable expertise at the intended destination. The patient may need regular expert review to detect organ rejection, and logistically there may be problems related to supplies and monitoring of immunosuppression. Such issues should be discussed with the transplant team. There is no contraindication for patients fed enterally via a tube to undertake air travel, but it must be borne in mind that if the tube becomes displaced it may require revision or replacement. Patients with cancer who have undergone major surgery are at increased risk of thromboembolic complications. Indeed, all such patients are at risk of a deep vein thrombosis, and should seek advice with respect to prophylactic measures prior to a long flight.

PATIENTS WITH STOMAS

Patients with stomas are a special group, not least because of the potential difficulties arising from immobility, dehydration, changing cabin pressures and cramped and often unsuitable lavatory facilities. Gas in the gastrointestinal tract expands at the cabin altitude, and this may cause embarrassment because of noise and odour. Eggs, onions and spicy foods, as well as fizzy drinks, are best avoided. Frequent emptying of the stoma bag may help, as might the attachment of a 'flatus filter' device to the stoma prior to departure. Patients with an ileostomy may dehydrate rapidly due to excessive output and so adequate fluid intake is important. Dietary restrictions to reduce effluent and anti-diarrhoeal medication prior to departure or on the flight may be advisable. Abstention from alcohol will reduce the possibility of dehydration.

Patients should take ample supplies of stoma equipment and any prescribed medication and ensure that some is in their hand luggage just in case the main luggage goes astray. It may also be helpful to obtain the contact details of an overseas appliance supplier before departure. Some devices may contain metal attachments and ground staff will need to be notified with respect to metal detector security checks. The stoma bag should be changed just prior to departure and, if possible, an aisle seat close to the lavatory should be chosen. Some airlines will provide additional baggage allowance for any extra medical equipment that is needed. Adequate and appropriate travel insurance is advised, and patient associations can provide a travel certificate in case of any problem. Some patients may require anti-diarrhoeal medication such as codeine, which may be restricted in some countries.

REFERENCES

Laine L and Peterson WL. Bleeding peptic ulcer. *N Engl J Med* 1994; **331**: 717–27.

Longstreth GF. Epidemiology of hospitalization for acute upper gastrointestinal haemorrhage: a population based study. *Am J Gastroenterol* 1995; **90**: 206–10.

Rockall TA, Logan RF, Devlin HB and Northfield TC. Selection of patients for early discharge or outpatient care after acute gastrointestinal haemorrhage: national audit of acute upper gastrointestinal haemorrhage. *Lancet* 1996; **347**: 1138–40.

von Sonnenburg F, Tornieporth N, Waiyaki P *et al*. Risk and aetiology of diarrhoea at various tourist destinations. *Lancet* 2000; **356**: 133–4.

Thillainayagam A. Diarrhoea. *Medicine* 1998; **26**: 57–64.

FURTHER READING

Feldman M, Scharschmidt BF and Sleisenger MH. *Sleisenger and Fordran's Gastrointestinal and Liver Disease*, 6th edn. Edinburgh: WB Saunders, 1997.

Kumar P and Clark M. *Clinical Medicine*, 4th edn. Edinburgh: WB Saunders, 1998.

19

Renal medicine

PAUL E STEVENS

Although less common than cancer or cardiovascular disease, more than 100 diseases affect the kidneys. The point prevalence of chronic renal failure (defined as a serum creatinine level (≥ 150 μmol l^{-1})), is at least 2000 adults per million population. The increased availability of international air travel, together with a more enlightened attitude of doctors towards patients with renal disease undertaking air travel, requires an understanding of the potential problems such patients may encounter. The same general principles apply to patients with renal disease as with any other. Those with rapidly evolving disease processes should be discouraged from travelling unless treatment facilities are available in-flight, for example, the aeromedical evacuation of a patient with acute renal failure. Conversely, some patients with what may appear to be quite alarming blood biochemistry may readily undertake a journey provided they have chronic, stable disease.

HAEMATURIA AND PROTEINURIA

Haematuria is a sign of underlying disease; it may be macroscopic or microscopic, transient or persistent. Although the most common causes are infection or inflammation of the prostate or bladder, other causes include renal stones, malignancy, and glomerular disease. Haematuria occurring in association with proteinuria (>500 mg d^{-1}) is indicative of glomerular bleeding. Isolated proteinuria may be transient, orthostatic, or persistent. Transient proteinuria is by far the commonest, occurring in 4 per cent of men and 7 per cent of women on a single reagent strip examination with subsequent disappearance on repeat testing (Robinson 1980). Orthostatic proteinuria usually occurs in adolescents and is characterized by increased proteinuria in the upright position, but a normal protein excretion in the supine position. Persistent proteinuria is a sign of underlying disease and may be glomerular, tubular, or 'overflow' in origin. Tubular proteinuria is not detected by the reagent strip test, which primarily detects albumin. Neither does the reagent strip detect light chains (the usual cause for overflow proteinuria).

When haematuria and/or proteinuria are discovered just prior to travel, there are a number of key questions to be answered (Table 19.1). The answers to these questions will determine whether or not it is advisable to continue with the planned journey, and whether investigation and treatment are required prior to embarkation. The distinction between glomerular and non-glomerular urinary tract bleeding will determine the direction of future investigation, nephrological or urological. The

Table 19.1 *Key questions in the evaluation of haematuria and proteinuria*

- Is there a history of other disease such as diabetes, congestive cardiac failure, or a history of previous renal disease?
- Is there a family history of renal disease?
- What medications is the patient taking?
- Are there associated symptoms and signs of other organ involvement suggesting a multisystem disorder, or are symptoms and signs confined to the urinary tract?
- Is the haematuria macroscopic or microscopic?
- Is the haematuria glomerular or extraglomerular?
- Is the haematuria or proteinuria isolated?
- What kind of protein is present?
- How much protein is present?
- Is the underlying renal function normal or abnormal?
- Is the underlying disease process acute or chronic?

degree of haematuria (macroscopic or microscopic) may be unhelpful in making this distinction, although macroscopic glomerular bleeding may present a 'coca-cola' or smokey-brown coloured urine, and clots are not normally present in glomerular bleeding. Urine microscopy may reveal dysmorphic red cells and the presence of red cell casts, indicating glomerular bleeding.

Both transient and orthostatic proteinuria are benign and of no consequence for airline travel. Isolated glomerular microscopic haematuria in a normotensive patient with normal renal function is also likely to be benign. Proteinuria in association with nephrotic syndrome is considered separately below. Provided renal function is either normal or stable and there is no acute phase response, all other levels of glomerular proteinuria, either isolated or in association with microscopic haematuria, do not contraindicate travel and no special precautions are necessary. Acute-phase response may be simply assessed by measurement of C-reactive protein or plasma viscosity. Patients with haematuria and/or proteinuria who have abnormal renal function, macroscopic glomerular haematuria, or proteinuria >3 g d^{-1} require further evaluation with total protein and albumin estimation, full blood count, blood and urine electrophoresis, measurement of acute-phase response, renal ultrasound, and referral for a nephrology opinion. They should be discouraged from travel until adequately assessed.

NEPHROTIC SYNDROME

Nephrotic syndrome is characterized by peripheral oedema, hypoalbuminaemia (<30 g dl^{-1}), heavy proteinuria (albuminuria ≥ 3 g per 24 h), and by hypercholesterolaemia. There may be associated renal insufficiency, which can be acute or chronic, depending on the underlying disease process. Nephrotic syndrome may occur in association with systemic disease, such as diabetes mellitus or systemic lupus erythematosus, or may be due to primary renal disease. In children, minimal change glomerulonephritis remains the commonest cause. In adults, a recent study found that 35 per cent of cases was due to focal glomerulosclerosis, 33 per cent due to membranous glomerulonephritis, and 15 per cent due to minimal change glomerulonephritis (Haas *et al.* 1997). Other causes include IgA glomerulonephritis, membranoproliferative glomerulonephritis, post-infectious glomerulonephritis and amyloidosis. Although albumin is the principal protein lost in the urine, other proteins such as clotting inhibitors, transferrin, and hormone-binding proteins may be lost as well, with important consequences in terms of complications and manifestations (Table 19.2). The most relevant to aviation medicine are oedema and thromboembolic disease.

All patients with nephrotic syndrome who have not been properly assessed should be discouraged from travel. After assessment and diagnosis, all patients will require treatment directed against the manifestations and complications of nephrotic syndrome, together with specific treatment directed against the underlying cause in a number of cases. In the early stages, there is a requirement for close monitoring with both clinical and laboratory assessments and it follows that travel is contraindicated until a degree of stability has been attained.

One of the problems with the treatment of oedema in nephrotic syndrome is that oedema may be associ-

Table 19.2 *Complications and manifestations of nephrotic syndrome*

- Hypovolaemia
- Acute renal failure
- Protein malnutrition
- Infection
- Endocrine dysfunction

ated with an elevated circulating blood volume, or circulating blood volume may be diminished – so-called 'underfill' oedema. The latter group usually have a glomerular filtration rate of at least 75 per cent of normal and are more likely to have had acute onset of nephrotic syndrome or severe hypoalbuminaemia (Vande Wall *et al.* 1995), but this is by no means proscriptive. The degree of oedema can be massive; the last patient to present to our unit with nephrotic syndrome still retained evidence of mild peripheral oedema despite losing 41 kg fluid weight during treatment. Treatment comprises that of the underlying condition, which generally involves high-dose steroids and treatment directed towards resolution of oedema.

The majority of patients will have an elevated circulating blood volume and these patients respond well to loop diuretics. Usually the excess fluid can be removed without inducing blood volume depletion (Geers *et al.* 1985). Some patients may be resistant to loop diuretics, requiring higher doses and the addition of a thiazide diuretic such as metolazone. In markedly hypoalbuminaemic patients (<20 g dl^{-1}) intravenous frusemide given together with salt-poor albumin infusions may be required during the early stages. Once patients begin to respond to treatment, the diuresis may be dramatic. The patient referred to above lost 18 kg fluid over a weekend and illustrates both the importance of close monitoring and of deferring travel plans until the clinical situation is stable.

Thromboembolism

The risk of thromboembolism from air travel has recently received considerable interest both in the press and the scientific literature. Thromboembolism is also an important complication of nephrotic syndrome with an increased incidence of both arterial and venous thrombosis, especially deep vein thrombosis and renal vein thrombosis. It has been suggested that even asymptomatic patients have evidence of ongoing coagulation (Chen *et al.* 1993) and this is therefore an important consideration in pre-flight preparation. Renal vein thrombosis is most common in the nephrotic syndrome due to membranous glomerulonephritis. It may be unilateral or bilateral and may extend into the inferior vena cava. Acute renal vein thrombosis presents with loin pain, haematuria, increased proteinuria, and deterioration in renal function, together with an increase in renal size on ultrasound scanning. More usually the onset is insidious, producing little in the way of symptoms referable to the kidney, and patients may present with pulmonary embolism. Where thrombosis occurs, patients should be anticoagulated and remain on anticoagulants until the nephrotic syndrome is in remission. There are no randomized controlled trials of prophylactic anticoagulation in nephrotic syndrome. Our practice is to consider prophylactic anticoagulation in patients with severe hypoalbuminaemia (<20 g dl^{-1}), and in those with additional risk factors such as a history of deep venous thrombosis. Unless the patient is in remission prior to flight, air travel should be considered to be a risk factor.

Patients should be warned prior to travel to expect a certain amount of increased leg oedema and reassured that this will resolve post-flight and does not represent relapse of the nephrotic syndrome. Normal subjects studied during simulated 12-hour long-distance flights were shown to retain an average of 1150 ml fluid, which corresponded to the simultaneous swelling of the lower legs (Landgraf *et al.* 1994). All patients should be advised to stand up frequently during flight and to perform leg-stretching exercises. Those not taking prophylactic anticoagulation, and patients with remaining oedema, should consider compression stockings. Non-steroidal anti-inflammatory drugs should be avoided in nephrotic syndrome, especially for patients with minimal change disease (Whelton 1995), and if antiplatelet agents are required, other drugs such as clopidogrel may be considered.

RENAL STONE DISEASE

Renal stone disease is common; in industrialized societies stone disease accounts for between 7 and 10 of every 1000 hospital admissions (Kreutzer and Folkert 1993). The precise incidence varies with the population studied, but rates of stone disease are higher in men and increase with age in all populations. Patients may be asymptomatic or present with classical symptoms of renal colic radiating to the groin and haematuria. Atypical symptoms include non-specific abdominal pain, penile and testicular pain, and dysuria. Calcium-based stones occur in 80 per cent of cases; other types include uric acid, struvite and cystine stones. Stone formation occurs when the normally soluble constituents of the stone supersaturate the urine and begin to crystallize out of solution. The crystals aggregate and become anchored (normally at the end of the collecting ducts) and then subsequently slowly increase in size. There is a hereditary element to stone disease; those with a family history of stone disease are said to have a relative risk 2.57 times greater than the general population (Curhan *et al.* 1997). A past history of calcium-based stone disease confers the highest risk of future stone formation, the estimated risk being 14 per cent at 1 year, 35 per cent at 5 years, and 52 per cent after 10 years (Uribarri *et al.* 1989). The major risk factors for the formation of calcium-based stones are shown in Table 19.3.

The main consideration for the airline passenger presenting with renal stone disease is whether or not the stone, or stones, have passed through the urinary tract. It is reasonable to assume that asymptomatic stones found within the kidney on a routine radiological examination are unlikely to cause a problem. In a study of 107 patients with asymptomatic stone disease followed up for a mean of 31.6 months, 73 patients remained asymptomatic (Patel and Fuchs 1998). Of the remainder, 16 passed a stone without intervention, 9 received extracorporeal shock wave lithotripsy (ESWL), 6 underwent endo-ureteral removal, and 3 had percutaneous nephrolithotomy (PCNL). More usually, stones are found following investigation of blood in the urine or sudden onset of pain. If a stone lies within the urinary tract, its size and

Table 19.3 *Main risk factors for calcium-based stones*

Previous calcium-based stone episode
Family history of stone disease
• Increased promoters of stone formation
• Low fluid intake and low urine volume
• Hypercalciuria
• Hyperoxaluria (due to high dietary intake of oxalate or low dietary calcium intake)
• Enteric hyperoxaluria
• Hyperuricosuria
• 'Junk food' diet (rich in protein and sodium)
Reduced inhibitors of stone formation
• Hypocitraturia
• Hypomagnesuria
Medullary sponge kidney
Hyperparathyroidism
Type I renal tubular acidosis
Sarcoidosis
Primary hyperoxaluria

anatomical position will determine whether or not the stone is likely to cause problems during the journey. Stones less than 5 mm in diameter that have passed into the ureter will generally pass within a few days given adequate hydration and pain relief. Stones between 5 and 9 mm may also pass without intervention but larger stones rarely pass spontaneously. After symptoms abate, further radiological investigation should be undertaken to ensure complete passage of the stone, and an absence of further stones. Hospital admission may be required for severe pain, for those unable to tolerate oral fluids, or for intervention. When a stone impacts in the ureter, there are two potential problems: obstruction leading to loss of function, and the possibility of infection behind the stone.

Wherever possible, it is advisable for the airline passenger to undergo any stone disease interventions prior to travel. Options for treatment include ESWL and PCNL. There are also a number of other minimally invasive surgical procedures including endoscopic ultrasonic, laser and electrohydraulic lithotripsy. The most frequently used procedure is ESWL. Recovery time is short and most patients resume normal activities within a few days. Bruising and minor discomfort of the back and a low-grade fever are frequent after effects but complications are rare. Usually the stone fragments pass easily through the urinary tract and there is a low incidence of obstruction. Where large stones that are thought likely to cause a problem are being treated, most urologists will electively stent the ureter prior to ESWL. When stones are large or in a difficult position, PCNL may be used. This requires the creation of a tunnel into the kidney through a small incision in the back and generally patients stay in hospital for several days. Patients with or at risk from further stones should undergo subsequent investigation for underlying risk factors. Appropriate therapy should be introduced and dietary advice given. All patients should increase their fluid intake to a level sufficient to produce clear, colourless urine.

Deep vein thrombosis has been described after long-distance air travel in a patient following PCNL for a staghorn calculus (Cottrell 1988) and airline passengers who have recently undergone stone removal procedures are advised to employ general measures to prevent thromboembolic complications during flight. If there is a possibility of acute renal colic occurring in-flight, it is advisable to travel with adequate analgesia. Renal colic may be severe enough to provoke nausea and vomiting and pain relief is paramount. Diclofenac 75 mg by intravenous or intramuscular injection or 100 mg rectally may prove more effective than the oral route of administration. Alternatively, oral pethidine tablets may be carried, but if any narcotic agent is used, a covering letter detailing the reason for the prescription should also be provided.

OBSTRUCTIVE UROPATHY

Urinary tract obstruction is also common. The cause and the site of the obstruction vary according to gender and age. Obstruction may be partial or complete, acute or chronic, unilateral or bilateral. In young adults, the cause is most likely to be stone disease. In middle-aged to elderly men prostatic outflow tract obstruction becomes more prevalent. Other causes include pelvi-ureteric junction obstruction, retroperitoneal fibrosis, and retroperitoneal and pelvic malignancy. Whilst acute urinary tract obstruction may result in pain, chronic urinary tract obstruction may be symptomless. Whatever the cause, and whether acute or chronic, untreated urinary tract obstruction will lead to impairment of renal function. Investigation, diagnosis and treatment therefore take precedence over travel in the airline passenger found to have urinary tract obstruction. Although relatively complete recovery of function can occur after total ureteral obstruction of 1 week's duration, if relief of obstruction is delayed by 12 weeks little or no recovery of function occurs.

After relief of obstruction, a post-obstructive diuresis generally occurs, the extent of which is again dependent on the severity and duration of obstruction. Most of the functional recovery occurs in the first 10 days and tubular function may be impaired as well as glomerular function. This may result in impaired concentrating ability, salt wasting and an acquired renal tubular acidosis with hyperkalaemia. From a practical point of view, the significance of this to the airline passenger is that, as with other diseases, the disease process should be stable before travel is contemplated.

CHRONIC RENAL FAILURE

These patients by definition have chronic disease and whilst functional deterioration in the patient with chronic renal failure (CRF) may be inexorable, it is slow and occurs over a period of months or years. By convention, CRF is defined by a glomerular filtration rate (GFR) of less than 50 ml min^{-1} (normal range 109–152 ml min^{-1} 1.73 m^{-2} body surface area in males and 101–133 ml min^{-1} 1.73 m^{-2} body surface area in females), roughly corresponding to a serum creatinine level of $\geq$150 μmol l^{-1}. End-stage renal failure (ESRF) is defined by a GFR of <10 ml min^{-1} and these patients will normally be receiving regular dialysis treatment.

The level of underlying renal function in the patient with CRF and ESRF will be the main determinant of potential problems these patients may encounter when they become airline passengers. Although symptoms such as tiredness, diminished well-being and reduced work capacity begin to appear when the GFR falls below 45 ml min^{-1}, it is not until it drops below 30 ml min^{-1} that potential problems arise. Below this level of function, anaemia, acidosis and disorders of calcium and phosphate metabolism begin to occur. As the GFR diminishes further, additional problems such as hyperkalaemia and oedema become more prevalent. Below 15 ml min^{-1}, nausea, vomiting and gastritis begin to appear and below 10 ml min^{-1}, cardiac failure, neuropathy, sleeping difficulties and mental changes become manifest. Patients with levels of GFR $\leq$10 ml min^{-1} who are not receiving regular dialysis treatment should not be allowed to travel.

Where possible, it is advisable to give every patient travelling a letter advising the diagnosis, past history, complications and current treatment. This letter should clearly state contact details of the unit primarily responsible for their care. All patients at potential risk should have the benefit of assessment prior to flight. At a cabin altitude of 5000 feet (see Table 19.4), the partial pressure of oxygen is considerably less than at sea level (Figure 19.1); thus, flying at altitude can cause significant hypoxia. This may be exacerbated by anaemia and pulmonary oedema, especially in patients with coexistent pulmonary disease. Any cardiac failure and/or volume overload must therefore be corrected and

Table 19.4 *Cabin altitudes in commercial aircraft*

Aircraft	Cabin altitude (feet)
DC-8	5000
DC-9	7300
DC-10	5400
BAC-111	7900
B-727	5400
B-737	8000
B-747	4700
B-757	5400
B-767	5400
A-300	6100
A-320	6000

Adapted from Cottrell (1988).

hypertension controlled. Up-to-date haematology and biochemistry should be obtained and haemoglobin level optimized.

Regulation of salt and water balance is usually maintained until the GFR falls below 15 ml min^{-1}. Nevertheless, even patients with mild-to-moderate renal failure are prone to fluid overload because they are less able to respond rapidly to salt and water loading. In dialysis-dependent patients, the risk of volume overload may be ameliorated by the presence of significant residual renal function. Loss of residual function occurs more rapidly with patients on haemodialysis (HD) as compared with continuous ambulatory peritoneal dialysis (CAPD) (Rottembourg 1993). However, patients treated with CAPD are often chronically fluid overloaded

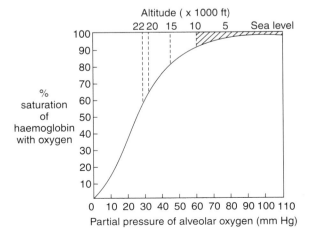

Figure 19.1 *Partial pressure of alveolar oxygen at altitude.*

(Coles 1997), the risk of fluid overload increasing with the length of time patients have been on this treatment modality. Recognition of fluid overload in the absence of oedema, raised jugular venous pressure and pulmonary signs can be difficult and hypertension may be the only pointer. Strict attention to fluid balance must be part of the pre-flight preparation of all dialysis-dependent patients.

In those patients with residual renal function, the introduction of diuretic treatment may be of benefit. Either a loop diuretic such as frusemide (up to 500 mg alternate days or daily) or a combination of loop diuretic and metolazone (5–10 mg daily) may be used (Tzamaloukas 2000). In the absence of residual renal function, peritoneal dialysis patients may require higher-strength glucose dialysate or the introduction of icodextrin to achieve the necessary increase in ultrafiltration. Patients on HD should be dialysed within 24 hours of the flight departure time. All patients should be counselled to restrict their fluid intake, particularly when the flight time is long and/or there is risk of delay.

The availability of recombinant human erythropoietin (rHuEPO) has been one of the major advances in the treatment of renal failure. Both the American National Kidney Foundation Dialysis Quality Outcomes Initiative (NKF-DQOI) and the European Renal Association guidelines recommend that the target range for haemoglobin should be at least 11 g dl^{-1} for both pre-dialysis and dialysis patients. Using rHuEPO treatment these levels can be readily achieved in the majority of patients. Although air travel may not be contraindicated at lower levels of haemoglobin, where possible the recommended target levels should be reached prior to travel to reduce the risk of hypoxia.

Plasma potassium concentration is determined by the relationship between dietary intake, distribution between cells and extracellular fluid, and urinary excretion. Normally, ingestion of a potassium load leads initially to increased uptake into cells, with subsequent elimination through the kidney over a period of 6–8 hours. In the patient with CRF/ESRF, renal elimination may obviously be compromised, but additional factors also serve to increase levels of potassium in the blood. In the presence of metabolic acidosis, buffering of hydrogen ions into cells leads to movement of potassium out of cells. Non-selective β-blockade interferes

Table 19.5 *Drugs implicated in hyperkalaemia*

Drug	Mechanism
Non-selective β-blockers	Reduction of β_2-adrenergic mediated uptake of potassium into cells
Angiotensin-converting enzyme inhibitors	Reduction of AII-mediated and potassium-stimulated aldosterone release
Angiotensin II blockers	Reduction of AII-mediated and potassium-stimulated aldosterone release
Non-steroidal anti-inflammatory drugs	Reduction in renin secretion
Cyclosporin	Aldosterone resistance
Amiloride	Aldosterone resistance
Spironolactone	Aldosterone resistance
Triamterene	Aldosterone resistance
Trimethoprim (high dose)	Aldosterone resistance
Pentamidine	Aldosterone resistance

with β_2-adrenergic facilitated uptake of potassium into cells. Any cause of hypoaldosteronism in the presence of CRF will reduce potassium excretion. This may be associated with renal disease, for example, hyporeninaemic hypoaldosteronism in diabetic nephropathy and aldosterone resistance in tubulointerstitial disease, or may be related to drug therapy (Table 19.5). Angiotensin-converting enzyme inhibitors and angiotensin II antagonists decrease both angiotensin II-mediated and potassium-stimulated aldosterone release. Non-steroidal anti-inflammatory drugs lower renin secretion and aldosterone resistance is associated with cyclosporin, amiloride, spironolactone, triamterene, high-dose trimethoprim (especially in the elderly), and pentamidine. Any change in treatment prior to flight should either be avoided or followed up by monitoring of biochemistry.

Before travelling, it is essential that dialysis-dependent patients have made arrangements for dialysis at their destination. Information about holiday dialysis can be obtained from the parent unit, from the various kidney patient associations, and from the worldwide web. There are a number of sites providing advice about travel insurance, paying for holiday dialysis (including areas of the world with reciprocal agreements with the UK), and about availability of holiday dialysis with contact details of the various units (Table 19.6). Deliveries of peritoneal dialysis fluid can be made to most holiday destinations throughout the world provided sufficient notice is given to the supplier. Normally your own renal unit will do this for you. It is advisable to warn hotels about deliveries of fluid and to make arrangements for disposal of waste. Availability of holiday haemodialysis depends on the destination. Your own unit will want to know where and when you intend to undergo holiday haemodialysis. There are many dialysis centres in the world where there is a high risk of transmission of blood-borne disease. Any holiday unit that does not request up-to-date information about hepatitis B and C and HIV status should be viewed with suspicion. Many units now routinely vaccinate patients against hepatitis B and this is worth enquiring about several months in advance of travel.

The subject of immunization is considered elsewhere. The contraindications to immunization in patients with CRF and dialysis-dependent renal failure are no different from those for patients with normal renal function, but it should be remembered that immunization in patients with advanced renal failure is less likely to be successful (Girndt *et al.* 1995). Successful protection may require the use of imm-une globulin. Where malaria prophylaxis is required, patients with significant renal failure

Table 19.6 *Useful websites for holiday dialysis*

www.globaldialysis.com
www.eurodial.org
www.kidney.org.uk
www.kidneypatientguide.org.uk
www.nephron.com
www.nephronline.com

(GFR <50 ml min^{-1}) should avoid proguanil because of the risk of bone marrow depression. In patients with a GFR of <10 ml min^{-1}, the dose of chloroquine should be reduced by 50 per cent. The drug is only minimally removed by dialysis. No dosage adjustments are necessary with mefloquine. Patients with a GFR <10 ml min^{-1} taking doxycycline as prophylaxis should not take more than 100 mg d^{-1}. Mefloquine and doxycycline represent a safer combination for the patient with impaired renal function.

Essential medication should always be carried in cabin baggage together with multiple copies of required prescriptions. Peritoneal dialysis patients may wish to carry equipment sufficient for a couple of fluid exchanges if there is a scheduled break between flights or there is a risk of diversion or delay. Where indicated, fluid intake should be restricted during the flight and consumption of alcohol avoided. In-flight catering arrangements vary widely between the different carriers and although none of the major carriers was able to advise what the electrolyte content of their respective meals is, nevertheless some offer special diets provided sufficient notice is given.

HD patients should have undergone dialysis prior to travel. Peritoneal dialysis patients are better advised to have undergone a period of intensive dialysis in the days leading up to departure and to have drained out prior to flight embarkation. Not only are conditions on board commercial aircraft ill suited to peritoneal dialysis fluid exchanges, but also Boyle's law predicts that gases trapped in confined spaces expand as altitude increases. The associated abdominal distension may make peritoneal dialysis uncomfortable and may also contribute to hypoxia through splinting of the diaphragm.

FUNCTIONING RENAL TRANSPLANT

Few nephrologists are happy to allow newly transplanted patients undertake air travel away from the centre until patients are at least 1 year post-transplantation. Although most episodes of acute rejection occur in the first 6 months, nevertheless a first episode of acute rejection occurs in up to 8 per cent of patients after 1 year. In the immediate post-transplantation period, there are also additional problems such as ureteric stent removal, the possibility of acute infectious problems such as cytomegalovirus, and the requirement to stabilize levels of anti-rejection drugs. Travel is therefore absolutely contraindicated in the first 6 months and actively discouraged for the remainder of the first year.

As with patients on dialysis or with advanced CRF, it is vitally important that transplant patients travel with a letter documenting their past history, complications, treatment and up-to-date transplant biochemistry and haematology. Contact details of the unit responsible for their care should also be carried. All transplant medication should be carried as cabin baggage. Live vaccines are contraindicated in immunosuppressed patients and have to be avoided. Hepatitis B vaccination in transplant patients has a variable response (18–73 per cent), not much is known about the response to hepatitis A vaccination and where indicated human immune globulin is recommended. The main consideration governing malaria prophylaxis is the underlying transplant function and the same advice as with CRF patients applies.

ACUTE RENAL FAILURE

Acute renal failure (ARF) may be defined as a potentially reversible loss of renal excretory function occurring over a period of hours or days. It is a syndrome with a wide range of morphological counterparts dictated by the underlying cause and its genesis is frequently multifactorial. The practical difficulties of aeromedical evacuation of patients with ARF include the nature of the underlying illness, electrolyte abnormalities, fluid overload and low haemoglobin. As already indicated, the hazards of fluid overload and anaemia may be potentiated by altitude.

Aeromedical evacuation of these patients should only be undertaken if no local facility for their treatment is available, or if they require specialized life-saving treatment in another centre. The key to safe travel is to have stabilized the patient prior to transfer. Patients with ARF are frequently highly catabolic and hyperkalaemia is a serious consideration, often exacerbated by the coexistent metabolic acidosis. These patients should receive renal replacement therapy to correct fluid and electrolyte abnormalities prior to aeromedical transfer. Blood transfusion, if available and safe, may be used to bring haemoglobin levels up to 10 g dl^{-1}. Where there is a serious risk of hypoxia, intermittent positive pressure ventilation should be instituted in an appropriate facility on the ground and continued in-flight. Up-to-the-minute blood biochemistry and haematology, together with blood gas analysis, must be obtained before departure. Arrangements for immediate treatment at the destination facility should be made before any transfer is undertaken.

Equipment for in-flight monitoring and treatment has undergone considerable development. The equipment required for monitoring and resuscitation is the same as that for any other patient with, or at risk from, multiple organ failure (see Chapter 24). In ARF, a major advance in the safe transfer of casualties has been the use of in-flight haemofiltration. Use of arteriovenous techniques avoids the need for sophisticated equipment that takes up space in what may be cramped conditions. Haemofiltration allows control of intravascular volume and continued administration of intravenous fluids throughout the duration of the flight. Use of intravenous glucose and insulin together with haemofiltration enables good control of blood potassium levels (Stevens *et al.* 1986). The rate of haemofiltration required is governed by the amount of intravenous fluid administered, the patient's intravascular volume status, the duration of the flight and the degree of catabolism. In practice, rates of 200–500 ml h^{-1} are used. Higher rates or continued haemofiltration during longer flight times requires the use of haemofiltration replacement fluid.

OTHER PROBLEMS IN THE RENAL PATIENT

Many of the potential emergencies which may be generated by the airline passenger with renal disease may also occur in patients with other diseases. These include myocardial infarction and cardiac arrest, acute pulmonary oedema, gastrointestinal bleeding, and convulsions. Additional problems in the passenger with advanced renal failure include pericarditis and hyperkalaemia. A full range of drugs and equipment for the emergency management of these conditions should be available. There should also be appropriate analgesia for treatment of acute renal colic (diclofenac and pethidine injections) and the necessary equipment to relieve acute urinary retention.

REFERENCES

Chen CY, Huang CC and Tsao CJ. Haemostatic markers in nephrotic syndrome. *Am J Haematol* 1993; **44**: 276–9.

Coles GA. Have we underestimated the importance of fluid balance for the survival of PD patients? *Perit Dial Int* 1997; **17**: 321–6.

Cottrell JJ. Altitude exposures during aircraft flight. Flying higher. *Chest* 1988; **93**: 81–4.

Curhan GC, Willet WC, Rimm EB and Stampfer MJ. Family history and risk of kidney stones. *J Am Soc Nephrol* 1997; **8**: 1568–73.

Geers AB, Koomans HA, Roos JC and Doorhout-Mees EJ. Preservation of blood volume during oedema removal in nephrotic subjects. *Kidney Int* 1985; **28**: 652–7.

Girndt M, Pietsch M and Kohler H. Tetanus immunization and its association to hepatitis B vaccination in patients with chronic renal failure. *Am J Kidney Dis* 1995; **26**: 454–60.

Haas M, Meehan SM, Karrison JG and Spargo BH. Changing aetiologies of unexplained adult nephrotic syndrome: a comparison of renal biopsy findings from 1976–1979 and 1995–1997. *Am J Kidney Dis* 1997; **30**: 621–31.

Kreutzer ER and Folkert VW. Etiological diagnosis of renal calculus disease. *Curr Opin Nephrol Hypertens* 1993; **2**: 949–55.

Landgraf H, Vanselow B, Schulte-Huerman D, Mulmann MV and Bergau L. Economy class syndrome: rheology fluid balance and lower leg edema during a simulated 12-hour long-distance flight. *Aviat Space Environ Med* 1994; **65**: 930–5.

Patel A and Fuchs GJ. Air travel and thromboembolic complications after percutaneous nephrolithotomy for staghorn stone. *J Endourol* 1998; **12**: 51–3.

Robinson RR. Isolated proteinuria in asymptomatic patients. *Kidney Int* 1980; **18**: 395–406.

Rottembourg J. Residual renal function and recovery of renal function in patients treated by CAPD. *Kidney Int Suppl* 1993; **40**: S106–10.

Stevens PE, Bloodworth LL and Rainford DJ. High altitude haemofiltration. *Br Med J* 1986; **292**: 1354.

Tzamaloukas AH. Avoiding the use of hypertonic dextrose dialysate in peritoneal dialysis. *Semin Dial* 2000; **13**: 156–9.

Uribarri J, Oh MS and Carroll HJ. The first kidney stone. *Ann Intern Med* 1989; **111**: 1006–9.

Vande Wall JG, Donckerwolcke RA, van Isselt JW, Derks FH, Joles JA and Koomans HA. Volume regulation in children with early relapse of minimal change nephrosis with or without hypovolaemic symptoms. *Lancet* 1995; **346**: 148–52.

Whelton A. Renal effects of over-the-counter analgesics. *J Clin Pharmacol* 1995; **35**: 454–63.

Diabetes

VINCENT McAULAY AND BRIAN M FRIER

When people with diabetes travel by air, particularly on long flights that cross several time zones, the management of this condition requires careful planning and provision to avoid potential metabolic abnormalities associated with diabetes. Metabolic disturbance may be aggravated by intercurrent illness, travel sickness, the stress and anxiety associated with travel, the disruption to normal meal times caused by flight delays, and by unexpected adversity such as accidents or loss of medication. With detailed preparation before travelling, ensuring the maintenance of adequate supplies of medications and carbohydrates, frequent self-monitoring of blood glucose during the journey and a pragmatic understanding of how to deal with unpredictable and potentially disruptive contingencies, people with diabetes can pursue long-distance travelling for business or pleasure with confidence.

Metabolic problems that may occur during air travel include the development of hypoglycaemia (predominantly in people treated with insulin), or persistent hyperglycaemia, which in extreme circumstances may progress to diabetic ketoacidosis or a hyperosmolar non-ketotic state with the risk of coma. People with diabetes may have concurrent complications affecting both small and large blood vessels, which may pose problems and jeopardize their safety during long-distance air travel.

Because of the metabolic complexity of diabetes and its management, and the frequent coexistence of other medical disorders such as hypertension and dyslipidaemia (particularly in type 2 diabetes), the traveller with diabetes may require several concurrent medications in addition to their treatment for diabetes. The availability and efficacy of these treatments may be important to maintain their health during air travel. The fundamental importance to the management of diabetes of maintaining an appropriate diet and adequate oral intake of fluids may also be compromised during air travel. Before considering these aspects in detail, the nature and classification of diabetes is described, standard treatment regimens are outlined, and the underlying pathophysiology of metabolic decompensation and the effects of vascular complications are discussed.

Diabetes mellitus is the generic name for a group of disorders that are characterized by the development of chronic hyperglycaemia, which is associated with defective regulation of carbohydrate, lipid and protein metabolism (Table 20.1). This results from an absolute or relative deficiency of insulin, which may be associated with insulin resistance. The metabolic disturbances of diabetes range from asymptomatic hyperglycaemia to life-threatening metabolic decompensation. Exposure to chronic

Table 20.1 *Classification of diabetes mellitus*

Type 1 diabetes (pancreatic β-cell destruction, usually leading to absolute insulin deficiency)
   Immune mediated
   Idiopathic
Type 2 diabetes (may range from predominant insulin resistance with relative insulin deficiency to a predominant
  secretory defect with mild insulin resistance)
Other specific types
   Genetic defects of β-cell function, e.g. maturity-onset diabetes of youth (MODY) syndromes
   Genetic defects in insulin action
   Diseases of the exocrine pancreas, e.g. pancreatitis, haemochromatosis
   Secondary to endocrinopathies, e.g. acromegaly
   Drug or chemical induced, e.g. glucocorticoids, thiazide diuretics
   Infections, e.g. cytomegalovirus
   Genetic syndromes associated with diabetes, e.g. Down's syndrome
Gestational diabetes

hyperglycaemia over many years results in functional and structural changes in many tissues, and in particular predisposes to the development of vascular disease, with both microvascular and macrovascular damage. Microangiopathy commonly affects the eye, kidney, heart and peripheral nerves, and is manifest as the classical diabetic complications of retinopathy, nephropathy, specific heart disease of diabetes, and peripheral and autonomic neuropathies. Macrovascular disease with widespread and often premature atherosclerosis affects the coronary arteries, the cerebral and peripheral circulation, and manifests with ischaemic heart disease, cerebrovascular disease and peripheral vascular disease, which contribute to the excess morbidity and mortality of diabetes.

TYPE 1 DIABETES

Type 1 diabetes is an autoimmune disorder in which selective destruction of the insulin-producing β-cells of the pancreatic islets occurs in genetically predisposed individuals. This process develops slowly over several years, but clinical presentation is usually acute with a short history (days to weeks) of weight loss and severe fatigue with osmotic symptoms of polyuria and polydipsia. Insulin is required to sustain life. If untreated, ketoacidosis will develop. This condition develops mostly in children, adolescents and young adults, and usually before the age of 40 years, although it can occur at any age.

Treatment with insulin

Insulin therapy is essential in people with type 1 diabetes and daily treatment using various insulin regimens is required to control blood glucose. A wide variety of insulin types and formulations is available for therapeutic use and regimens are usually tailored to meet the needs of the individual. Although a large number of insulin preparations are available in clinical practice, their utilization and prescription are relatively straightforward. Insulin preparations can be classified according to their species type, duration of action, preparation, method and mode of delivery.

Human insulin is the most commonly used and is manufactured by recombinant DNA technology. Animal insulins (*porcine* and *bovine*) are still manufactured and available for clinical use, though this is diminishing. More recently, fast-acting insulin analogues, insulin lispro (Humalog, Eli Lilly) and aspart (NovoRapid, Novo Nordisk), have become available. By a small modification of the position of amino acids in the insulin molecule, the absorption of insulin occurs more rapidly, allowing an earlier onset of biological action, a more rapid peak effect and a shorter duration of action.

Insulin can be subdivided into short, intermediate and long-acting types based on the pharmacokinetics of different preparations (Table 20.2). Minor differences in the pharmacokinetics are evident with different insulin species, the onset of action being fastest for human insulin, with porcine and bovine insulins having a slower onset and a later peak activity. Other factors that influence the time-action profile of insulins

Table 20.2 *Insulin preparations in current use for the treatment of diabetes*

Preparation	Onset (min)	Time action profile	
		Peak (h)	Duration (h)
Fast-acting insulin analogues Lispro/aspart	10–20	1–2	3–5
Short-acting soluble (regular)	30	1–3	4–8
Intermediate-acting isophane (NPH)	60–120	3–8	7–14
Long-acting (Ultralente)	180–240	6–12	12–30
Long-acting insulin analogue (Glargine)	90–120	None	24

include the site and depth of injection, the ambient temperature, and the volume of insulin injected. Smaller volumes of insulin are absorbed more rapidly. Local mechanical effects such as increased skin temperature, muscle exercise and massage of the injection site increase the rate of absorption.

To obtain an optimal hypoglycaemic effect that matches the post-prandial rise in blood glucose, short-acting insulin should be injected 30–45 minutes before a meal, but in practice this prerequisite is ignored by many people. The fast-acting insulin analogues can be injected immediately before, or after, the ingestion of food, which confers a practical benefit with respect to convenience of administration and a closer match between the post-prandial rise in blood glucose and insulin bioavailability. The insulin analogues, insulin lispro and insulin aspart, have a rapid onset of action. Therefore, they are particularly useful in situations where it is difficult to determine the likely interval between injecting insulin and eating a meal, or when a decision on insulin dose has to await an assessment of the carbohydrate and caloric content of an unknown meal – a common situation during air travel. The capacity to inject insulin immediately before (or after) a meal enhances the flexibility of insulin usage and so improves the quality of life for people with type 1 diabetes. The availability of these fast-acting insulin analogues has simplified the administration of insulin during long-distance air travel and the treatment of intercurrent illness.

Various insulin regimens are available, and insulin can be administered using plastic syringes, pen devices (reusable or disposable) or pre-programmable insulin pumps (continuous subcutaneous insulin infusion). Insulin administered once daily is seldom used for people with type 1 diabetes, but may be used in the treatment of people with type 2 diabetes, usually in combination with oral hypoglycaemic agents, or occasionally in elderly people in whom strict glycaemic control may be neither necessary nor desirable. Many people with insulin-treated diabetes use a combination of short-acting, soluble (regular) insulin with intermediate-acting, isophane (NPH) insulin, which is administered twice daily, before breakfast and before the evening meal. These insulins can be mixed in the same syringe (free mixing) or given as a pre-mixed combination (fixed mixture), the most commonly used containing 30 per cent soluble and 70 per cent isophane insulins. Some people take soluble insulin alone before the evening meal and administer the isophane insulin at bedtime.

Multiple insulin injection therapy requires administration of short-acting insulin (or a fast-acting insulin analogue) before meals, supplemented by one or more injections of isophane insulin (usually given at bedtime). This is often called a basal-bolus insulin regimen and offers greater flexibility in time of administration and dose adjustment before meals. The injection of a single insulin or a fixed mixture enables the use of a pen device which provides relative ease of measuring the dose of insulin and the use of cartridges of insulin, obviating the need to draw up insulin from a vial. The transport of insulin pens and spare cartridges of insulin (or disposable pens) is easier than carrying disposable syringes and vials of insulin, and pen devices are well suited for travel.

Most English-speaking countries now use U-100 strength insulin (100 U ml^{-1}), but U-40 (40 U ml^{-1}) and U-80 (80 U ml^{-1}) strengths of insulin are still supplied in some parts of the world. The use of a different strength of insulin in a syringe marked for U-100 insulin requires calculation of the dose using a conversion factor. This risks error but may be necessary in an emergency.

TYPE 2 DIABETES

Type 2 diabetes is the most common primary type of diabetes, but comprises a heterogeneous group of disorders with a spectrum of abnormality involving varying degrees of defective insulin secretion associated with insulin resistance. The relative contributions of these defects varies between individuals, but obesity is common and there is often a family history of this condition. The disease is preceded by a period of impaired glucose tolerance that progresses at a variable rate, but is often present for several years before the development of frank diabetes. Most patients with type 2 diabetes are diagnosed at a relatively late stage of this process and because the condition is often asymptomatic, many people with type 2 diabetes remain undiagnosed for years. It may be revealed by chance when an individual seeks medical attention for an unrelated condition, or is found coincidentally to have an established complication of diabetes such as retinopathy or peripheral neuropathy.

Classical symptoms include the typical osmotic features of hyperglycaemia – thirst, polyuria, nocturia and fatigue, and some people suffer fungal infections such as genital candidiasis. Recent weight gain is more common than weight loss (a prominent feature of uncontrolled type 1 diabetes) and ketonuria is absent. Microvascular complications are present at the time of diagnosis in 25 per cent of people with type 2 diabetes. This reflects the tissue damage that results from protracted exposure to preceding hyperglycaemia (for up to 10 years before diagnosis) and some individuals present with a major macrovascular event such as a myocardial infarction or a stroke.

On a global basis, type 2 diabetes accounts for more than 85 per cent of diabetes, although prevalence rates vary between different populations. It is a disease of ageing with 10 per cent of people over the age of 65 years in the UK having type 2 diabetes. A global pandemic of type 2 diabetes is in progress with the prevalence predicted to double in the next 10 years, partly through increasing longevity, but other contributory factors include obesity, a diet high in saturated fat and refined carbohydrate, sedentary lifestyle and increasing industrialization of many countries. This now presents a formidable public health problem throughout the world.

Treatment of type 2 diabetes

The cornerstone of therapy is diet, supplemented by regular exercise. In addition to restricting the intake of refined sugars and saturated fats, many obese people require caloric restriction to attempt weight reduction. Type 2 diabetes progresses in severity with time and the majority of people require the introduction of oral medication and/or insulin to achieve optimal glycaemic control. Oral antidiabetic drugs can be classified as hypoglycaemic agents or antihyperglycaemic agents (Table 20.3), based on their mode of action and propensity to promote hypoglycaemia as a side effect. The mainstay of treatment for many years has been the sulphonylureas and metformin, and acarbose (an α-glucosidase inhibitor) may be of value in some patients. Several new classes of drugs for the treatment of diabetes have been introduced with which clinical experience is limited at present. These include the thiazolidinediones, rosiglitazone and pioglitazone, which enhance the action of the endogenous secretion of insulin and reduce insulin resistance. They can be prescribed in combination with either a sulphonylurea or metformin, or with insulin (although they are not yet licensed for use with insulin in the UK). The meglitinides, e.g. repaglinide, and amino acid derivatives such as nateglinide, are further new classes of oral medication (prandial glucose regulators) which stimulate insulin secretion and are given before meals.

Oral antidiabetic drugs are usually effective for a while, but with increasing duration of type 2 diabetes, the dose tends to escalate, multiple agents may be required and it becomes increasingly difficult to control hyperglycaemia and achieve good control of diabetes. A gradual deterioration in glycaemic control indicates the development of

Table 20.3 *Oral medications used to treat type 2 diabetes*

Drug	Mode of action	Risk of hypoglycaemia

Sulphonylureas
  Chlorpropamide
  Glibenclamide
  Gliclazide
  Glimepiride
  Glipizide
  Gliquidone
  Tolbutamide
	Insulin secretagogues	Yes

Biguanide Metformin	Reduces insulin resistance Reduces hepatic glucose output	No

Alpha-glucosidase inhibitors
  Acarbose
  Miglitol
	Slow carbohydrate absorption	No

Meglitinide Repaglinide	Insulin secretagogue	Yes
Amino acid derivative Nateglinide	Insulin secretagogue	Yes

Thiazolidinediones
  Pioglitazone
  Rosiglitazone
	Insulin enhancers
	Reduces insulin resistance
		No

secondary failure of oral medications and the need to introduce treatment with insulin. This is sometimes started as a single daily injection of isophane insulin at bedtime while oral medications are continued, but this combination therapy is not effective indefinitely and complete conversion to treatment with insulin is eventually required. In some situations, such as during intercurrent illness, perioperative stress, or the use of drugs such as corticosteroids that antagonize the action of insulin, it is necessary to treat with insulin temporarily until the individual has recovered or the insulin antagonist is withdrawn.

AIR TRAVEL OF PEOPLE WITH DIABETES

Epidemiology

What sort of problems are encountered in air travellers who have diabetes? There has been a paucity of clinical research with very little scientific evidence being published on this topic, although anecdotes are plentiful. In a prospective study of the causes of medical emergencies presenting at Seattle-Tacoma International Airport over one year,

only one-quarter of travellers' problems occurred during air flights and most took place on the ground (Cummins and Schubach 1989). Of the 13 problems ascribed to diabetes (2 per cent of the total), 10 occurred within the airport and were divided equally between people with insulin-treated diabetes who had either forgotten or mislaid their insulin, and those who thought they were experiencing hypoglycaemia. Gastrointestinal problems such as nausea, vomiting, diarrhoea and abdominal pain (which could affect the management of diabetes) were relatively common in this survey and occurred in 16 per cent of all travellers. Similarly, symptoms of cardiac disease (chest pain, angina and suspected myocardial infarction) were reported by 11 per cent of all travellers.

In a 6-month retrospective review of in-flight medical emergencies among passengers arriving at Los Angeles International Airport, 11 per cent had gastroenteritis and 9 per cent had developed unstable angina (Speizer *et al.* 1989). Although the Los Angeles survey did not report diabetes-specific diagnoses, 39 per cent of cases were placed in an 'other' diagnostic category, consisting of 33 different but unspecified diagnostic groups as reported by three or fewer travellers. It is likely that some of these had involved a medical problem associated with diabetes.

Finally, in a 1-year retrospective evaluation of the in-flight use of emergency kits on United Airlines flights, 2.8 per cent of all cases were defined as being related to the management of diabetes or hyperglycaemia (Cottrell *et al.* 1989).

Preparation for air travel

PERSONAL IDENTIFICATION

Careful planning and preparation prior to air travel is to be recommended for most people with diabetes. A letter from the specialist clinic or general practitioner stating that the individual has diabetes, and the nature of the treatment required (particularly when this is insulin), should be obtained. This helps to allay the suspicions of immigration and customs officials who may (not unreasonably) suspect drug addiction when syringes and needles are found on examining hand luggage. If a prolonged period of travel abroad is intended, it is useful to carry a copy of a prescription letter with a list of medications (including the generic names in addition to brand names of medications which often vary between countries), insulin prescription, syringes, and blood-testing items.

In addition to standard items of personal identification such as a passport, visa or driving licence, people who have diabetes should carry some form of identification providing information on their condition, particularly if they are treated with insulin. 'Medic Alert' provides stainless steel bracelets or necklaces containing personalized medical information. These are recognized world wide. In many countries people can apply to associations concerned with the health of those with diabetes to provide an identification card showing their photograph, doctor's name and contact telephone number, and a statement that they type 1 diabetes printed in different languages.

INSURANCE

Air travellers who have diabetes should obtain comprehensive medical insurance cover for accidents and illness requiring medical assistance, and insurance which covers loss or theft of their personal medical equipment and medications. On taking out insurance, it is particularly important to check that the medical insurance policy covers pre-existing medical conditions and especially diabetes, otherwise the individual may find that they are not covered for any subsequent claim relating to these disorders. Many insurers insist that the presence of diabetes must be declared in advance of the travel/vacation, otherwise any subsequent claim will not be allowed. Most travel policies contain exclusions so proposed medical insurance policies should be read scrupulously because diabetes is a frequent exclusion. If a medical insurance policy specifies diabetes as an exclusion, the individual may not be covered for conditions such as a stroke or a myocardial infarction for which diabetes is a recognized medical risk factor, or treatment of such conditions which have been complicated by pre-existing diabetes. The traveller must therefore ensure that the medical insurer records the diagnosis of diabetes at the time the policy is purchased. Travellers with diabetes should check that insurance cover is adequate if potentially dangerous sporting activities are intended, and that emergency air transport to convey the individual home (or at least back to their country of residence) will be provided in the event of a serious accident or illness.

Travel in the European Community and USA

When travelling in countries in the European Community (EC), emergency medical attention is usually provided free to people from member states, although immediate payment for treatment may be demanded in some countries such as France. Travellers should obtain a specific form (E111). This entitles them to emergency medical care that is either free or at a reduced charge in most EC countries, although full medical travel insurance is still necessary. If patients plan to stay in an EC country for more than 6 months, an E112 form is required. Some non-EC countries such as Australia and Russia offer free or reduced rate medical care for EC members. Leaflet SA 30 ('Medical Costs Abroad') gives details of the care available in non-EC countries and can be obtained from travel agents and appropriate government departments. Emergency medical treatment in the USA can be extremely expensive and people who have diabetes and intend travelling to North America may have to pay a high insurance premium. A list of insurers who do not load the premium of applicants who have diabetes can be obtained from patient associations.

Finally, irrespective of the medical insurance cover obtained, it should be appreciated that the quality of emergency medical care available in some countries is substandard at best, and in some developing countries may be poor or potentially dangerous to the individual with a diabetes-related medical emergency. There are parts of the world where insulin is not readily available and intravenous fluids for emergency use may be in short supply. Whilst this should not deter air travel *per se*, it may influence the choice of destination.

Drugs and equipment

Essential items that the air traveller with diabetes should carry are listed in Table 20.4. Those who are treated with insulin should carry an ample supply of insulin in their hand luggage, in two different bags (one can be carried by a relative or friend) in case of loss or theft. When travelling by air, the supply of insulin that is not in current use should not be packed in baggage to be transported in the hold of

Table 20.4 *Essential items for travel for people with insulin requiring diabetes*

Equipment
Insulin as vials or cartridges
Syringes and needles/pens and spare pen needles
Flask/cool bag for insulin storage
Blood glucose meter; spare meter; spare batteries
Finger pricker and spare; lancets; container for used
  needles
Blood glucose strips (visual reading)

Hypoglycaemia treatment
Fast-acting carbohydrate:
  glucose drinks (screwtop container)
  glucose tablets/confectionery (foil wrapped; powder
    form in hot humid climate)
Slow-acting carbohydrate:
  biscuits; cereal bars

Fluids
Glucose-free drinks (screwtop container)
Bottled water (plastic container)

Documents
Diabetes identity card/bracelet
Document stating that individual has diabetes including
  description of therapy, necessity to carry syringes,
  needles, etc.
Blood glucose monitoring diary

the aircraft. Although the cargo hold of most commercial airlines is heated and pressurized, in some parts of the world luggage may be exposed to subzero temperatures at altitude which will freeze and denature the insulin, and luggage often goes astray. Insulin should be carried in hand luggage in a cool bag or a pre-cooled vacuum flask. Extremes of temperature and high altitude can also disable blood glucose meters and the accuracy of glucose test strips, so blood monitoring equipment should also be carried in hand luggage, where it is immediately available for in-flight use. The air pressure within the cabins of passenger aircraft is equivalent to an altitude of up to 8000 feet, which should not affect the accuracy of most blood glucose meters (Gautier *et al.* 1996). Availability of visually read glucose strips provides a useful backup if the glucose meter fails in transit, and it is prudent to take a spare meter when travelling abroad.

The use of short-acting soluble insulin or fast-acting insulin analogues during long flights may be most conveniently given by a pen device (which could be disposable in type). For those who have only ever used a syringe for insulin injection, instruction on the use of a pen device may be required before departure. Air travellers with insulin-treated diabetes should be advised that their usual daily insulin requirement may be significantly altered by the timing or content of meals provided in-flight, enforced inactivity on the plane with lack of physical exercise and changes in temperature.

When managing glycaemic control during flights, those prone to motion sickness should carry a supply of antiemetic tablets to avert the problems caused by nausea and vomiting. In addition, antidiarrhoeal agents should be carried along with a supply of a broad-spectrum antibiotic, particularly if travelling within parts of the world where the risk of acquiring gastroenteritis is high. Analgesics, e.g. paracetamol for pain or pyrexia, may be useful and an antihistamine may be valuable to treat itchy insect bites. People who have peripheral sensory neuropathy should pack comfortable and appropriate footwear for travel by plane.

Crossing time zones

A common problem faced by the air traveller with insulin-treated diabetes who is traversing several time-zones in the course of a long air flight is how to adjust their timing and dose of insulin to cope with disrupted meal times and the effects on circadian rhythm, yet be in synchrony with lócal time on arrival at their destination. There is virtually no scientifically based information published on this topic. Recommendations are derived from theoretical assumptions and the opinions of health-care professionals, which probably accounts for the variability of the advice that is dispensed to patients. Some specialists advocate detailed and complicated alterations to meal patterns and the time of administration of insulin even for relatively short flights across North America where the time difference from coast to coast is only 5 hours (Benson and Metz 1984). One survey confirmed the diversity of opinion and advice concerning adjustment of insulin therapy among diabetes specialists in the UK. It is disconcerting that 14 per cent of responses recommended giving excessive doses of insulin either in-flight or on arrival, which would be liable to induce hypoglycaemia (Gill and Redmond 1993). On a more reassuring note, in 70 per cent of specialist clinics only experienced staff (consultant diabetologist or specialist diabetes nurse) provided advice on this important topic.

The problem of in-flight insulin schedules has been greatly simplified by the availability of fast-acting insulin analogues and the ease of administration with pen devices. This avoids the use of isophane or other intermediate-acting insulins during air travel, which increase the risk of a mismatch between insulin dose and prevailing blood glucose. However, a few general points of advice can be given. To plan in-flight management of diabetes, the patient should ascertain in advance the anticipated flight times, duration of the flight and the local time of arrival and discuss with the diabetes specialist team details of how they will take their insulin before and during air travel. Plans for insulin dose and type to be administered before and after the flight can be made and, depending on the length of the flight, additional short-acting (or fast-acting) insulin may be necessary. They should be advised to check their blood glucose frequently (at least 4-hourly) while in transit and when changing time zones. Excessively strict glycaemic control should be avoided while in-flight, and it may be prudent to allow slightly higher blood glucose values than usual to avoid the risk of developing hypoglycaemia.

A personal supply of carbohydrate should be carried at all times, in addition to emergency treatment for hypoglycaemia. The time that in-flight meals are intended to be served after take-off can usually be obtained from the airline, and these can either be regarded as snacks or as main meals, depending on the travel schedule. Some airlines provide so-called 'diabetic' meals, but these are often small, are mainly intended for people with type 2 diabetes, contain an insufficient content of carbohydrate (Johnston *et al.* 1986) and may risk incipient hypoglycaemia. Patients may wish to supplement the in-flight meal with their own stock of suitable carbohydrate, but it is impractical to carry large quantities. Alternatively, extra bread rolls may be requested (although travellers must not rely on this). In our experience, the 'vegetarian' meal choice is worth investigating as it is often suitable for people with type 1 diabetes, containing pasta-based dishes or rice. Allowances may have to be made for unpredictable contingencies such as delayed flights or long intervals between meals. Travel fatigue may blunt appetite, and travel sickness will reduce the consumption of adequate carbohydrate.

Most commentators opine that extension of the day when flying westerly, necessitates an additional dose of short-acting insulin. Conversely, when flying easterly, the day is shortened, and a reduction in insulin dose before flying or during flight may be required. The situation is complicated by the numerous insulin regimens that are in use. The frequent administration of short-acting insulin or a fast-acting insulin analogue before meals is much simpler to manage than attempting to modify the times of administration and dosage of intermediate-acting insulin. With this approach, intermediate-acting lente or isophane insulins need not be administered before or during flights and the insulin requirement is provided entirely in a short-acting form. Some guidance on insulin dose is required and this will depend upon size, content and frequency of meals, and the results of blood glucose testing. An additional advantage of a fast-acting analogue is that its administration can be delayed until the food on offer is available and can be assessed for carbohydrate content (or palatability), or it can be injected after the airline meal, thus providing greater flexibility of time of administration and dosage.

An extended day will necessitate additional meals and insulin. For example, an *east to west* flight from

London to New York will add 5–6 hours to the traveller's day (not including possible flight delays). If the outward flight leaves at 12 noon, the British traveller would expect to arrive at around 1400 hours local time in New York. For the person on a basal-bolus insulin regimen (e.g. soluble insulin before meals and isophane insulin at bedtime), the usual morning dose of insulin would be taken, lunch with preprandial insulin would be consumed on the flight, and on arrival, an additional dose of short-acting insulin would be taken with a snack or a small meal. The evening meal would be eaten later with the usual insulin dose. For those using a fixed insulin mixture, e.g. 30 per cent soluble with 70 per cent isophane insulins, the usual dose of insulin would be taken at breakfast. Upon arrival in New York, a small additional dose of short-acting (soluble or analogue) insulin (which should be obtained by prescription beforehand) can be administered before food until the usual mealtime in the early evening.

On the return *west to east journey*, 5 or 6 hours of the normal day are lost as a result of the direction of travel. Most of these flights leave during the evening and fly during the night, which is truncated. For patients taking a basal-bolus insulin regimen, the usual intermediate-acting insulin can be omitted, and substituted with short-acting insulin to cover the in-flight meal. On arrival in the UK, the usual dose of short-acting insulin can be taken before breakfast. Table 20.5 describes a rational approach to the management of insulin during the crossing of time zones. Some passengers with insulin-treated diabetes prefer a seat near a toilet for ease of insulin injection, but with pen devices this may not be necessary. However, this is a matter of personal preference and desire for privacy when injecting insulin, and most airlines will try to accommodate such a request. People with type 2 diabetes who are taking oral agents should not experience these problems. Additional doses of tablets are usually not required to cover an extended day, although the use of a drug like repaglinide may be valuable for an additional meal. A dose may have to be omitted on a truncated day in the case of a long west to east air journey.

Table 20.5 *Management of diabetes during long-distance air travel – advice for travellers with diabetes*

- Obtain advice from the diabetes clinic before travelling
- Obtain essential information including the local time of departure, flight duration and local time of arrival
- Inform the airline that you have diabetes, especially if treated with insulin
- Ensure facility for frequent self-monitoring of blood glucose during travel
- Carry adequate supplies of extra carbohydrate; anticipate that delays may occur
- The time of the usual meal and insulin before departure and after arrival should be ascertained, and the time between these injections calculated. If this time is in excess of 12 hours then additional in-flight insulin with food may be needed
- For people taking premixed insulin, some (but not all) eastward flights involve a shortened duration between injections. If less than 8 hours, a reduction in pre-flight insulin doses should be considered
- Time-zone travel may necessitate two consecutive morning or evening insulin doses, before and after the flight
- Do not strive for meticulous control of blood glucose during air travel

HYPOGLYCAEMIA

Hypoglycaemia is the most serious and disruptive side effect of the treatment of diabetes and it is a recognized clinical consequence of the use of insulin and also of sulphonylureas in all age groups taking such therapy. In people with type 1 diabetes, many factors can influence the absorption and action of exogenous insulin. A mismatch between plasma insulin concentration and blood glucose occurs frequently so that hypoglycaemia is a common side effect of treatment. Although hypoglycaemia is considered to be relatively uncommon with oral hypoglycaemic agents (UK Prospective Diabetes Study Group 1998), many sulphonylureas can promote hypoglycaemia of varying frequency and severity. The increasing use of oral hypoglycaemic agents combined with a single dose of isophane insulin to treat type 2 diabetes may augment the frequency of hypoglycaemia in an older population, and the risk of exposure to insulin-induced hypoglycaemia in people with type 1 diabetes is also rising as a consequence of policies of using intensive insulin therapy to achieve strict glycaemic control .

Physiological responses to hypoglycaemia

The brain is dependent upon glucose as its principal source of fuel and requires a continuous supply of glucose via the cerebral circulation. Depriving the brain of glucose rapidly causes neuroglycopenia, which has various effects, including impairment of cognitive function. In humans, a decline in blood glucose concentration activates the secretion of counter-regulatory hormones (particularly glucagon and adrenaline), and the subsequent development of characteristic warning symptoms which alert the informed individual to the development of hypoglycaemia (Cryer 1993). This allows early and appropriate action (the ingestion of carbohydrate) to be taken to assist recovery. These responses are usually effective in maintaining the arterial blood glucose concentration within the normoglycaemic range (arbitrarily defined as a blood glucose above 3.8 mmol l^{-1}), and they protect the brain from exposure to prolonged neuroglycopenia.

Symptoms

Hypoglycaemia generates symptoms as a direct consequence of depriving cerebral neurones of glucose and also by activation of the autonomic nervous system (Cryer et al. 1989). Symptoms of hypoglycaemia are classified as neuroglycopenic, autonomic or non-specific in type and are age-specific (Table 20.6). Elderly subjects often experience transient neurological features which may be misinterpreted by observers as transient ischaemic attacks, whereas children may exhibit behavioural changes which may be interpreted as being naughty or irritable, rather than the manifestations of a low blood glucose. Cognitive function is progressively impaired during hypoglycaemia as blood glucose declines. Following treatment with glucose, most patients rapidly feel better, but despite apparent recovery it can take as long as 40–90 minutes after the blood glucose has returned to normal for cognitive function to be fully restored (Blackman et al. 1992, Lindgren et al. 1996).

Table 20.6 *Common symptoms of hypoglycaemia in different age groups*

Adults	Autonomic	Neuroglycopenic	Non-specific
	Sweating	Weakness	Headache
	Trembling	Visual disturbance	Nausea
	Pounding heart	Difficulty speaking	
	Anxiety	Tingling	
	Hunger	Dizziness	
		Difficulty concentrating	
		Tiredness	
		Drowsiness	
		Confusion	
Children	**Autonomic**	**Neuroglycopenic**	**Behavioural**
	Hunger	Weakness	Tearful
	Trembling	Dizziness	Confused
	Pallor	Poor concentration	Irritable
	Sweating	Drowsiness	Aggressive
			Naughty
Elderly	**Autonomic**	**Neuroglycopenic**	**Neurological**
	Sweating	Weakness	Unsteady
	Shaking	Drowsiness	Poor coordination
	Pounding heart	Poor concentration	Double vision
	Anxiety	Dizziness	Blurred vision
		Confusion	Slurred speech
		Lightheadedness	

Sulphonylurea-induced hypoglycaemia

Long-acting sulphonylureas such as chlorpropamide and glibenclamide are associated with inducing severe hypoglycaemia in people with type 2 diabetes (Tessier *et al.* 1994, Stahl and Berger 1999) and asymptomatic biochemical hypoglycaemia is also common (Brodows 1992). However, one of the newer long-acting sulphonylureas, glimepiride, stimulates insulin production primarily in response to meals, and the incidence of hypoglycaemia reported with this preparation is low (Schneider 1996, Campbell 1998).

The use of long-acting sulphonylureas should be avoided in elderly people with type 2 diabetes and in people with renal impairment because delayed excretion prolongs their hypoglycaemic activity. The risk of hypoglycaemia is probably underestimated in people with type 2 diabetes taking sulphonylureas, especially in the fasting state and after the consumption of alcohol (Burge *et al.* 1999). Alcohol is the commonest cause of hypoglycaemia in the non-diabetic population and when drunk in excessive amounts is a potential source of trouble during long flights. The importance in people with diabetes is discussed later. People with type 2 diabetes cannot be relied upon to recognize hypoglycaemia. Knowledge of symptoms of hypoglycaemia is poor (McAulay and Frier 2000) and many people taking sulphonylureas do not know that they can cause hypoglycaemia (Browne *et al.* 2000).

Unusual presentations of hypoglycaemia

Hypoglycaemia does not always present with characteristic symptoms, and the nature of the presentation may vary with the age of the affected individual. In addition, acute hypoglycaemia provokes a profound haemodynamic response secondary to sympatho-adrenal activation, which may compromise an ailing cardiovascular system (Fisher and Heller 1999). When the effects of hypoglycaemia in provoking catecholamine-mediated hypokalaemia are combined with the profound haemodynamic changes, the potential for acute hypoglycaemia inducing a serious cardiac arrhythmia or myocardial ischaemia is enhanced. This degree of haemodynamic stress seldom causes any pathophysiological problem to the young person who has normal cardiac function, but in the older individual with diabetes who may have established coronary heart disease, hypoglycaemia may have serious or even fatal consequences.

Lengthening of the QT interval on the electrocardiogram has been demonstrated during hypoglycaemia both in non-diabetic and in diabetic subjects (Marques *et al.* 1997). When QT dispersion, a marker of spatial difference in myocardial recovery time, is increased, this indicates an enhanced risk of ventricular arrhythmias and sudden death. QT dispersion significantly increased during acute insulin-induced hypoglycaemia in 13 people with type 2 diabetes aged 48–63 years (Landstedt-Hallin *et al.* 1999). Cardiac arrhythmias have been observed during experimentally induced hypoglycaemia and in anecdotal case reports in diabetic individuals who had no overt clinical features of heart disease (Lindström *et al.* 1992, Fisher and Heller 1999). Sudden death during hypoglycaemia-induced cardiac arrhythmia has also been described (Frier *et al.* 1995, Burke and Kearney 1999). Acute myocardial infarction and congestive cardiac failure may also be precipitated by acute hypoglycaemia (Fisher and Heller 1999).

Psychological and neurological manifestations of acute hypoglycaemia are varied and can affect sensory and motor functions. Transient ischaemic attacks and hemiplegia can result from severe neuroglycopenia. In a retrospective review of 778 cases of drug-induced hypoglycaemia, a permanent neurological deficit was described in 5 per cent (Seltzer 1972). The neurological sequelae of hypoglycaemia may result from different mechanisms, such as direct focal cerebral damage from neuroglycopenia; acute thrombotic occlusion associated with the haemodynamic, haematological and haemorrheological changes that are associated with hypoglycaemia; or by cerebral ischaemia provoked by changes in regional blood flow in the brain (Perros and Deary 1999).

Diagnosis and treatment

Hypoglycaemia is only one of several differential diagnoses in a person who presents in a confused or comatose state, but a known diagnosis of diabetes should arouse suspicion that the cause may be metabolic. Clues to the diagnosis will often be found in the hand luggage of the ill passenger (blood glucose meter, testing strips, insulin, etc.) and this should be examined as part of the assessment of the passenger who has reduced consciousness. Although manifestations of cerebrovascular disease may be suspected, hypoglycaemia should be excluded by measurement of the blood glucose if this is possible. However, even when the blood glucose is low, other common causes such as stroke, intracerebral or subarachnoid haemorrhage, head injury, either deliberate or accidental drug overdose and excessive alcohol ingestion should not be overlooked. A failure either to respond rapidly, or at all, to treatment with intravenous dextrose should raise the possibility that the coma has a different cause.

In the conscious individual with insulin-treated diabetes, acute hypoglycaemia is treated with rapid-acting oral carbohydrate, usually in the form of glucose tablets, confectionery such as sweets or chocolate, or beverages with a high glucose content, such as fresh orange juice. Some form of long-acting carbohydrate (bread, biscuits, cereal or other alternatives) should then be consumed to prevent recurrence of the hypoglycaemia.

In the drowsy or unconscious adult who cannot swallow safely, an intravenous injection of dextrose (20–50 ml of a 50 per cent solution) will reverse neuroglycopenia rapidly. Glucagon (1 mg by intramuscular injection) is also effective if administered to a hypoglycaemic individual who is semiconscious or comatose, but it can induce nausea and/or vomiting as a side effect. Because it acts by breaking down hepatic glycogen to produce glucose, it is sometimes ineffective in patients with protracted hypoglycaemia whose stores of glycogen are already exhausted, in people with advanced liver disease or alcohol abuse and in those with malnutrition or inanition.

Mild sulphonylurea-induced hypoglycaemia is treated in a similar way to insulin-induced hypoglycaemia. Hypoglycaemic coma requires intravenous dextrose and treatment in hospital because hypoglycaemia from sulphonylureas (particularly following overdose) is often prolonged with frequent relapses (Gale 1980, Marks 1981a, Ferner and Neil 1988). Following a bolus intravenous injection of 20–50 ml of 50 per cent dextrose, many patients require a prolonged intravenous infusion of 10 per cent (or even 20 per cent) dextrose to maintain a blood glucose concentration above 5.0 mmol l^{-1}, and these solutions are unlikely to be available on a commercial

flight. Suspicion of sulphonylurea-induced hypoglycaemic coma would require diversion of the flight to arrange early hospital treatment for the affected passenger. Cerebral oedema, a further complication of severe hypoglycaemia, causes depressed consciousness, has a high morbidity and mortality and requires urgent medical treatment. Because glucagon stimulates insulin secretion, it is therefore said to be contraindicated in the treatment of sulphonylurea-induced hypoglycaemia (Marri et al. 1968) in people with type 2 diabetes, many of whom have residual pancreatic β-cell function, but the evidence for this is sparse.

Alcohol

The role of excessive consumption of alcohol during air travel has aroused considerable concern, mainly because of the effect of drunken behaviour of passengers in the confined space of an aircraft, and alcohol abuse has been implicated in cases of 'air rage'. However, both in non-diabetic and diabetic passengers, the consumption of pre-flight and in-flight alcoholic drinks can affect the blood glucose during travel and predisposes to an increased risk of hypoglycaemia. The net effect of alcohol on blood glucose depends on numerous factors, including the quantity and the type of alcoholic beverage consumed, the relation to previous meals, the nature and quantity of food consumed, the circulating plasma insulin concentration and the hepatic store of glycogen.

Whilst alcohol (7 kcal g^{-1}) in beverages may also contribute to total caloric intake, the important and potentially dangerous metabolic effect is inhibition of hepatic gluconeogenesis, even at blood alcohol concentrations that are not usually associated with intoxication. In people with type 1 diabetes, alcohol impairs the ability to perceive and interpret the symptoms of hypoglycaemia (Kerr et al. 1990) and, unfortunately, many of the neuroglycopenic features of hypoglycaemia may be mistaken for alcohol intoxication. During a flight, this misinterpretation could have potentially serious consequences if the wrong treatment is given in error.

By a similar mechanism (inhibition of hepatic gluconeogenesis), hypoglycaemia may also occur in non-diabetic persons if a substantial quantity of alcohol is consumed, while fasting or after eating insufficient food. Alcohol intoxication is the commonest cause of hypoglycaemia observed in the community setting in the non-diabetic population (Marks 1981b). The risk of hypoglycaemia is greatest when hepatic glycogen stores are depleted by fasting, or after periods of starvation or malnutrition, so it may be aggravated in people with chronic alcoholism or states of inanition associated with other diseases. In addition, alcohol may increase the severity of iatrogenic hypoglycaemia and may cause brain damage when associated with insulin-induced hypoglycaemia (Arky *et al.* 1968). A risk of early reactive hypoglycaemia may occur if mixers with a high sugar content stimulate the secretion of insulin in people who have residual endogenous insulin secretory capacity (many people with type 2 diabetes). Alcohol consumption before and during air travel is inadvisable in people with diabetes, in view of the problems that may be caused with glycaemic control, and the potential risk of inducing hypoglycaemia. The ingestion of water or non-alcoholic drinks is preferable as this avoids dehydration, whereas alcohol has the opposite effect as it induces a diuresis. Dehydration may have indirect effects such as encouraging the development of deep venous thrombosis (see Chapter 15).

HYPERGLYCAEMIA AND DETERIORATION IN GLYCAEMIC CONTROL

Deterioration in glycaemic control may occur during air travel, aggravated by taking insufficient insulin, inappropriate food, inadequate fluid intake and intercurrent illness, such as gastrointestinal disturbance, nausea, vomiting (travel sickness) and diarrhoea. In more extreme situations, the life-threatening metabolic disturbances of diabetic ketoacidosis (DKA) and hyperosmolar non-ketosis may develop, particularly in association with intercurrent illness. The former could potentially develop during a long-haul flight in a person with type 1 diabetes who has an intercurrent illness such as a urinary tract or respiratory infection or gastrointestinal upset, and rarely it could be the initial presentation of undiagnosed type 1 diabetes. Unusual and opportunistic infections (such as fungal infection) and tropical diseases may occur in the traveller with diabetes, particularly if they have poor glycaemic control.

Diabetic ketoacidosis

DKA is a state of uncontrolled catabolism associated with an absolute or relative deficiency of insulin. Elevated plasma concentrations of counter-regulatory hormones contribute to the condition and the pathophysiological processes shown in Figure 20.1. With insufficient insulin, hepatic glucose production is increased, and peripheral utilization of glucose by tissues such as muscle is reduced, leading to uncontrolled hyperglycaemia. This causes an osmotic diuresis, with polyuria promoting the loss of fluid and electrolytes, leading to severe dehydration. Plasma osmolality rises and renal perfusion falls. At the same time, lipolysis is stimulated, leading to elevated plasma concentrations of free fatty acids, which are metabolized within the liver, with the production of ketone bodies. Their accumulation produces a metabolic acidosis. These metabolic abnormalities are typically associated with nausea and vomiting, leading to further loss of fluid and electrolytes. The excess ketones are excreted in the urine (ketonuria) and are exhaled in the breath, producing a distinctive smell of pear drops, similar to acetone. Respiratory compensation for the acidosis leads to hyperventilation, described as 'air hunger' or Kussmaul respiration. Progressive dehydration impairs renal excretion of hydrogen ions and ketones, further aggravating the acidosis. If un-treated, severe DKA is invariably fatal, *and this is a medical emergency that requires an immediate diversion and urgent hospital treatment.*

In addition to features of uncontrolled diabetes (polyuria, polydipsia, fatigue and lethargy), there may be associated nausea and vomiting, hyperventilation (air hunger), and abdominal pain (mainly in children) which can confuse the diagnosis. In severely ill patients, confusion and stupor may be present. Coma is a late manifestation and is unlikely to be the presenting problem of DKA in the air traveller with diabetes. To reach this stage of DKA during a flight would be very unusual, as it is likely that the affected person would have been too ill to embark on the aircraft! Most cases of impending DKA are likely to be encountered at a relatively early stage, when a patient is becoming unwell as a result of intercurrent illness. A rapid clinical examination may reveal dehydration, with features such as dry tongue, decreased skin turgor and tachycardia with the characteristic odour of acetone being detected on the breath.

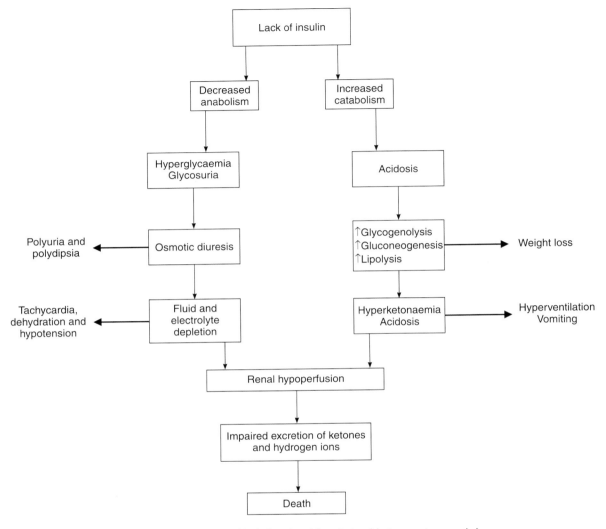

Figure 20.1 *Pathophysiology of diabetic ketoacidosis (DKA) and its relationship to symptoms and signs.*

Metabolic decompensation can be confirmed by demonstrating hyperglycaemia (with measurement of a blood glucose if possible) and a metabolic acidosis can be inferred by the presence of ketonuria if this can be measured. However, ketonuria can also be present after fasting and may be found in individuals with alcoholic intoxication. The actual level of blood glucose is not a reliable guide to the severity of the metabolic disturbance in DKA, and occasionally hyperglycaemia may not be prominent, especially when DKA complicates a diabetic pregnancy. Deterioration in the clinical condition can occur rapidly, and unnecessary delays in arranging emergency medical treatment could have serious consequences, including the development of life-threatening cerebral oedema.

Emergency management of early DKA

A reasonable approach to the emergency management of early DKA during a flight is outlined in Table 20.7, but will be restricted by the availability of testing and treatment materials. It may be possible to manage early cases if the individual can drink relatively freely. An adequate intake of fluid with small doses of short-

Table 20.7 *Management of hyperglycaemia and vomiting during air flight – advice for insulin-treated passengers*

- Aim to drink 4–6 pints of sugar-free liquid over 24 hours
- If unable to eat, replace the carbohydrate in food with alternatives such as milk, ice cream or fruit juice
- Insulin should NEVER be withheld. Test the blood glucose every 2–4 hours. If the blood glucose is 7–11 mmol l^{-1}, continue with the usual insulin dose. If blood glucose is less than 7 mmol l^{-1}, the insulin dose may be marginally reduced to avoid precipitating hypoglycaemia
- If blood glucose is between 11 and 15 mmol l^{-1}, take an extra 4 units of short-acting insulin (soluble insulin, insulin analogue, or fixed mixture if this is the only insulin available) at each injection
- If blood glucose is greater than 15 mmol l^{-1}, take an extra 6 units of above insulin
- If blood glucose is persistently at levels of 15 mmol l^{-1} or greater in association with ketonuria, active medical care and further assessment may be necessary

acting insulin may avoid the progression to severe metabolic decompensation. Few aircraft carry a sufficient supply of intravenous fluids, so parenteral replacement of fluid is not an option. The drowsy or semi-unconscious patient requires urgent medical treatment and this will require diversion of the aircraft to the nearest large city for emergency medical care.

HYPEROSMOLAR NON-KETOTIC SYNDROME

Hyperosmolar non-ketotic syndrome is characterized by pronounced hyperglycaemia (often in excess of 50 mmol l^{-1}), with no acidosis but with severe dehydration and pre-renal failure, leading to drowsiness and depression of consciousness. It usually occurs in middle-aged and elderly subjects with uncontrolled (and often undiagnosed) type 2 diabetes and has an insidious onset. Progressive thirst and polyuria have often led to the consumption of beverages high in refined sugars, and dehydration may have been aggravated by profuse sweating in high temperatures in a hot, humid climate. These individuals are very sensitive to insulin and do not require large doses to lower the blood glucose. However, the fluid depletion requires urgent intravenous fluid replacement, and this condition has a much higher mortality than DKA.

CONCOMITANT MEDICAL CONDITIONS AND DIABETIC COMPLICATIONS

Individuals with diabetes may suffer both from microvascular and macrovascular complications of diabetes and may be taking several concurrent medications. Some diabetic complications may cause problems during air travel. During flights, the Valsalva manoeuvre is commonly used by passengers to overcome the effects of barotitis media. However, this form of straining may increase the risk of vitreous haemorrhage occurring in people who have untreated proliferative retinopathy and have new vessels visible on ophthalmoscopy. The Valsalva manoeuvre should be avoided in people who have active diabetic eye disease. If they have clinical evidence of recent vitreous haemorrhage on indirect ophthalmoscopy, or have untreated proliferative retinopathy with neovascularization, they should be advised not to fly. People with diabetes should not fly immediately after eye surgery including resection of cataracts and vitreoretinal surgery.

Cardiovascular disease

Cardiovascular disease and hypertension are common in people with diabetes, particularly in older patients with type 2 diabetes. Mortality and morbidity following myocardial infarction is greater in people with diabetes, with development of a higher frequency of cardiac failure. Recent myocardial infarction, unstable angina, poorly controlled congestive heart failure and recurrent cardiac arrhythmias are contraindications to air travel in people with diabetes. Those who have a history of cardiovascular disease should carry a detailed history of their previous problems and current therapy, keep a supply of medications on their person or in their hand luggage, and avoid carrying this in baggage stored in the hold of the aeroplane.

Venous thromboembolism

Although this potential complication of air travel has not been reported to occur with greater frequency in travellers with diabetes, the increased viscosity and hypercoagulability associated with chronic hyperglycaemia may enhance the risk of venous thrombosis. Prophylactic measures are no different from people who do not have diabetes and are discussed elsewhere in this book. Diabetic patients with nephrotic syndrome secondary to diabetic nephropathy may be at increased risk of venous thromboembolism due to a loss of fibrinolytic factors in urine, increased synthesis of clotting factors, thrombocytosis and over-diuresis.

Diabetic neuropathy

Some travellers who have peripheral neuropathy may develop dependent oedema in-flight, and people with neuropathic feet should wear appropriate and comfortable footwear during flights. In people who have autonomic neuropathy, postural hypotension may occur, particularly in patients who may also be taking antihypertensive medication. It may be necessary for them to lie down on the floor of the aircraft to maintain their cerebral circulation. Limited cabin space may make this difficult and commercial aircraft do not have areas that can be used as a sickbay. Postural hypotension may be exacerbated by dehydration, so adequate intake of fluid and avoidance of alcohol are essential, and the use of elasticated stockings may be beneficial.

CONCLUSION

The air traveller with diabetes has the potential to present with a variety of problems related to this complex condition, its complications and treatment. Many of the metabolic problems, such as hypoglycaemia, are rapidly reversible, although others may be less amenable to emergency therapeutic measures. However, with careful planning, professional advice on treatment and attention to self-management, the potential for disturbance of metabolic control can be avoided, allowing people with diabetes to pursue long-distance air travel without personal adversity.

When asked to assist an unwell passenger in-flight, the health-care professional should be mindful that the problem may be related to a complication of diabetes or its treatment, especially in passengers with a reduced conscious level. Aggressive or odd behaviour should arouse suspicion of hypoglycaemia and corroboratory evidence should be sought, such as a medical identity bracelet or the finding of syringes, pens, insulin or blood glucose testing equipment in hand luggage. Many acute metabolic problems relating to diabetes can be managed in-flight without the need for diversion of the flight to obtain emergency medical treatment, but suspected diabetic ketoacidosis may require intensive therapy and unnecessary delays could have serious consequences.

REFERENCES

Arky RA, Veverbrants E and Abramson EA. Irreversible hypoglycemia. A complication of alcohol and insulin. *J Am Med Assoc* 1968; **206**: 575–8.

Benson E and Metz R. Management of diabetes during intercontinental travel. *Bull Mason Clin* 1984; **38**: 145–51.

Blackman JD, Towle VL, Sturis J, Lewis GF, Spire JP and Polonsky KS. Hypoglycemic thresholds for cognitive dysfunction in IDDM. *Diabetes* 1992; **41**: 392–9.

Brodows RG. Benefits and risks with glyburide and glipizide in elderly NIDDM patients. *Diabetes Care* 1992; **15**: 75–80.

Browne DL, Avery L, Turner BC, Kerr D and Cavan DA. What do patients with diabetes know about their tablets? *Diabetic Med* 2000; **17**: 528–31.

Burge MR, Zeise TM, Sobhy TA, Rassam AG and Schade DS. Low-dose ethanol predisposes elderly fasted patients with Type 2 diabetes to sulfonylurea-induced low blood glucose. *Diabetes Care* 1999; **22**: 2037–43.

Burke BJ and Kearney TK. Hypoglycaemia and cardiac arrest. *Pract Diab Internat* 1999; **16**: 189–90.

Campbell RK. Glimepiride: role of a new sulfonylurea in the treatment of Type 2 diabetes mellitus. *Ann Pharmacotherapy* 1998; **32**: 1044–52.

Cottrell JJ, Callaghan JT, Kohn GM, Hensler EC and Rogers RM. In-flight medical emergencies. One year of experience with the enhanced medical kit. *J Am Med Assoc* 1989; **262**: 1653–6.

Cryer PE. Glucose counterregulation: the prevention and correction of hypoglycemia in humans. *Am J Physiol* 1993; **264**: E149–55.

Cryer PE, Binder C, Bolli GB *et al*. Hypoglycemia in IDDM. *Diabetes* 1989; **38**: 1193–9.

Cummins RO and Schubach JA. Frequency and types of medical emergencies among commercial air travelers. *J Am Med Assoc* 1989; **261**: 1295–9.

Ferner RE and Neil HA. Sulphonylureas and hypoglycaemia. *Br Med J* 1988; **296**: 949–50.

Fisher BM and Heller SR. Mortality, cardiovascular morbidity and possible effects of hypoglycaemia on diabetic complications. In Frier BM and Fisher BM (eds), *Hypoglycaemia in Clinical Diabetes*. Chichester: John Wiley and Sons, 1999; 167–86.

Frier BM, Barr StCG and Walker JD. Fatal cardiac arrest following acute hypoglycaemia in a diabetic patient. *Pract Diab Internat* 1995; **12**: 284.

Gale EAM. Hypoglycaemia. *Clin Endocrinol Metab* 1980; **9**: 461–75.

Gautier JF, Bigard AX, Douce P, Duvallet A and Cathelineau G. Influence of simulated altitude on the performance of five blood glucose meters. *Diabetes Care* 1996; **19**: 1430–3.

Gill GV and Redmond S. Insulin treatment, time-zones and air travel: a survey of current advice from British diabetic clinics. *Diabetic Med* 1993; **10**: 764–7.

Johnston RV, Neilly IJ, Lang JM and Frier BM. The high flying diabetic: dietary inadequacy of airline meals. *Diabetic Med* 1986; **3**: 580A (abstract).

Kerr D, Macdonald IA, Heller SR and Tattersall RB. Alcohol causes hypoglycaemic unawareness in healthy volunteers and patients with Type I (insulin-dependent) diabetes. *Diabetologia* 1990; **33**: 216–21.

Landstedt-Hallin L, Englund A, Adamson U and Lins PE. Increased QT dispersion during hypoglycaemia in patients with Type 2 diabetes. *J Intern Med* 1999; **246**: 299–307.

Lindgren M, Eckert B, Stenberg G and Agardh CD. Restitution of neurophysiological functions, performance, and subjective symptoms after moderate insulin-induced hypoglycaemia in non-diabetic men. *Diabetic Med* 1996; **13**: 218–25.

Lindström T, Jorfeldt L, Tegler L and Arnqvist HJ. Hypoglycaemia and cardiac arrhythmias in patients with Type 2 diabetes mellitus. *Diabetic Med* 1992; **9**: 536–41.

Marks V. Drug-induced hypoglycaemia. In Marks V and Rose FC (eds), *Hypoglycaemia*, 2nd edn. Oxford: Blackwell Scientific, 1981a; 357–86.

Marks V. Alcohol-induced hypoglycaemia. In Marks V and Rose FC (eds), *Hypoglycaemia*, 2nd edn. Oxford: Blackwell Scientific, 1981b; 387–98.

Marques JLB, George E, Peacey SR *et al*. Altered ventricular repolarisation during hypoglycaemia in patients with diabetes. *Diabetic Med* 1997; **14**: 648–54.

Marri G, Cozzolino G and Palumbo R. Glucagon in sulphonylurea hypoglycaemia? *Lancet* 1968; **i**: 303–4.

McAulay V and Frier BM. Hypoglycaemia. In Sinclair AJ, Finucane P (eds), *Diabetes in Old Age*, 2nd edn. Chichester: John Wiley and Sons, 2000; 133–52.

Perros P and Deary IJ. Long-term effects of hypoglycaemia on cognitive function and the brain in diabetes. In Frier BM, Fisher BM (eds), *Hypoglycaemia in Clinical Diabetes*. Chichester: John Wiley and Sons, 1999; 187–210.

Schneider J. An overview of the safety and tolerance of glimepiride. *Horm Metab Res* 1996; **28**: 413–18.

Seltzer HS. Drug-induced hypoglycemia: a review based on 473 cases. *Diabetes* 1972; **21**: 955–66.

Speizer C, Rennie CJ and Breton H. Prevalence of in-flight medical emergencies on commercial flights. *Ann Emerg Med* 1989; **18**: 26–9.

Stahl M and Berger W. Higher incidence of severe hypoglycaemia leading to hospital admission in Type 2 diabetic patients treated with long-acting versus short-acting sulphonylureas. *Diabetic Med* 1999; **16**: 586–90.

Tessier D, Dawson K, Tetrault JP, Bravo G and Meneilly GS. Glibenclamide vs gliclazide in Type 2 diabetes of the elderly. *Diabetic Med* 1994; **11**: 974–80.

UK Prospective Diabetes Study Group. Intensive blood-glucose control with sulphonylureas or insulin compared with conventional treatment and risk of complications in patients with Type 2 diabetes (UKPDS 33). *Lancet* 1998; **352**: 837–53.

The neurological patient

MICHAEL D O'BRIEN

There are few contraindications to commercial flights for passengers with neurological disease. Most of these relate to the degree of disability and can be divided into problems that may arise at airports and those which may arise in flight. Large airports throughout the world tend to have the necessary facilities for disabled travellers as they have been built since the needs of the disabled have been more widely recognized. These include wheelchair access and toilet facilities, and many airports provide wheelchairs or will transport patients with mobility problems in special buggies. Smaller airports, particularly in less developed countries, may not have these facilities though the buildings may be on a single level.

However, there will be the problem of access to the aircraft, if the only way of getting aboard is up a flight of steep steps. Sometimes the food truck has a lift that can be used. Nevertheless, many travellers who are unable to walk the distances of large airports are able to climb a flight of steps into the aircraft, with assistance. Airports and airlines are helpful, but they must be consulted in advance. Modern aircraft are often crowded and cramped places, and the choice of seat may be important for some disabled passengers. Again, the airline should be consulted well in advance so that an appropriate reservation can be made. An aisle seat near the lavatories is often preferable, particularly if there is gangway space in front of the seat. Sometimes these seats cannot be used by disabled passengers because the gangway provides access to the emergency exit. Passengers unable to get to a lavatory unaided should travel with a companion.

DEFICIT WITHOUT RISK OF PROGRESSION

Patients in this group who are not affected by the hypoxia of the cabin environment are the easiest to advise because the problem can be assessed before flight and appropriate steps taken. Such conditions include stable neurological disorders such as a traumatic paraplegia, congenital abnormalities (spina bifida), old strokes, the consequences of subarachnoid, subdural and extradural haemorrhages, and the sequelae of head injury and neurosurgical procedures. However, it is a matter for individual judgement when a condition has become stable. This is not a problem for distant events, but the question often arises when the decision has to be made about how soon after an event, which may have occurred abroad, is it safe for the patient to return home. The decision must be related to the length of the journey and whether the condition might be affected by the cabin hypoxia. Patients who need transport when potentially unstable usually travel with a medical assistance company. The carriage of the seriously ill is dealt with in a later chapter.

In some patients their condition may be affected by the hypoxia of the cabin. The cabin of a modern jet aircraft is pressurized to the equivalent of 5000–8000 feet and this leads to a significant reduction in alveolar oxygen tension, though limited changes in saturation. In the vast majority of neurological problems this will have no adverse effect, but in certain circumstances it may be sufficient to cause deterioration in function, although this may be only temporary. The brain stores neither oxygen nor glucose and so depends on a constant delivery of blood to supply these needs. There are complex and sophisticated methods of maintaining a constant blood supply. Over quite a wide physiological range of systemic blood pressures, cerebral blood flow is maintained constant by a variation in blood vessel diameter. The vessels constrict to rising pressures – a process known as autoregulation. Cerebral blood flow autoregulates to both changes in pressure and to changes in oxygen and glucose content of the blood.

If the blood pressure falls below the level at which this compensatory vasodilation fails, the next step is an increase in the oxygen extraction. When this fails, the cerebral metabolism is affected and the subject goes through pre-syncope and then syncope. The thresholds at which this occurs are raised in the elderly whose blood vessels are less elastic and particularly in patients with a long history of hypertension. Oxygen saturation may also be affected by pulmonary disease, which may aggravate the problem, and hypoglycaemia in patients with diabetes would also contribute to these processes. The reduction in cabin oxygen pressure results in a compensatory vasodilation, using up some of the reserve. This may be sufficient to produce clinical manifestations in certain patients.

A susceptible group of patients is those with evidence of small vessel disease producing widespread white matter change. Patients who are already showing signs of cognitive impairment might become more confused, whilst patients without obvious evidence of cognitive impairment could also be affected, particularly on long overnight flights where the cabin lights are dimmed. These patients are mostly elderly and with hypertension usually of long standing. There may also be a problem with patients who have had a recent cerebrovascular event or a recent head injury. The precise interval after which it is safe to fly is, of course, dependent on the severity of the event. Patients with sickle cell disease may also be affected.

DEFICITS WITH RISK OF PROGRESSION

Very few neurological conditions in which there is a risk of progression are likely to deteriorate within the time scale of even a long-haul flight. The length of the flight is much more a problem for patients with impaired mobility. However, some rare conditions such as cerebral arteriovenous malformation, cerebral lupus and primary cerebral arteritis may show deterioration within this time scale. Neurological conditions tend to be relatively chronic and although the underlying condition is progressive, a significant change during the flight is unlikely. This would include multiple sclerosis, Parkinson's disease, motor neurone disease, the inherited ataxias, peripheral neuropathy, most muscle diseases both acquired and the dystrophies, and cervical myelopathy. For these patients the problem is that of their disability rather than any risk of a new problem arising during flight.

EPISODIC EVENTS

Patients known to suffer from episodic events may well have attacks either at the airport or in the aircraft. Common conditions include migraine, epilepsy, syncope, panic attacks, vertigo and transient ischaemic attacks.

Syncope

Syncope may occur for a number of reasons. Simple syncope is unlikely to occur while sitting without clear provocation and can be dealt with by lying the subject as flat as possible. Syncope is much more likely to occur in the context of claustrophobia and panic attacks. Patients who are known to be claustrophobic or to have experienced the problem on a previous aircraft can seek advice from a clinical psychologist about how to handle this phobia. Many patients with mild symptoms manage with a tranquillizer taken an hour or so before the flight. A benzodiazepine such as diazepam or lorazepam is often suitable. Patients with a recent history of transient ischaemic attacks should be appraised before a flight and, although the risk is small, only flights in an emergency should be undertaken without such an assessment.

Epilepsy

Epilepsy is much more a problem, particularly if the passenger is liable to major convulsive seizures. There are several reasons why a patient with epilepsy may have an attack during a flight. These include missing their medication. Their medication may have been forgotten or packed with the checked luggage. Sometimes patients become confused about the timing of the medication, which may be important with some short-acting drugs. Fits may also occur because of lack of sleep, irregular meals and alcohol. Patients with poorly controlled major seizures should seek advice from a neurologist before embarking on a flight.

Patients with reasonably well controlled or completely controlled epilepsy should ensure that they have their medication with them, that they take their drugs throughout the flight on the same schedule that they were using before the flight and only consider changing the timing of dosage once they arrive at their destination. Again advice should be sought from their neurologist as to whether it is more appropriate to take a slightly increased dose or a slightly reduced dose in a period of 24 hours. This is the choice with patients who take their medication twice a day and then undertake a 6-hour flight. Patients with epilepsy should avoid alcohol throughout the flight and maintain good hydration. Those who are sensitive to sleep deprivation may benefit from a benzodiazepine such as clobazam or clonazepam for an overnight flight. Patients with a liability to major seizures should, of course, travel with an appropriate companion who can handle these situations. Only under exceptional circumstances would it be appropriate to carry a supply of rectal diazepam.

Migraine

Patients liable to attacks of migraine will be familiar with their problem and its management. Once again, it is better to avoid alcohol, to maintain hydration, to try to sleep on overnight flights, and to use their medication. Patients particularly prone to severe attacks should carry a tryptan, having ascertained before the flight that this is an effective treatment.

Vertigo

Passengers prone to episodic vertigo may also have attacks on flights and this can be quite disabling. Such patients should travel with a supply of an antiemetic drug such as prochlorperazine or cinnarizine and consider taking some medication prophylactically. Prochlorperazine is available as a tablet, by injection or by suppository.

Rarer conditions

Much rarer conditions include cluster headaches, familial periodic cerebellar ataxia, periodic paralysis, and the narcolepsy/cataplexy syndrome. Patients with these conditions will be well aware of their problems and should seek advice on how to deal with these events. There is no particular reason why any of these conditions is likely to be triggered by flying, but of course any of them could occur during a flight. Patients should be informed on how to handle such events, and many carry appropriate medication. In an aircraft an effective treatment for cluster headache is readily available, and that is oxygen.

IN-FLIGHT NEUROLOGICAL EVENTS

Assuming that other factors such as head injury and hypoglycaemia can be excluded, episodes of loss of consciousness are likely to be due either to epilepsy or to syncope. It can be difficult to distinguish these events, since a brief episode of loss of consciousness without any other associated features may be due to epilepsy, and syncope may be associated with some jerky movements, particularly if it is prolonged. Sometimes syncope will precipitate a major epileptic seizure.

Epileptic seizure

It is very unlikely for a first fit to occur during a flight. A passenger having a fit will almost certainly have a liability to epilepsy and this would probably be known by a travelling companion. Passengers travelling by themselves may not have sought advice before travelling and may not have alerted the carrier in advance. Sometimes patients carry armbands (Medic Alert) or some other identification. They may also carry medication indicating that they are taking medication for epilepsy and, more usefully, the nature of the medication. A major epileptic seizure occurring during a flight is likely to be over in a few minutes. The patient should be put in the recovery position, though turned onto one side with the seat fully reclined might be sufficient. Oxygen is unlikely to be useful, unless it is an anoxic fit. An airway is very seldom needed. Nothing should be put in the mouth, except perhaps the end of rolled handkerchief or serviette. If the attack is over within a minute or two, no further action is required and the patient will recover. Diazepam should not be given in these circumstances, since it would do nothing for the fit and makes a subsequent assessment more difficult.

If the fitting continues or a second fit occurs without full recovery, diazepam should be given and is now available in most aircraft medical kits. Diazepam 20 mg as Diazemuls (10 mg in 2 ml) should be given intravenously, the first 10 mg as a bolus and the second 10 mg by slow infusion over 10 minutes. Rectal diazepam may also be effective, but might not be easy to administer on an aircraft. Intramuscular diazepam is not very effective and should be avoided. If fitting continues, a second dose of diazepam may be given, but certainly no more because of the danger of respiratory depression.

A second fit without full recovery could well herald the onset of status epilepticus and the patient should be given intravenous phenytoin without further delay provided they are not already taking phenytoin. Phenytoin should be given intravenously in a dose of 15 mg kg^{-1} (500–900 mg) and it is essential that this is given very slowly (50 mg min^{-1}) to avoid cardiac effects. Phenytoin must not be given intramuscularly or subcutaneously. If a cardiac monitor is available, it should be used while phenytoin is injected. In these circumstances, the aircraft should divert to the nearest airport with facilities close by capable of handling this type of problem. Less severe epileptic attacks do not require any special management and when the patient recovers possible reasons for the fit should be determined from the patient or companion. If this is due to missing antiepileptic medication, then their usual medication should be taken. Other factors such as alcohol, missed meals and missed sleep cannot be instantly rectified.

Syncopal attack

There will be little confusion about a syncopal attack that follows classic features with an aura stage of feeling faint and dizzy, pallor, rapid pulse, often rapid deep breathing leading to blurring of vision and distortion of sounds before loss of consciousness. A simple faint will respond rapidly to appropriate positioning, although this may be difficult in an aircraft. The patient may have to be put on the floor since many seats do not recline sufficiently. Any delay in achieving this will prolong and aggravate the syncope. Oxygen may be given, but no other intervention is required. It may be that the initial stages of a faint are unnoticed and that the patient is observed simply to lose consciousness. Sometimes syncope will produce jerky movements of the limbs, which may be mistaken for epilepsy. Appropriate positioning will quickly restore consciousness and these patients should not be given diazepam. In older patients, the possibility of cardiac syncope may need to be considered.

Head injury

Head injury occurs quite often in aircraft, due to heavy items such as computers and bottles falling out of the overhead luggage bins. Head injury may also occur from sudden and unexpected turbulence if the passenger is not wearing a seatbelt or is walking about the cabin. Minor head injury without loss of consciousness does not require any special intervention except analgesia, if requested. Head injury with brief loss of consciousness and rapid recovery can be managed in the same way. Head injury with prolonged loss of consciousness, blood in the ear indicating a skull base fracture, deteriorating consciousness levels after initial recovery, or the development of physical signs such as pupillary inequality are all indications for diversion to the nearest airport with appropriate facilities. This may well be the planned destination. There is, of course, no point in diverting to an airport without appropriate facilities. Sedation should be avoided unless confusion causes a management problem.

Headaches

Headaches occur quite commonly in-flight and most can be treated with reassurance and mild analgesia. It is unlikely that migraine will occur during a flight for the first time, and, in any case, patients subject to migraine should be carrying their usual medication. If not, a combination of an analgesic such as aspirin or paracetamol (acetaminophen) together with an antiemetic such as metoclopramide or prochlorperazine may be all that is necessary. Sudden severe headaches, particularly if associated with loss of consciousness, may suggest a subarachnoid haemorrhage – although in one survey only 10 per cent of patients presenting in primary care with sudden headache had a subarachnoid haemorrhage. This rose to 40 per cent of those attending hospital. Neck stiffness may take hours to develop and its absence initially does not exclude subarachnoid haemorrhage. Subhyaloid haemorrhages are a good marker. If the suspicion of subarachnoid haemorrhage is strong enough, the aircraft should be diverted to the nearest airport with appropriate facilities. There is little that can be done on the aircraft except to give analgesics (codeine phosphate can be effective) and general support measures.

Ischaemic attacks and stroke

Strokes can vary from relatively minor transient ischaemic attacks to major lobar infarcts. A major problem is that within a few minutes of the onset it is not possible to tell whether it is a transient ischaemic attack or a completed stroke since the time course will not be evident at that stage. A judgement can therefore only be made on the extent of the deficit at or shortly after onset. A hemiparesis including face, arm, hand and leg with a hemianopia and dysphasia, if it is on the appropriate side, is clear indication of an extensive infarct involving most of the territory of the middle cerebral artery. There is little that can be done in these circumstances except to maintain an adequate airway and supply oxygen. Steroids are of no proven benefit. Since such patients may deteriorate due to brain swelling, it would be advisable to divert to the nearest airport with appropriate facilities, even though there is very little in the way of intervention that is profitable at that stage. These patients are not appropriate for thrombolysis. Nor is it appropriate to load such patients with aspirin since the risk of bleeding at this stage is quite high and it may not be possible to differentiate between a deep-seated cerebral haemorrhage and a more extensive infarct. At the other end of the spectrum, a patient who develops a relatively minor deficit, perhaps including the face and hand only but without a field defect and without loss of consciousness, can be managed expectantly. A patient like this, not already on aspirin, can be given 600 mg, though it is perfectly reasonable to postpone this until arrival, particularly if there is any suspicion of haemorrhage. Most patients with stroke fall somewhere between these extremes and it is then a matter of judgement as to whether diversion is appropriate or not. This might depend on the general condition, the need for the maintenance of an airway, the location of the lesion and the time to destination.

22

Mental health: pre-flight and in-flight

E GRAHAM LUCAS

The World Health Organization definition of health is 'a state of mental, physical and social well-being' (1980), and this highlights the fact that the mental and physical components of any individual cannot be considered in isolation. The unity of health applies particularly in-flight, and encouraging 'health' in passengers and harmonious interpersonal relationships between crew and passengers is vital to the safety and well-being of all on board. Indeed, flight security can be compromised by passengers with irrational behaviour whether of psychological or physical origin. The well-adjusted and healthy person is flexible and can adapt to predictable and unpredictable stressors. On the other hand, the vulnerable person is less able to adapt and can easily overreact. In few places is this more critical than in an aircraft and this chapter deals with relevant aspects of personality, and the pre-flight assessment and in-flight management of specific conditions.

PSYCHOLOGICAL ASPECTS OF AIR TRAVEL

Initially it is worth looking at which aspects of air travel may affect the psychological well-being of the pas-
senger, particularly the first-time flier. The journey may, itself, have particular significance. It could be a much-coveted holiday, an important business meeting, or a reluctant relocation. It could involve separation from loved ones, visiting a seriously ill relative, or coping with a bereavement. Some passengers may be travelling alone, or to an unfamiliar destination. The journey to the airport and the checking-in procedures could have been involved and tiring, and those in economy accommodation may be exposed to irritations from which those in more privileged situations are spared. Nevertheless, flight delays, lack of information and separation from luggage affect everyone.

Once aboard the aircraft, the aisles of the economy cabins are likely to be congested as the passengers often struggle to find their seats. Some passengers may find the safety demonstration worrisome, and then be disturbed by the unexplained noises of the take-off, air turbulence, and by illumination of the seat belt sign without adequate explanation. In such a confined space, the behaviour of other passengers may be irksome. Despite limits to on-board luggage, the hand luggage of other passengers may cause obstruction, other passengers may be noisy or smelly, and some may cause disturbance by behaving irrationally or by being anxious. Children and other passengers may be kicking the seat from behind. Finally, some may have fear of a sudden illness in circumstances that lack adequate medical attention. Such a scenario can easily affect personal vulnerability.

Although travel by air is less hazardous than that by train or car, the memory of rare, but terrifying, accidents is never far from the minds of some passengers whether they are reluctant occasional travellers or veterans of the sky. For them the risk of flying is exaggerated, and this is compounded by the fact that air disasters, as well as the potential for accidents, occupy a special place in the hearts of newspaper editors. From the Hindenburg explosion in 1937 to the Concorde accident over 60 years later, the uncertainties of air travel can stir the emotions. The memory of the horror of the suicide hijacking of September 11, 2001, which has added another dimension, illustrates the legacy of such traumatic events. Every air incident or accident receives wide media coverage, where speculation abounds. Television and newspapers spare few details and the explicit features and descriptions feed our voyeurism and anxieties. Newspaper articles such as 'One million good reasons to fly' and 'Happy landings for flying phobics' are difficult to find.

However, whilst flying is safer than the alternatives, this swift method of travel does not suit everyone for a variety of reasons. Even in the case of the sophisticated frequent flier, travel by air may be both mentally and physically a very different experience from travel by any other mode. A flight implies a degree of surrender of control greater than that of any other negotiable situation. Once on the aircraft there is no escape. For some, this situation fosters intense anxiety. Many well-known people, including footballers, are loth to fly. Generally, men are thought to be less able than women to admit fear in a variety of situations, and so within the context of flying they may react by becoming demanding and aggressive, and attempt to attain control.

BEHAVIOURAL EMERGENCIES

Anxiety related to flying does not necessarily signify morbidity, though the consequences are distressing and need to be identified and addressed. Any acutely disturbed behaviour sufficient to disrupt the flight or endanger other passengers or the crew calls for prompt attention. In extreme cases it may even be necessary to consider diverting the flight. The most common behavioural emergencies are panic attacks, alcohol- or drug-induced disruptions and confusion in the elderly. Air rage, the ultimate loss of self-control in an aeroplane, where surrender to circumstances is implicit, can erupt in those who are basically irritable with a low threshold for impulsive and angry behaviour, whether or not fuelled by alcohol. Occasionally, depressed passengers have committed suicide in flight. There is also the occasional in-flight death from natural causes, and witnessing such events can be distressing for passengers and cabin staff. In some cases such an event can trigger post-traumatic stress.

Prophylactic measures entail psychological techniques to minimize flight-related anxiety. These include psychotherapeutic programmes of anxiety management, or lay courses dealing with fear of flying. Help can also be provided and improvement facilitated by a relative or friend who is familiar with the condition. Cabin staff, trained in the basic techniques of anxiety management, are adept at coping with a wide range of behaviours. Hopefully, passengers with anxieties will confide in their medical practitioner or their occupational health physician, and sometimes a psychiatrist should be consulted. Pre-flight assessment with comprehensive direct questioning is crucial to the prevention of disruptive behaviour, and this will ultimately contribute to the safety and comfort of the flight. It must also be borne in mind that apart from diagnosable psychiatric illness, flight stress and anxiety can aggravate a range of physical conditions including psoriasis, headache, musculoskeletal pain, irritable bowel syndrome, asthma, tinnitus and vertigo.

MENTAL ILLNESS AND DISABILITY

The psychological aspects of physical illness and disability also need attention. Those who normally cope with such impairments may experience stress and anticipatory anxiety due to the potential effect of air travel on their underlying condition. These include pain of whatever origin, and other conditions dealt with elsewhere in this book. As with the elderly, disabled travellers frequently experience a range of stressors, even from kerbside and concourse, long before boarding. However, even though sensitively handled, they can suffer a sense of helplessness due to uncertainty regarding a possible emergency. Vertigo, tinnitus, impaired hearing and vision are not always easy to identify but may nevertheless be aggravated, and there is the need for tactful questioning and reassurance.

Apart from those whose disabilities are easily recognized, a significant proportion of passengers has health-related anxiety which can be exacerbated by air travel, and which is often associated with restricted access to facilities and medical assistance. These include the uncertainty of a recent medical investigation, diagnosis of a non-life-threatening illness, or an even more serious condition. Musculoskeletal pain, particularly in the back and neck, with impaired mobility, is a problem, and ischaemic heart disease, cardiac arrhythmias and recent bypass surgery may lead to stress and anxiety which may, in turn, precipitate angina. Those with asthma and chronic obstructive airways disease need careful monitoring. Menorrhagia, prostatism, irritable bowel syndrome, ileostomy or colostomy can all create anxiety when there are limited toilet facilities, and such people may need advice by an appropriate specialist. The risk of deep vein thrombosis is certainly a problem and has been widely featured by the media. As far as diabetes is concerned, dietary provision allays anxiety and self-help groups can contribute greatly. With skin diseases and those who wear contact lenses, discomfort may be exacerbated by the dryness of the air. Removal of contact lenses and insertion of artificial teardrops is helpful. General well-being is promoted by adequate water intake.

With these patients, pre-flight assessment needs to take into account their mental vulnerability. Anticipatory anxiety may easily be exacerbated. Asthma is particularly relevant as the control of breathing is the key to all anxiety management. Breathing techniques can be taught and practised before the flight and can prevent hyperventilation which can predispose to panic. As far as the flight is concerned, each illness and disability may require specific therapeutic support. As β-blockers are contraindicated in asthma and chronic obstructive airways disease, diazepam 1–5 mg is a useful anxiolytic and can be repeated.

SLEEP

Sleep is also crucial for mental and physical well-being, and long-haul flying can certainly exacerbate poor sleep. This is particularly common in stress and anxiety, and with the early morning waking of depression. The nightmares of post-traumatic stress disorder are also associated with sleep impairment and excessive nocturnal movements. Certainly, irritability and disorientation, particularly during long-haul flights, can be aggravated by sleep deprivation. Sleep disturbance is, therefore, of particular relevance in anxiety, depression and dementia. The basic management of any sleep-related disturbance is that sleep hygiene should be practised before and during the flight. This includes avoidance of heavy meals, alcohol, caffeine and not dealing with stressful business or domestic matters late in the evening. Relaxation techniques, soothing imagery and music can be used. Pre-flight short-acting hypnotics such as temazepam (10–20 mg) or zolpidem (5–10 mg) may be useful, whilst a small dose of promazine (25 mg) is preferable for the elderly. However, caution must be exercised with the use of hypnotics in flight as they may lead to immobility, and interact with alcohol.

PERSONALITY

Personality and the psychosocial aspects of flying determine the behaviour of all individuals on an aircraft. In turn, it is the individual's personality that will dictate their reaction to stress. Air passengers constitute a representative cross-section of the general population with concomitant ranges of personality traits and styles of behaviour. Traits and symptoms such as anxiety, sensitivity, cyclothymia (tendency to mood swings) and obsessionality can all become manifest or exaggerated, and can contribute to impulsive behaviour, to the detriment of the individual, crew and fellow passengers. In-flight, people of widely varying personality, age, language, ethnicity, intelligence and socioeconomic status are inevitably herded together. No matter how sensitively flight attendants address individual needs, there is no comparable group of people in which a person is so prevented from distancing himself or herself from an adjacent fellow being. Stress is the inevitable consequence. Therefore, it is helpful to identify people experiencing unacceptable stress, and so anticipate and effectively handle their various foibles. Acute interpersonal difficulties may arise due to different needs, reactions to unpredictable situations, and respective coping strategies.

Anger can be a function of unfulfilled high expectations. The frustration of the thwarted long-haul holiday traveller can create problems, and it is likely that the longer the journey and the more exotic the destination, the greater the expectation of enjoyment with the risk of disappointment and resentment if schedules are altered for whatever reason, marring the eagerly anticipated holiday. At the same time, the long-haul business traveller flying to a crucial meeting is also vulnerable, and if the tranquillity, empathy and cooperation expected from the attendants and promised by the airline does not materialize, resentment builds. In this way, the services of the cabin staff are frequently misunderstood. Their role is primarily that of safety, but they are, at times, ruthlessly exposed to passenger pressure. Such a job interfacing with a demanding and potentially aggressive section of the community is stressful. The primary role of cabin staff in safety must be emphasized.

Vulnerable personality traits alone or combined with minor psychiatric morbidity plus physical illness, all contribute to uncertainty, loss of control and anxiety. These can aggravate fear of flying and precipitate disturbed impulsive behaviour, panic attacks, alcohol or drug abuse and even air rage. In any pre-flight assessment, identification of these personality characteristics is essential. It is necessary to decide what is within the normal range and whether psychotherapeutic intervention is necessary to be fit to fly. In-flight it is best to avoid detailed dialogue, which may be perceived as confrontation. 'I do understand, how best can I help?' is the preferred approach. Simple language must be used, understanding demonstrated, and the passenger assured of the accessibility of the flight staff: 'I do understand how you feel, Sir, and I'll watch your overhead signal throughout the flight.'

Anxiety is associated with overreaction to a manageable situation, and with apprehension and foreboding regarding the worst scenario. Such individuals seek control and are distressed by its apparent loss. Social anxiety traits are very common and are often inappropriately labelled as 'shyness'. They predispose to withdrawal and isolation, and in extreme cases can result in social phobia. This can develop in particular situations such as flying where an unpleasant sensation such as choking can cause embarrassment. Individuals may feel that their fellow passengers are unsupportive.

Low self-esteem is associated with enhanced social anxiety. Such individuals are unable to trust themselves or others, or to tolerate risk, having a heightened need to control events and people. The obligatory surrender of control involved in air travel is severely testing. They, like others with anxiety, may seek reassurance by studying the facial expressions of the cabin staff, and are aware of unexpected movement, constantly listening for unusual noises. A paranoid person thrown into an unknown milieu can become suspicious, with a sense of self-importance, and perceive non-intended criticism from an innocuous remark. 'I'll be with you in a minute, Sir' can result in an irrational, exaggerated response based on paranoid thoughts. Obsessional and hypochondriacal (health-related anxiety) traits exist in individuals who may demand extra attention from the cabin staff and compliance from other passengers. They will react adversely if thwarted.

It is necessary to identify patients whose health may be adversely affected by air travel, and those whose ill health could adversely affect the flight. Passengers are required to inform the airline of any significant illness so as to facilitate pre-flight assessment. A copy of current psychotropic medication and dosage should be carried as this facilitates in-flight medical management either by a doctor on board or through a ground medical adviser. Nevertheless, psychiatric morbidity, apart from flying-related anxiety, is often not declared. This could be considered, in some ways, as indicating restoration of confidence with attenuation of the illness.

ANXIETY

Anxiety may not be recognized pre-flight as it frequently presents with somatic complaints. Anxiety, as well as depression, predisposes to excessive use of alcohol, caffeine, smoking and comfort eating. Sleep impairment, particularly in getting off to sleep, is a key feature, and is further aggravated by these agents, and by excessive eating late at night. Anxiety (free-floating) may well predispose to fear of flying. Panic attacks are a separate entity, although inevitably there is some overlap. Anxiety is characterized by unrealistic and excessive worry about any life situation. It may be flying, lifts, or heights, or interacting with others (social anxiety). The mood of anxious passengers is further aggravated by annoyances such as noise, especially crying babies. Any encroachment such as kicking or tilting of the seat in front compounds irritation. Many passengers consider that turbulence signifies that the pilot is not in complete control, however temporarily. Thus switching on the seat-belt sign with an announcement of impending turbulence may awaken a latent fear in someone previously calm during the flight.

The management of anxiety commences pre-flight with sleep hygiene, appropriate time structuring and practical advice on stress and anxiety management. Teaching the individual to identify 'What if…?' thinking, and regular exercise is helpful. However, if the flight is imminent and cannot be postponed, a simple explanation of turbulence can be reassuring. The use of the lowest effective dose of a benzodiazepine such as diazepam 1–5 mg at an appropriate time prior to the flight can be useful. Alternatively, provided there is no history of asthma, a β-blocker can be used. In-flight it is useful for passengers to remind themselves of the pre-flight explanation of turbulence, avoid alcohol and caffeine, and practise previously acquired breathing and relaxation techniques including imagery, thought-stopping, and the use of films and music. An anxiolytic during the flight may also be helpful.

PANIC DISORDER (EPISODIC PAROXYSMAL ANXIETY)

There is a well-established overlap between anxiety and depression. Their prevalence is somewhere between 15 and 30 per cent of the population. They are often unidentified and untreated. However, panic disorder, defined as two or more panic attacks, seems to be a separate entity from generalized anxiety. Associated physical (autonomic) symptoms are common and severity varies. Panic is associated with such symptoms, and the individual's perception of them. In these circumstances, behaviour can be grossly impaired, and urgent intervention is indicated.

A panic attack consists of a sudden, unexpected discrete episode of heightened anxiety. It may last for seconds or minutes, often causing fear of physical disease due to misinterpretation of symptoms. It can be triggered by a previous related stressful event in flight such as vomiting or observing someone else do so. Once a passenger has had a panic attack during a flight they are sensitized to another on a subsequent flight, and embarrassment compounds the situation.

The catastrophic misinterpretation of somatic autonomic symptoms creates a vicious circle. There is hypervigilance and repeated scanning for physical sensations. Safety-seeking behaviour, avoidance and demands for reassurance ensue. They are unable to understand that the cause of their fear is unfounded. The autonomic response to an anxiety-provoking situation is the release of adrenaline and this may cause dizziness, sweating, palpitations and hyperventilation.

Palpitations are misinterpreted as a heart attack, hyperventilation as suffocation, chest tightness as dying, dizziness as fainting or collapsing, and a feeling of unreality as losing control or going mad. Physiological symptoms can also include disorientation, confusion, sweating, trembling and shaking, headache and hyperarousal. There may be attempts to escape, hold on to something or somebody, seek reassurance, be demanding and irritable, fidget, and nail bite. Men, who notoriously hide feelings, may be aggressive.

Cognitive behavioural therapy is effective in the pre-flight management of panic attacks (see Appendix A). It facilitates exposure to and challenging of such irrational negative thoughts, and reduction of anxiety without counterproductive avoidance, which merely reinforces apprehension. In-flight, a calm attitude is essential, but bland reassurance by flight attendants or companions can inadvertently reinforce the severity of panic attacks. The sufferer is barely aware of what is being said and feels that the agony being experienced is not understood. In this way the individual feels isolated and helpless. A range of helpful strategies can be used to relieve a panic attack. Initially, it is important to exclude an underlying medical or surgical emergency. A complaint of difficulty in breathing, or of palpitations, could signify an acute cardiorespiratory condition, notwithstanding obvious associated severe anxiety. The individual needs to be assessed. It is important to remember that anxiety cannot be assumed to be of psychological origin – it may be physical.

The passenger should, if at all possible, be moved to an isolated area. This will alleviate embarrassment and prevent a potentially contagious panic from spreading, particularly if there appears to be a genuine cause such as unusual noise or the smell of smoke. The flight attendant should talk through the problem sensitively, and acknowledge the distress and the sensations being experienced. This relaxes, and facilitates the practice of controlled breathing. It is also useful to explain that the condition is common and transient. It need not embarrass the passenger and will not cause mental illness or death. This discourages a catastrophic scenario. The individual should be distracted by conversation, offered water or food, observed and supported during the remainder of the journey. A simple factual explanation of turbulence can be given. Prior to recent new security regulations, a visit to the flight deck often aided a better understanding and diverted anxiety-related thoughts, with relief of claustrophobia and reassurance that the captain was in control.

FEAR OF FLYING (AVIOPHOBIA)

Between 10 and 20 per cent of people have a phobia at some point during their lives, more commonly in childhood and in females. A phobia is a persistent, excessive or unreasonable fear cued by the presence or anticipation of a specific object or situation, such as heights, closed spaces or flying. All these elements are present in flight. Aviophobia is the third most common phobia after fear of spiders and snakes. Anxious or phobic subjects can suffer a panic attack in any situation, but are able to escape from the supermarket, shopping mall, motorway, bridge or tunnel. There is nowhere to go at 35 000 feet. Untreated aviophobia can affect in-flight behaviour and is unlikely to improve spontaneously. Some who fear flying may not have experienced a panic attack before and will board a plane without having had previous treatment for anxiety. After a panic attack in-flight, unwillingness to fly may ensue. People are loth to return to the circumstances of their previous discomfort. Other situations allow gentle exposure, but flying is all or nothing. Besides affecting subjects with a flying phobia, panic attacks can also predispose to, or are associated with, alcohol and drug abuse, both of which provide short-term relief of anxiety, but then cause its exacerbation.

Fear of flying is a manifestation of anxiety and its early recognition can avert a panic attack. It is not, necessarily, an indication of psychiatric morbidity and is essentially curable. Nevertheless, it is commoner in those with vulnerable personalities or identifiable psychiatric morbidity, whether or not

currently undergoing psychotherapeutic or medicinal treatment. A degree of fear of flying occurs in more than 90 per cent of otherwise normal adults, and 10 per cent of airline passengers experience intense fear. Probably about 20–50 per cent are mildly distressed, mainly by turbulence, and these effects are commoner in females. If possible, fear of flying is best approached pre-flight by a dedicated programme, and such facilities are available world wide. They are based on psycho-education, anxiety management, exposure to a flight simulator and, finally, a test flight. Understanding the feared consequence facilitates progress which can be tracked using a Panic Diary. This lists the details of the panic-related experiences and helps to initiate behavioural exposure to challenge misinterpretations of physical symptoms with alternatives, to reinforce learning, and encourage self-help. Once successful flights are undertaken, whether simulated or real, trust and self-confidence improve.

Interventions of a 1-day 'fear of flying' course have a high success rate when the condition is essentially anticipatory anxiety without any underlying established panic disorder or other psychiatric morbidity. Such programmes include familiarization with respect to aircraft noises, movements, banking, stacking and cabin crew chimes, to prevent overreacting. The nature of anxiety is explained: it is a normal process experienced in daily life. Coping strategies preventing the misinterpretation of somatic symptoms are taught. Anxiety-management techniques are taught so that it is confronted effectively. This is preferable to quoting air accident statistics compared with those of other forms of transport. It is also important to promote awareness of in-flight procedures interacting with predictable physiological and autonomic responses, i.e. whole-body relaxation, correct breathing (breathe and squeeze), and self-talk (distract and count). It is essential to explain that a safe flight may not include a perfectly smooth take-off and landing, and this will counteract anxiety and resentment. Also, it must be accepted that it is not feasible for passengers to control the aeroplane, but that they can control their own anxiety by understanding its causes and mechanisms. In this way, it is possible to prevent potential panic attacks even in those with pre-existing panic disorder. Treatment of underlying depression, anxiety, alcohol or drug abuse is also relevant.

Panic disorder is certainly a serious manifestation of fear of flying and can occur before or during the flight. Regimens for its treatment should also include cognitive behavioural therapy (CBT). Such a programme targets fear of flying at source and varies between five and ten sessions. It clarifies the mechanisms of anxiety and its relation to physical sensations. Details of CBT are given in Appendix A.

Medicinal treatment options include the selective serotonin re-uptake inhibitors (SSRIs), paroxetine (20–50 mg) or citalopram (10–60 mg). The tricyclic antidepressants clomipramine (50–150 mg daily) and imipramine (75–200 mg daily) can be very effective, although sometimes less well tolerated, and their onset of action is slower. Anticipatory anxiety and phobic avoidance of flying are equally effectively reduced in the long term by these medications. However, it is emphasized that psychotropic medication in flight must be merely an adjunct to a comprehensive pre-flight psychotherapeutic regimen and, alone, is not the treatment of choice.

To relieve anticipatory anxiety when there is not enough time to complete a full course in 'fear of flying', or CBT, lorazepam 0.5–1 mg or diazepam 1–5 mg are useful, or a β-blocker, provided the passenger is not asthmatic. However, caution is advisable with benzodiazepines, particularly for the business traveller or the elderly. Timing of self-administration to allay fear without impairing cognition has to be learned. It necessitates careful titration and rehearsal. Caffeine and alcohol should not be taken before or during the flight. Adequate hydration should be ensured.

In-flight, the fear of flying is aggravated by events such as lurching, banking and engine noise which occur without a reference point. It contrasts with driving, or being driven, and being able to watch what is happening. A running commentary or a timely PA are useful, though not often feasible. If fear results in a panic attack, then strategies for its management should be followed. Reporting fear of flying on boarding ensures cabin staff awareness, communication and effective response by identifying the onset of abnormal anxiety and demonstrating understanding and confidence in dealing with the condition. The attendant can explain and monitor slow, deep breathing, which is the key to controlling panic, and re-emphasize the technique of visualization or other coping strategies learned pre-flight.

POST-TRAUMATIC STRESS DISORDER

Post-traumatic stress is a normal reaction to a grossly abnormal event causing near-death experience to self or a loved one. It is characterized by re-experiencing the event, avoiding similar situations, and hyperarousal. However, minor flight events associated with intrusive and speculative media attention may be seen as a 'life-threatening experience' to the susceptible, thereby predisposing to acute post-traumatic stress features. Further, the condition may pre-exist due to childhood abuse, a road traffic accident, mugging or other traumatic events. Appropriate handling of any acute stress reaction can prevent the development of post-traumatic stress disorder by effective resolution of the reaction to the traumatic event. However, the routine use of critical incident post-event briefing is now seriously questioned.

Prior to flying, the effect of any previously experienced in-flight incidents that could be exacerbated should be discussed. Cognitive behavioural therapy is the treatment of choice together with antidepressant medication, if there is associated depression. This comorbidity is common. Eye movement desensitization and reprocessing can be an effective treatment, although not yet fully validated. It entails full-range horizontal tracking eye movements combined with refocusing on, and cognitive processing of, the dominant traumatic memory. It is then replaced by the recall of a selected positive experience – the so-called 'safe haven' (Shapiro 1996). Post-traumatic stress disorder can be aggravated by further traumatic in-flight events predisposing to a range of manifestations of anxiety, including panic attacks, and may aggravate depression and alcohol abuse. In-flight management is essentially the same as for anxiety and panic, including the carefully monitored use of anxiolytic medication (if available).

DEPRESSION

Depression is common at all stages of life from adolescence to old age. In assessing a patient, the objective account of a key relative or friend is particularly important prior to air travel. Psychosocial factors may exist, including bereavement. Features include spontaneous weeping, withdrawn behaviour, low mood, irritability, guilt, suicidal thoughts, impaired energy, sleep, appetite and libido, loss of self-confidence, indecision, reduction in cognitive function, isolation and excessive use of alcohol, caffeine and nicotine. Depression occurs in up to 25 per cent of those with physical illness, and can lower the pain threshold. It is difficult to predict those who will succumb to depression, and it occurs in strong, capable people.

Marital relationships, social networks, basic personality, psychiatric history and previous traumatic flight events are all relevant in a comprehensive pre-flight assessment. Counselling is indicated in mild depression, which is known to be less responsive to antidepressants. In more severe cases, counselling is valuable in conjunction with antidepressant medication, which should rarely be used in isolation. In-flight, despite their own misery, which may or may not be manifest, the only risk is impulsive behaviour and suicidal attempts, though they are a rare occurrence. Nevertheless, it is important to be vigilant with respect to changes in behaviour and mood, and to be aware that alcohol and stimulant drugs may modulate the mood of the individual and react adversely with prescribed medication.

POST-NATAL DEPRESSION

Post-natal depression develops in approximately 10 per cent of women after an uneventful pregnancy with delivery of a healthy infant. Puerperal psychosis only occurs in 1–2 per 1000 deliveries and so is relatively rare. The features of post-natal depression often include poor social support. The patient has a low mood and often feels guilty because of comments such as 'Aren't you lucky to have such a lovely baby?', a sentiment which the patient does not herself experience. There are feelings of inadequacy, loss of appetite, libido and self-confidence, with irritability, tiredness, impaired cognitive function and obsessive ideas of harming the infant, though suicidal thoughts are less common. Assessment is aided by the Edinburgh Post-natal Depression Scale (Cox *et al.* 1987).

Pre-flight, the patient with post-natal depression may need an antidepressant, in addition to a full range of psychosocial support and counselling. Breast-feeding need not necessarily be stopped during antidepressant treatment provided the correct medication, such as lofepramine, is used and the infant is thriving. However, this has to be monitored during lactation. In-flight, those with post-natal depression are particularly vulnerable to stress. Mothers who wish to breast-feed need tactful help and comfortable facilities when available. If the aircraft is not full, it may be possible to offer a more secluded seat. In general terms, one should follow the in-flight management strategies outlined for depression.

PSYCHOSES

These are severe mental illnesses. Acute psychotic depression, hypomania/mania or schizophrenia can present with irritability, impulsive behaviour and attempted suicide and can constitute in-flight clinical emergencies, albeit rarely. Features may also include impaired insight and cognitive function, loss of touch with reality, paranoid thoughts, delusions, hallucinations, ideas of reference and influence and confusion. These conditions may result from organic, toxic, or metabolic states, or be drug-induced. However, the media focus most commonly on manic-depressive illness, and schizophrenia. Once diagnosed, most patients are stabilized by antipsychotic medication and psychotherapeutic community monitoring. It must also be remembered that the malaria prophylactic, mefloquine hydrochloride (Larium), used by travellers bound for certain 'at-risk' regions can also cause confusion or psychosis.

Pre-flight, there should be a routine assessment of mental state with reference to behaviour, orientation, mood, cognitive function, thinking, perception, judgement and suicidal risk. Assuming that the prospective passenger is stabilized and compliant with psychotropic medication, there is no specific psychiatric contraindication to flying independently. Passengers with psychotic illness should always carry details of their psychotropic medication, and of a clinical contact, together with an adequate supply of medication for the journey, and advice on dosage of 'as-required' medication. Such written instructions are augmented by ground-based medical advice where necessary. For those who are relocating, appropriate clinical arrangements at the destination should be organized well ahead of the flight. The current dosage may require adjustment in flight. Haloperidol (10 mg), olanzapine (10 mg), lorazepam (1–5 mg) or diazepam (5–15 mg) are effective in the emergency control of acute psychotic illness. Neuroleptics are unlikely to cause confusion.

Some psychotic patients will be in transit with a psychiatric nurse. It is important to confirm that those who need such supervision are fit to fly. Every effort must be made to avoid embarrassment to the patient or apprehension in the crew and other passengers. Pre-flight, the medication must be stabilized, and it is important to continue the regimen at the home time rather than that of the destination. If the patient becomes distressed or agitated, the dosage should be increased, and ground-based advice sought. If pre-flight assessment identifies any active or incipient psychoses, the flight should be postponed. If it is essential, then a specialized carrier service is mandatory to ensure appropriate equipment and psychiatric nursing staff. The following medication may then be considered. Haloperidol (10–30 mg) over 24 hours, procyclidine (5–10 mg) oral or intramuscular for extrapyramidal signs, if indicated, provided all relevant resuscitation equipment is available.

DEMENTIA

It is now common for elderly people to fly, often on distressing occasions. They may well be physically and mentally healthy. On the other hand, there may be some physical illness or disability such as impaired mobility, or they may be suffering from anxiety and depression, resulting from the realization that memory is deteriorating. Dementia occurs in 10 per cent of the population over 65. The differential diagnosis between dementia and pseudo-dementia is important. The latter is depression mimicking dementia and, appropriately diagnosed, it is eminently treatable with antidepressants (and even ECT, although this remains controversial). Memory assessment is helpful; impaired cognitive function is the key to assessing dementia, but it can also be impaired in depression. On questioning, the depressive may respond 'I don't know' when unable to answer correctly. In dementia there is confabulation, that is, making up answers or merely the frequent repetition of the question posed. Visuospatial impairment in dementia is identified by the inability to draw a clock face. A 'Mini-Mental State Examination' score of less than 23 is said to signify dementia (Folstein *et al.* 1975). In over-70s who

left school before age 15 years, a score of 20 or less is significant (Appendix B).

Pre-flight, the elderly may become agitated by the anticipation of travel. In these circumstances, risperidone (0.5–1 mg) two hours prior to travel is useful. It is helpful if the travelling companion is already known and is acquainted with the use of the medication and, where possible, the elderly passenger has been familiarized with the airport and concourse, and reassured that a wheelchair will be available, and that post-flight arrangements are in place. In-flight, the elderly may well be affected by the hypoxia and dehydration that can compound or precipitate confusion and agitation. Identification ensures monitoring and specific cabin staff awareness. On long-haul flights, confusion, agitation and wandering can be particularly disruptive.

ALCOHOL AND DRUG ABUSE

Alcohol and drug abuse will be considered together as there are commonalities with reference to their central action and consequent effects on behaviour, orientation and, in some cases, levels of consciousness. Alcohol and drugs can impair cognitive function and sleep and can cause disinhibition, confusion, impulsive, disruptive and violent behaviour. In pre-flight assessment it is important to elicit the relevant history and to involve a reliable third party. Objective assessments include liver function tests, determination of mean corpuscular volume and urinalysis. The latter only detects the majority of illicit drugs for up to 10 days after administration. The active ingredient of cannabis, Δ^9-THC, is identifiable for approximately 30 days. They may interact with each other and with psychotropic and general medication, including hypnotics and analgesics. Being a diuretic, alcohol compounds the dehydrating effect of caffeine. Drugs, particularly cocaine, can cause severe psychotic illness. The onset of such an illness due to MDMA (Ecstasy) or cocaine can be very rapid, particularly when taken with alcohol. The physical and emotional stress of flying can exacerbate vulnerable personality traits and psychiatric morbidity which are compounded by alcohol and drug abuse, and by nicotine withdrawal. Smokers subjected to airline-imposed nicotine withdrawal may manifest irritable behaviour. Nicotine replacement is of dubious value, although some claim that it is effective. Alcohol may be consumed in an attempt to offset the effects of the enforced nicotine withdrawal.

The numerous pre-flight irritants, from the taxi from home to delays in the departure lounge, can be disconcerting. Anxious, fearful fliers and the socially phobic take their first dose of the universal 'tranquillizer'. Alcohol is used to relieve anxiety due to fear of flying, business or personal problems, or in response to peer pressure. Once in the aircraft, take-off may be delayed. Minor events can irritate or threaten. Restricted space, the compulsory seat belt restraint, the safety demonstration and the take-off with unexplained noises are irritants. Going on holiday calls for a party, with the opportunity and the excuse to drink in flight. With free alcohol, passengers are more likely to drink, be it for enjoyment or, understandably but misguidedly, for the relief of anxiety.

Alcohol is essentially a legal mind-altering drug, taken for stress relief or when celebrating. For some, it seems an obvious answer to the fear of flying. At first, it is anxiolytic, but soon causes exacerbation, especially of phobic anxiety. It is also a depressant, aggravating underlying depression.

Passengers travelling in groups and both men and women respond easily to peer group pressure when alcohol is so easily available. There are various patterns of drinking – occasional, binge, heavy and those who are psychologically and physically dependent on alcohol. The occasional or binge drinker often poses more of a threat in flight due to unpredictable behaviour. Such individuals are less likely to have received professional treatment, or even basic advice or education regarding 'sensible' drinking. Pre- and in-flight consumption of alcohol requires further scrutiny and health education.

Regulatory authorities have long-standing guidelines for pilots concerning the minimum interval for the ingestion of alcohol before flying, and it would seem that similar guidelines for passengers should be considered. Such 'intrusion on civil liberties' is accepted at sporting events where the risks are fewer. However, presumably such monitoring would entail breathalysation or random drug screening, which is not feasible. Meantime, a simple but explicit educational leaflet could be provided routinely at check-in, or on boarding. This would enhance sensitivity to, and emphasize the dangers of, excessive in-flight alcohol consumption or drug abuse, and hopefully encourage some limitation to in-flight consumption.

Features of alcohol intoxication such as slurred speech, garrulousness, changes in mood, loss of inhibition and self-control, irritability, lack of coordination, facial flushing, nausea, vomiting and impaired levels of consciousness make it important to appreciate that alcohol intoxication may coexist with drug abuse. Together they can mask a range of serious conditions including head injury, hypoglycaemia, or even cardiorespiratory insufficiency. Hence, there are dangers in labelling a person as drunk, without very careful assessment. It may be necessary to monitor levels of consciousness, and even resuscitation may be indicated in some cases.

Dealing with alcohol and drug-induced behavioural disturbance is difficult, as basic communication is impaired, or virtually impossible. The goal is to avoid impulsive behaviour, easily provoked by admonition, as this may well be perceived as a challenge, demanding an aggressive response, and such behaviour can be contagious. The problem can be contained by appropriate self-assertion without aggression, and avoidance of patronizing or heavy-handed confrontation. Further intake of alcohol is discouraged by offering alternatives, such as water and food. This will remain difficult to implement unless or until a fixed limit is imposed by agreement between airlines. Listening, and allowing petty infractions to pass unchallenged reduces the likelihood of a reaction, which would have an adverse effect on neighbouring passengers, and on the on-board community. The drunken passenger should be removed to another seat to separate them from those who may have been encouraging such behaviour, and from other passengers. Some airlines have adopted a 'yellow card' warning system, as in football.

AIR RAGE

In-flight interpersonal relationship problems may exist which involve breakdown of communication and cause stress and anxiety. It is often difficult to escape from such a perceived threat. Common irritants include a long toilet queue, noisy fellow passengers using provocative language, obstruction from hand luggage, and perceived slow service. In such situations, unresolved resentment and anger can escalate to uncontrollable proportions in the confined space of an aircraft cabin. Those who feel targeted also feel threatened and can become aggressive in self-defence. Failure of effective reasoning easily ensues. Voices are raised and, inevitably, others become involved. Listening and objective evaluation cease and judgement is impaired. Whether confined or spread into a larger group, there is a risk of verbal threats precipitating physical violence. The signs of air rage are now obvious. They include shouting, irritability, combative demeanour, anger, argumentative provocative stance, and verbal insults escalating to antisocial behaviour.

Passengers rarely reveal the possibility of such behaviour to their general practitioner. However, the doctor may well be aware of those with a previous history of uncontrollable anger, be it domestic, in the community, or even when driving. If so, anger management programmes are indicated and include interactive and assertive skills training. Cognitive behavioural therapy (see Appendix A) and psychotherapy are useful (time permitting). Prophylactic haloperidol (5 mg) may be used to reduce impulsivity. In-flight, intervention should only be attempted by those who possess the skills of listening and are capable of self-assertion without aggression. It is important to communicate calmly but not to patronize, to try to identify the trigger for the outburst, to acknowledge feelings, thoughts and sensitivities related to the trigger, which dictate the ultimate response. Air rage constitutes a serious threat to flight safety, and the use of physical restraint is acceptable if appropriate behavioural skills are of no avail. Diazepam (10 mg oral) is recommended, or parenteral if administered by a health professional. Even diversion of the aircraft may have to be considered in the extreme case.

Air rage is the most dramatic emergency, but there are a number of other well-established situations relevant to flight, affecting either the individual, or the whole aircraft. These include a first time or recurrence of a panic attack. However, it is important to exclude cardiorespiratory morbidity, as voluntary hyperventilation can cause dizziness and palpitations, and voluntary breath-holding can cause chest pains. Other conditions include alcohol intoxication, drug-induced psychosis, attempted suicide by a depressive, an acute psychotic episode, and confusion in the elderly with underlying dementia or delirium. An American study of all in-flight calls for physician consultations to MedAire were reviewed for psychiatric symptomatology (Matsumoto and Goebert 2001). Of 1375 consultations, 3.5 per cent were psychiatric, 90 per cent of these presenting as acute anxiety and 69 per cent of them requiring assessment on arrival; three cases necessitated diversion and landing. The potential value of a rapid onset anxiolytic for the on-board medical kit was recognized. Only two out of 48 psychiatric calls were for psychosis and none for 'air rage'. Apparently, disruptive on-board behaviour resulted in FBI rather than medical consultation.

CONCLUSION

At its inception, air travel was rudimentary, but it was also novel and for the privileged few. It is now a worldwide and in some respects a mass transport system. In its most modern manifestation it is of low cost, and low sophistication. Inevitably, there is a wide range of individual reactions to flying. On the one hand, the aircrew are an experienced and selected group of highly trained individuals who remain sanguine in the roughest spells of turbulence. On the other hand, the anxious first-time traveller may ruminate on the most recently recorded accident or hijacking. Inadequate preparedness and the behaviours that anxiety breeds in flight cannot be totally eliminated. Disruptive activity, even short of violence, can constitute an emergency whether due to air rage, simple anger or fear. It is equally hazardous whether the passenger is sober, drunk, on drugs, or suffering from acute stress of whatever origin, panic disorder, or an acute psychotic illness. The uncertainty ('what if...?') of air travel can induce intense anxiety by demanding an unparalleled surrender of control from those who are vulnerable. These risks can be mitigated by attention to health and behaviour pre-flight, on boarding, and in-flight. Guidance is available in the form of self-help, coping manuals, and more formal cognitive behavioural and desensitization initiatives.

Cabin staff promote safety and well-being by identification of distress, anxiety and provocative behaviour, and they can intervene with sensitivity, offer appropriate help and provide ongoing monitoring. By learning from how staff and passengers respond to situations, it is possible to design effective and workable procedures. These help to deescalate and defuse potentially violent incidents and to allay passenger fears about safety. Effective in-flight management is demanding, and entails sensitive self-assertion and flexibility to combat the whole range of behavioural emergencies, whether due to anger, abnormal mental and physical states, or alcohol and drug abuse. In this context, staff training in anxiety, stress, and anger management is very worthwhile.

In the longer term, education about air travel from childhood onwards would instil appropriate behaviour, enjoyment and safety. Understanding the procedures from initial booking, checking in, safe keeping of tickets and passports, the aircraft, the duties and professionalism of the whole crew can all be reassuring. In the most extreme circumstances, setting limits (the 'yellow card', which is the first warning prior to involvement of the police on arrival), with the threat of restraint and prosecution can be effective deterrents, though they must be conveyed in a non-threatening way to avoid generating the very type of behaviour that has to be avoided.

REFERENCES

Cox JL, Holden JM and Sagovsky R. Detection of postnatal depression. Development of the 10-item Edinburgh Postnatal Depression Scale. *Br J Psychiatry* 1987; **150**: 782–6.

Folstein MF, Folstein SE and McHugh PR. Mini-mental state. A practical method for grading the cognitive state of patients for the clinician. *J Psychiat Res* 1975; **12**: 189–98.

Matsumoto K and Goebert D. In-flight psychiatric emergency. *Aviat Space Environ Med* 2001; **72**: 919–23.

Shapiro F. Eye movement desensitization and reprocessing (EMDR): evaluation of controlled PTSD research. *J Behav Ther Exp Psychol* 1996; **7**: 1–10.

World Health Organization. Health aspects of well-being in working places: report on a WHO working group, Prague, 18–20 September 1979, Copenhagen: WHO (Euroreports & Studies 31), 1980.

APPENDIX A: COGNITIVE BEHAVIOURAL THERAPY

Many options can be considered in the management of anxiety, and anxiety-related conditions. These range from tea and sympathy, counselling, a lay course on the fear of flying, cognitive behavioural therapy and, when indicated, psychotropic medication. Behavioural and medicinal strategies are not mutually exclusive, and the medical practitioner with personal knowledge of the potential passenger is best placed to assess the indication for psychotropic medication.

Cognitive behavioural therapy explores the relationship between thought, behaviour and physiological response. It is an effective intervention for the individual who misinterprets stimuli such as increased heart rate and aircraft noises as perceived threats. An 'ABC' checklist structures the therapy. For example, the apprehensive passenger believes that his plane journey (**A**ctivating event) is unsafe (this is their **B**elief). These thoughts ('I won't survive the crash') lead to the physiological response (**C**onsequence). Thus anticipatory anxiety and the actual flying are the activating events which lead to the belief of a crash, suffocation or death, with anxiety, fear, and phobic avoidance as the consequences.

As a result of this process, there are various ways in which misinterpretation can be maintained. Attention to the threatening stimulus may be increased due to excessive scanning of the environment, thereby increasing the likelihood of further threat(s) being detected. Stimuli and the misinterpretation of threat enhance each other. Increased subjective anxiety arising from the original evaluation of threat complicates the relationship with 'I can't cope with this anxiety' and 'I can't fly because I know I am going to die'. Physiological responses to misinterpretation of stimuli are due to the systemic effects of adrenaline. Behaviour then maintains anxiety. First, the individual avoids the feared stimuli (airports, aeroplanes and/or flying), and this effectively reduces fear, but prevents the essential challenging of erroneous beliefs. Second, such behaviour can increase symptoms such as palpitations.

By exposing the subject to the symptoms of panic, their erroneous interpretations can be effectively challenged.

APPENDIX B: MINI-MENTAL STATE EXAMINATION

	Score	Points
Orientation		
1. What is the		
Year?	1	
Season?	1	
Date?	1	
Day?	1	
Month?	1	
2. Where are we?		
Country?	1	
County?	1	
Town?	1	
Hospital?	1	
Floor?	1	
Registration		
3. Name three objects, one per second (eg. BALL, FLAG, TREE). Then ask the patient all three after you have said them. Give one point for each correct answer. Repeat the words until patient learns all three	3	
Attention and Concentration		
4. Spell 'world' backwards: D L R O W	5	
Recall		
5. Ask for names of three objects learned in Q. 3. Give one point for each answer.	3	
Language		
6. Point to a pencil and a watch. Ask the patient to name them as you point.	2	
7. Ask the patient to repeat 'No ifs, ands or buts'.	1	
8. Ask the patient to read and obey the following: CLOSE YOUR EYES.	1	
9. Ask the patient to carry out a three-stage command: 'Take the paper in your right hand, fold it in half and put it on the floor.'	3	
10. Ask the patient to write a sentence of their own. (The sentence should contain a subject and an object and should make sense. Ignore spelling errors in scoring.)	1	
11. Ask the patient to copy a design (2 overlapping pentagons. Give one point if all sides and angles are preserved and the intersecting sides form a quadrangle.)	1	
	30	

23

The elderly and passengers with physical difficulties

FRANCIS G MISKELLY

The elderly and those with physical difficulties form a significant proportion of the population of the developed world. As far as the elderly are concerned, plenty of leisure time, families dispersed around the world, improving disposable incomes and cheap air fares encourage more and more to travel by air, while improved facilities for those with physical difficulties make possible journeys which only a few years ago would have seemed impossible. However, air travel is a double-edged sword. Significant advantages include speed and convenience whereas the alternative methods of transport by sea or train might take days or, perhaps, weeks. On the other hand, air travel is associated with its own risks of travel-related problems. Many factors influence the risk associated with travel. These include age, past medical history, length of flight, destination and the degree of disability.

As far as age is concerned, the elderly can be divided into two risk groups. The young elderly in the age group 65–75 fall into a lower risk category, whereas those 75 years and over are at greater risk. Risk can also be stratified according to past medical history, ranging from those with no previous illnesses to those with a series of medical problems. Whether any of these problems are active or the patient is currently medically unfit is particularly important. Disability may be due to a previous accident or disease such as arthritis or stroke. In an otherwise fit person, a mild disability with limited functional impairment may cause little difficulty in flight, but special provision will be needed for those requiring assistance with all the activities of daily living. The importance of these factors will, to some extent, depend on the duration of the flight. Transmeridian flights have a higher risk because of the additional problem of time-zone changes. Some destinations may also carry a higher risk. High-risk destinations involve polar or tropical environments with extremes of heat and humidity and areas at high altitude.

AGE-RELATED PHYSIOLOGICAL CHANGES

Reduction in physiological function with age affects the ability to withstand the inconveniences of travel. A precise description of the normal physiological changes with age is difficult because of the associated high prevalence of disease in the elderly, especially affecting the cardiovascular system. Respiratory function is similarly affected by a lifetime of accumulated damage from toxic gases, particulates, antigenic substances and micro-organisms. Nevertheless, reduction in cardiopulmonary reserve is a normal age-related phenomenon. Age-related changes in heart rate, blood volume and circulation time lead to a decrease in cardiac function of approximately 1 per cent per year. The change may not be apparent at rest, but becomes obvious on exercise when it can be measured using maximal oxygen consumption. There is a reduction in lung elasticity and chest wall compliance so that air trapping leads to a rise in residual volume and a fall in vital capacity. The arterial oxygen tension averages about 95 mmHg (12.6 kPa) at 30 years but may be as low as 75 mmHg (10.0 kPa) at 60 years.

Renal function can be reduced in the elderly to about 50 per cent of that of the young adult, decreasing 1 per cent per year from age 30 years. The aged kidney has impaired ability to both concentrate urine and to process an extra water load and this predisposes to fluid and electrolyte imbalance. The combination of renal ageing and systemic or renal disease may lead to the sudden onset of renal failure. Bladder function tends to deteriorate with age. Detrusor instability is more common in the elderly though bladder control may be retained unless additional factors are present, such as urinary tract infection. In men with prostatism the rigours of travel may precipitate urinary retention.

Neuronal loss, loss of synapses and possibly reduction in neurotransmitter function are part of the ageing process. Intelligence testing, learning ability, short-term memory and reaction time decline with age. However, there is usually a greater scatter than with younger subjects, possibly due to a greater prevalence of sensory motor or cognitive impairment. These changes are influenced by education and life experiences. Changes in mental function can be mild and, although not universal, 'benign senescent forgetfulness' is common. Dementia is a global impairment of intellect, memory and personality without alteration of conscious level and is present in 2 per cent over the age of 65, rising to 20 per cent over the age 80. These age-related changes in mental reserve combined with the fatigue, stress, noise and the melée of travel can exacerbate a chronic mild confusion. Other factors associated with travel such as acute infections, hypoxia, fluid or electrolyte imbalance, alcohol, hypothermia and hypoglycaemia can also precipitate an acute confusional state.

Approximately 1 per cent of individuals over 65 years are known to be partially sighted, and many more are visually disabled. Visual impairment is associated with diseases that tend to be more common in the elderly. These include glaucoma, macular degeneration, hypertension and diabetes. Hearing also changes with age. The wax of the external auditory canal becomes more viscous, and there is a loss of high-frequency hearing (presbyacusis), with deafness becoming more common. On formal testing, half of all elderly people have some hearing impairment and half of these would benefit from and accept a hearing aid.

AIR TRAVEL

The problems that elderly passengers may encounter with air travel can be conveniently divided into those on the ground, which include travel to and from the airport, and those in-flight. The most common problems encountered by the elderly or those with physical difficulties are steps, unhelpful staff and inaccessible toilets. Many are, of course, at risk of falls. On the ground, most difficulties arise either immediately before or immediately after the flight. Airports often appear as a mixture of noise, melée, confusion, poor communication, security procedures and delays, all of which contribute to travel fatigue, stress and, perhaps, disorientation. The distance to and from the airport can be considerable and parking arrangements may be inconvenient, involving long distances, maybe on foot, with baggage. Some airports have long walkways and trolleys for luggage may not always be readily available. Travellers with suitcases may have to carry them considerable distances. Special luggage-carrying equipment, some foldable, is worth consideration, though some may require extra assistance. Stairs can present formidable hazards to those with luggage. Passengers may be unprepared for the extremes of heat or cold that may be found at intermediate airports. Tight deadlines or long delays may add to the stress. Long periods of waiting in extreme temperatures can cause hypo- or hyperthermia.

Dehydration is commonly quoted as a consequence of air travel, but the actual fluid loss is no greater than that of any other form of transport. Nevertheless, an aircraft has a low relative humidity and this may create a sensation of dryness. However, real dehydration may occur in extreme heat or as a result of rushing around. Excessive consumption of alcohol can be a factor in some people and inadequate fluid intake can be a problem, particularly in the elderly. Urinary or faecal incontinence can occur in otherwise asymptomatic individuals if toilets are small or too few with poor access. The fear of incontinence persuades some travellers to avoid diuretics on long journeys, with implications for those with a tendency to fluid retention.

Exposure to other travellers who may be carrying infections is a risk common to all forms of public transport. The cabin environment is relatively safe as far as spread of disease is concerned and one advantage of air travel is that the air conditioning is fitted with high-efficiency particulate air (HEPA) filters designed to filter out infectious organisms. Time spent abroad increases the risk of infection with unfamiliar organisms, and the commonest of these infections is gastroenteritis. It may well be true that travel broadens the mind and loosens the bowels. At the destination, 'flu' can be a problem as it is endemic in many tropical countries, and is particularly common with fly/cruise holidays where considerable changes in the ambient atmosphere occur.

Jet lag is another problem and is due to disruption of the circadian rhythm. It causes difficulty going to sleep or remaining asleep, daytime sleepiness, reduced alertness and, sometimes, confusion. It is usually worse travelling west to east. On average, acclimatization occurs at the rate of about one time zone per day, but this is highly variable. The ability to adapt decreases with age. On long flights, inability to sleep in a standard seat adds to the problem, and hypnotics are contraindicated in the elderly due to the increased risk of adverse reactions including deep vein thrombosis when immobile for many hours. Other rhythms at work in the body affect not only sleep, but also appetite and bowel habit, and conflicts may arise between physiological cues such as the desire to eat and the provision of food.

Hearing loss can lead elderly travellers to misunderstand public address announcements and instructions and this is especially important as they may not understand the emergency drill instructions. The removal of excessive wax or the provision of a hearing aid may be of help, though speaking clearly and slowly may be all that is required. Visual impairment reduces the ability to read information and instructions from screens. Airline tickets and boarding cards may also be difficult to read because of print colour, quality and size, and may, in any case, be difficult to interpret because of the way the information is laid out. Simple measures to improve vision, such as clean spectacles and good lighting, can make a dramatic difference.

In-flight, it must be borne in mind that fear of flying is not uncommon among the elderly. Flying phobia is a psychological response out of proportion to the causative stimulus. Presenting symptoms are an acute anxiety state with any combination of sweating, tremor, shortness of breath, palpitations, tachycardia and pain. If there is sufficient time before the flight, behavioural therapy using desensitization may be attempted and some airlines run courses for this purpose. If time is short, then hypnotherapy combined with desensitization can be successful. The use of tranquillizers or β-blockers should be discouraged. If tranquillizers are used, then, ideally, they should be tried out beforehand. Benzodiazepines should be short acting. Particular care must be taken with β-blockers because of potential adverse effects on cardiorespiratory function.

The pressure inside the cabin is equivalent to 5000–8000 feet altitude on most flights and so the arterial oxygen tension drops from 98 mmHg at ground level to approximately 55 mmHg. This reduction, together with reduced cardiopulmonary reserve related to ageing and associated disease of these systems, predisposes to arterial hypoxia which is, therefore, a danger for older travellers with cardiac, respiratory or cerebrovascular disease. The physical restraint associated with long periods seated in confined positions and with limited leg room is likely to increase the risk of peripheral oedema, deep venous thrombosis and pulmonary embolism. Symptoms of arthritis such as pain and stiffness can be exacerbated. It should be noted that the problem of restricted space is not confined to air travel. Extra space may be required by passengers with disabilities and this may be particularly so on economy flights. Furthermore, narrow aisles can be a problem.

As far as motion sickness is concerned, this is now much reduced on large aircraft, but may still be a problem with smaller aeroplanes used for shorter flights. However, for some unknown reason, motion sickness is not usually a problem for people over 50 years of age. Confusion is common in the elderly and can be encountered both on the ground and in-flight. It may be precipitated or exacerbated in vulnerable patients by the hostile environment or by in-flight factors such as reduced oxygen levels. It can appear unpredictably at any time either before, during or after the flight.

CONTRAINDICATIONS TO AIR TRAVEL

Absolute contraindications to air travel are few and often a short delay will enable the passenger to travel. Airlines within the International Airline Travel Association (IATA) require medical clearance for passengers whose fitness to fly is in doubt, but in any case advice should be sought from the airline before the flight. Particular attention must be paid to passengers with chronic cardiorespiratory problems. Problematical areas are recent myocardial infarction especially if complicated by arrhythmias, shock or failure, uncontrolled heart failure with dyspnoea at rest or mild exertion, and respiratory failure with arterial hypoxaemia. Consideration must also be given to cerebrovascular infarction or haemorrhage, acute infectious diseases, acute otitis media and sinusitis, recent gastrointestinal haemorrhage, severe anaemia <7.5 g dl^{-1}, unstable mental illness, confusion or dementia, and recent surgery. Many of these issues, as they concern adult passengers, are covered in detail earlier in this volume, but the same principles apply to the elderly.

It must also be borne in mind that the use of electrically powered medical equipment is unlikely to be permitted during take-off and landing. This includes respirators, of which certain types can be carried, though cabin power cannot be guaranteed. A portable respirator with a dry or gel cell battery is to be preferred. Portable dialysis machines may be carried but cannot be used in the cabin. Passengers using chronic ambulatory peritoneal dialysis are regarded as standard passengers. Heart pacemakers may be affected by the electrical security equipment of some countries, and so the instructions issued with the pacemaker should be carefully followed. It is always advisable to consult the security officials of the departing and destination airports, though clearance is not required for heart pacemakers.

MANAGEMENT

The in-flight management of the elderly or passenger with physical difficulties can be conveniently considered in two phases: in-flight, including transit flights and coach shuttles, and on the ground, including travel from home and onwards on reaching the destination. It is important to evaluate the risk by careful consideration of the route and modes of transport, including departure, transits and destination. It is also useful to bear in mind when the journey may include a long car trip, whether the season at the destination may be excessively hot or cold and whether medical facilities will be available *en route* and on arrival. The passenger should always advise the travel agent about any disability and specialized equipment required. The travel agent should pass the information on to the airline so that special arrangements can be made, but it would perhaps be wise to ensure that the airline has been informed. Medical support includes, though often at a charge, on-board oxygen which is available with most airlines, extra space and mobility aids such as Zimmer frames (Figure 23.1) and wheelchairs. Special diets and special transport either at the departure, transit or destination will need to be arranged well in advance.

The medical problems of the elderly are similar to the medical problems of the young, although they are more common and often more severe. The elderly are frequently stoical and often deny or understate the severity of their condition. In this context, a pre-flight medical is recommended so that advice can be given on cabin altitude and pulmonary disease, precautions *en route* or at the destination, and prophylaxis and vaccination, and for diabetics, especially, advice on medication for the journey and on holiday. Where the traveller has an extensive list of medication, this should be reviewed. Vital medicines and equipment should be kept as hand baggage, especially for those

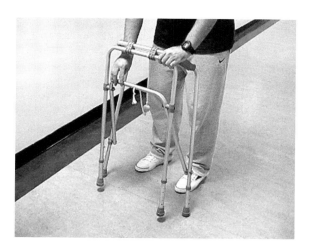

Figure 23.1 *Folding zimmer frame.*

with angina, diabetes and asthma. Medication boxes with compartments for separate doses may be helpful. Patients crossing time zones and on three- or four-times daily medication should continue with the same regimen arranged around sleep times. The elderly should also carry certificates and referral letters. These may include a medical clearance. Frequent travellers may have a card containing details of their requirements.

Good advice for the elderly and for passengers with physical disabilities is to avoid the smoking area, choose an aisle seat with good leg room, exercise regularly on the aircraft, maintain a reasonable fluid intake, avoid alcohol and rest for 24 hours on arrival at the destination. Passengers who have difficulty in walking should chose seats close to toilets. Special transit chairs are available on board aircraft to help less mobile passengers to reach the toilet and negotiate the narrow aisles. If assistance is required to use the toilet, then someone must travel with the passenger. Cabin staff are food handlers and must not assist with personal care. The elderly and those with physical difficulties usually board the aircraft first and leave last to avoid prolonged standing. If boarding the aircraft via steps can be a problem, it should be discussed with the airline beforehand.

Outside the aircraft, walking sticks, some folding and some with built-in seats, may be useful, and numerous types of crutches and walking frames, some telescopic or folding, can be made available depending on the degree of the disability. As far as the physically disabled are concerned, the facilities available at airports vary widely, so it is necessary to make detailed enquiries. These should include transit airports as well as the airports of departure and destination. Small remote airports may have very limited facilities.

Most major international airports have appropriate ramps for wheelchair access, but in smaller airports, in transit situations and during stopovers, wheelchair access may not be possible. Wheelchairs and walking frames are often stored in the aircraft hold, but are usually available until about to board the aircraft. It is worth considering whether to carry a repair kit, including a puncture repair kit, emergency tools and a pump. Wheelchairs that fold or dismantle easily can be very useful. Airline requirements vary considerably regarding electric wheelchairs and particularly the storage of batteries, and so enquiries must be made well in advance. The method of recharging the batteries at the new destination must also be considered.

Several pieces of equipment can assist travellers from a wheelchair into an aircraft seat. These include wooden boards with a polished surface, which facilitate sliding from one seat to another (Figure 23.2). There are also low friction fabric slides, which are ideal as they are very light and can be rolled up and stored in the hand luggage. Transfer belts and slings worn around the body can provide a firm grip for an assistant to help with transfers (Figures 23.3, 23.4), and a disc which is a turntable to stand on can allow the body to rotate while an assistant helps with the transfer. As far as incontinence is concerned, it must be appreciated that toilets in aircraft are often very small. Passengers unable to use them should consider alternatives such as

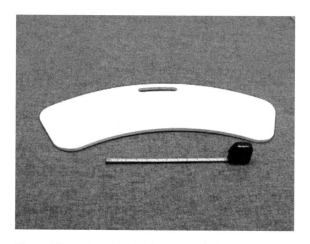

Figure 23.2 *Transfer board, gauge 12 inches.*

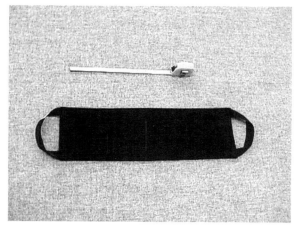

Figure 23.3 *Transfer strap, gauge 12 inches.*

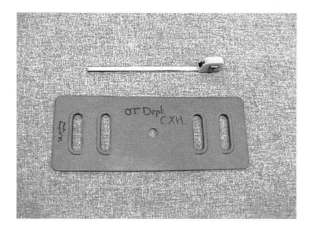

Figure 23.4 *Transfer strap, gauge 12 inches.*

penile sheaths, different types of urinals, temporary catheterization, protective garments, pads and pants, and medication. Using a suppository before the flight and a low-residue diet, perhaps with medication, can reduce bowel action for some time and may help avoid faecal incontinence.

It is advisable to wear loose, comfortable clothing. Those subject to ankle swelling should review their footwear. Shoes that can be removed easily or shoes with Velcro fastening may be more suitable. Portable seat units, pressure-relief cushions and lumbar supports can be carried for comfort, but inflatable devices should be avoided. Specialized seating systems such as vacuum support cushions or wedged cushions can be used, if necessary. As far as visual and hearing impairment is concerned, travellers may require assistance before flight with departure information and during flight with eating or safety instructions. Communication aids should be fully charged, especially for long flights, and portable induction loop systems are available. Comprehensive medical insurance without exclusions is vital for the elderly or those with physical difficulties, and equipment should be insured for its full replacement value.

CONCLUSION

Although air travel, like other forms of travel, is associated with an increased risk for the elderly and those with physical difficulties, age or disability are not absolute contraindications to air travel. Travel by air is possible when the flight is approached with realistic expectations, proper precautions and thorough planning. Indeed, air travel has significant advantages for the elderly or those with physical difficulties and allows them to undertake journeys that, until recently, were impracticable. However, facilities for the elderly or disabled vary substantially so they are advised to restrict, if possible, their travel to countries equipped to accommodate their needs. Facilities for the elderly and those with physical difficulties tend to be good to excellent in the developed world, but poor to non-existent in many parts of the developing world, Eastern Europe and Asia. Provided these risks are known, carefully evaluated and appropriate precautions taken, the benefits significantly outweigh the disadvantages.

FURTHER READING

Flying High: A Practical Guide to Air Travel for Elderly People and People with Liabilities. London: Disabled Living Foundation, 1994; 380–4.

McIntosh IB. *Travel and Health in the Elderly.* Dinton, Wilts: Quay Books, 1992.

McIntosh IB. Health hazards and the elderly traveler. *J Travel Med* 1998; **5**: 27–9.

24

Carriage of the seriously ill

COLIN AB McLAREN

Air transport to move the seriously ill was under discussion long before the first flight by the Wright brothers in 1903. Indeed, in 1892, the Dutch Surgeon General, de Mooy, produced sketches of aircraft and airships with underslung stretchers carrying the sick and wounded from the war zone (Vincent 1924). It has often been reported that aerial transport was used to move casualties during the siege of Paris in 1870 – a wonderful story, but not supported by the facts (Lam 1988). The first confirmed report of using an aircraft to move an injured patient was in 1920 when a military officer with necrosis of the middle toe of the left foot was flown to a field hospital. The journey took just 2.5 hours rather than the 48 hours overland with camels (Scholl and Geshekter 1989). During the years between the world wars, services were set up in areas of difficult terrain or where huge areas had limited medical facilities, and the Flying Doctor Service of the Australian outback was an example (Rosell 1939). However, it was during the Spanish Civil War that the improvement in morale brought about by flying the sick and wounded to base hospitals, rather than negotiating rail and sea journeys, became evident. Such flights used unpressurized and unheated aircraft, but the betterment in medical care was unequivocal (Kowalzig 1940).

CABIN PRESSURIZATION

Modern jet aircraft operate at altitudes up to and beyond 40 000 feet for reasons of speed, fuel economy and weather. As an aircraft ascends to its cruising level, the barometric pressure falls as a function of the height above sea level. In an unpressurized aircraft, as the altitude increases, gas in closed or semi-closed spaces expands, so that at 10 000 feet the volume of a gas will have increased by 50 per cent. Passenger aircraft are able to operate at high altitude because of the development of the pressurized cabin, which enables the cabin altitude to be maintained below 8000 feet. In certain circumstances, it is possible to operate at an ambient cabin altitude nearer to sea level, but there are severe penalties should this be needed. These include reduced speed and range, the need to fly around adverse weather and increased fuel consumption.

Although in the pressurized cabin of an aircraft the cabin altitude is kept to a maximum of 8000 feet, volume changes can, nevertheless, cause problems to patients with a pneumothorax, bowel obstruction or recent gastrointestinal surgery. In a patient with a known pneumothorax, a chest tube with either a Heimlich one-way valve or an underwater seal drain will have to be inserted. In an unsuspected case, changes in ambient pressure can give rise to respiratory and circulatory embarrassment due to the development of a tension pneumothorax. This requires an urgent decompression using a large-bore needle. It is, therefore, essential in all cases where there is a possibility of a pneumothorax, or even the suspicion of a pneumothorax, to take a radiograph prior to departure. It is far easier to insert a chest tube pre-flight than in-flight.

Expansion of gases in the intestinal tract can give rise to problems. Although the increase in gas volume is small, there is at least the risk of rupturing the suture lines of recent surgery. It has always been recommended that a patient should not be moved by air for at least 2 weeks after an operation, but as long as the bowel is decompressed with a nasogastric tube, a recent operation is no longer an absolute contra-indication (Dolev 1987). As far as paralytic ileus is concerned, treatment with hyperbaric oxygen has shown that high levels of inspired oxygen can reduce abdominal distension. It is, therefore, possible to move patients who have had recent operations, even suffering from paralytic ileus, as long as they receive 100 per cent oxygen via a mask or endotracheal tube before and during the flight (Loder 1977).

Problems can occur due to the expansion of small volumes of intracranial air in patients with closed cranial fractures or following neurosurgery. The air from diagnostic procedures such as air encephalograms, though rarely carried out nowadays, could present a serious hazard, making it necessary to allow time for gas to be absorbed before the flight. When a cavity is closed or semi-closed, positive or negative pressure can be painful if equilibrium with the cabin pressure cannot be achieved. A common cause is when the passenger has a minor cold, leading to difficulties in equalizing the pressures in the paranasal sinuses or the middle ear with the cabin pressure. Nasal decongestants in a spray form and a slower rate of climb and descent help to relieve symptoms. Pain is most likely to occur during the descent phase of the flight. A further group of patients to be considered is the ever-growing numbers of sub-aqua swimmers. A scuba diver can be in danger even in pressurized aircraft within 24 hours of completion of a dive in respect of the nitrogen in the tissues. Decompression to sea level or the ambient land barometric pressure may not have been completed. It is, therefore, possible for an individual exposed to altitude (even 5000–6000 feet) in a commercial aircraft to be suffering from decompression sickness ('the bends'), which can lead to neurological deficits. The danger is proportional to the cabin altitude and flight time to which the individual is exposed.

Changes in ambient pressure may also have an effect on the medical equipment. Almost all patients will be receiving intravenous fluids, and falling pressure in the cabin will tend to speed up the flow of fluids out of rigid containers. For this reason, it is recommended that all intravenous fluids should be carried in plastic bags. This also lessens the possibility of any risk during a sudden decompression. Further, although the volume of air in the cuff of an endotracheal tube is small, the change in volume at altitude can lead to necrosis of the tracheal mucosa, and it is essential that water or saline is used to inflate the cuff.

HYPOXIA

Changes in pressure are important, but it is the effect of a low pressure environment on the delivery of oxygen to the tissues which is crucial. The concentration of oxygen in the aircraft cabin remains the same as at sea level, i.e. about 21 per cent, but the partial pressure of oxygen (Po_2) in the cabin air will decrease in proportion to the decrease in cabin pressure. The Po_2 of air entering the lungs is diminished further by saturation with water vapour. The signs of hypoxia become obvious, even in healthy persons, when they are exposed to above 10 000 feet without supplemental oxygen. As the pressure falls, the amount of oxygen transported by the haemoglobin falls, though because of the sigmoid shape of the haemoglobin dissociation curve, the reduction is not linear. At sea level the alveolar oxygen tension is around 100 mmHg (13.3 kPa), with the arterial saturation between 94 and 96 per cent. In this way, as the cabin oxygen pressure falls there is initially a limited decrease in the amount of oxygen transported in the blood. However, at 8000 feet the arterial oxygen tension is reduced to 55 mmHg (7.3 kPa) and oxygen saturation is (below 90 per cent) around 87 per cent. With the sigmoid shape of the curve, a further increase in altitude leads to a precipitous fall in oxygen saturation. In view of the possible hypoxic effects of a low cabin pressure, a haemoglobin estimation should always be made prior to an air evacuation. The lowest acceptable haemoglobin level is 7.5 g dl^{-1}, though if the patient requires respiratory support it is advisable to have a haemoglobin level of, at least, 10 g dl^{-1}.

It is often not possible to tap into the main aircraft oxygen supply and in many aircraft supplemental oxygen is only available from oxygen cylinders, liquid oxygen (LOX) or on-board oxygen-generating systems (OBOGS). The commonest source of supplemental oxygen is cylinders that can provide sufficient oxygen for a 10-hour flight with a flow of 2 l min^{-1}. In large aircraft, there are few problems in carrying an adequate number of cylinders, but in aircraft with a limited payload, consideration may have to be given to using an alternative supply. For most patients who need oxygen in-flight, it is possible to raise the haemoglobin saturation to 94–95 per cent by providing 2 l min^{-1}, and this, together with the duration of flight, determine the requirement for oxygen (Cramer *et al.* 1996). When cylinders are used to operate ventilators, an accurate calculation of the oxygen needed must also be made, before departure, as airlines do not look kindly upon a diversion to pick up extra cylinders.

The advantage of liquid oxygen (LOX) is its light weight. A 30-litre unit will provide 22 000 litres of gaseous oxygen, though it is essential to include a heat exchanger into the system to avoid freezing as the liquid changes to a gaseous state. Unfortunately, aviation authorities often regard LOX as hazardous cargo and airlines decline to carry such supplies. On-board oxygen-generating systems (OBOGS) are already in use in military aircraft. Air from the engines is heated and filtered and then driven through a molecular sieve with zeolite crystals. This removes all nitrogen, leaving 95 per cent oxygen and 5 per cent argon. To date there have been no recorded adverse effects caused by the presence of argon in the respirable gas. The standard system can deliver 4 l min^{-1} and there is little or no difference in the weight penalty compared with LOX.

IN-FLIGHT STRETCHERS

The first requirement in aeromedical evacuation is the security of the stretcher and the patient. There are many types of stretcher available for in-flight use, and the variety can give rise to problems in locating the stretchers on the supports of different types of transport. The patient must be strapped securely into a harness to ensure little movement at any time during the transit. In designated aeromedical evacuation aircraft, there are fixed supports to minimize the acceleration and deceleration forces generated during the flight, especially during take-off and landing. In commercial flights, this facility will not be available and specially designed stretchers are spread along six seats. In this situation it is important to establish whether the patient is obviously injured or suffering from an infectious disease as other passengers will not take too kindly to having such patients in close proximity.

The transfer to the aircraft cabin of a stretcher case can give rise to problems due to the height of the aircraft cabin doors from the ground, as well as difficulties in getting the stretcher through the cabin door. In some cases there will be a ramp to assist the transfer, but it may be necessary to make use of a freight platform or even a catering vehicle with a lift facility. Many aeromedical evacuations use smaller aircraft with lesser problems of loading. However, there may still be problems in getting the stretcher through a small door. In some aircraft, the entry door may have been specially adapted with extending rails so that the stretcher can slide into the cabin and onto the supports directly from the ambulance.

Traditionally, the stretchers are placed longitudinally with the patient travelling head first, though the ideal position is transverse across the cabin, with fore and aft movements lessened during the various phases of travel. The location of the stretcher should, wherever possible, give all-round access to the patient, but, in many cases, especially with smaller cabins, this is not possible. Indeed, limited space can lead to difficult working conditions, especially for tall attendants. A low cabin can also make it difficult to generate the pressure head to ensure flow in the intravenous lines.

The transfer of patients with spinal or long bone fractures raises problems of some import. The aircraft will usually be flying above the weather conditions, but clear air turbulence can occur without warning, and, if the aircraft is bounced about, a traction weight of 10 lb (4.5 kg) maintaining the position of a fractured femur may cause problems. It is, therefore, essential to maintain the traction using splints fitted with horizontal spring tensioners instead of pulley weights. The maintenance of steady traction is of even greater importance in the transfer of spinal fracture cases, especially those with cervical fractures. In the latter case, the Povey Turning Frame (Povey 1968) overcomes the problems that occur with the Stryker Frame (Stryker 1939). The Povey Frame weighs only 70 lb (31.8 kg), and the traction weights are applied horizontally eliminating the effects of sudden forces. The whole frame can be turned through 360 degrees whilst maintaining the head and neck traction during nursing procedures. This facility is especially important for the quadriplegic, who needs frequent turning to avoid pressure sores. One of the potentially fatal and immediate complications of a spinal injury is acute dilatation of the stomach, and it is, therefore, important to pass a nasogastric tube before take-off to ensure stomach aspiration throughout the flight.

In some cases, a vacuum stretcher can be used instead of a normal stretcher. The vacuum stretcher is a mattress containing polystyrene beads. The patient is placed on the mattress in its softened state, and the mattress is moulded around the casualty, giving some support and a degree of comfort. The air is extracted from the mattress and the beads expand so that the mattress makes a total body splint. However, as the cabin pressure falls, support decreases, and this requires further removal of air. During descent, the converse occurs so that it is necessary to monitor the tension of the mattress to maintain the comfort of the patient. Similar problems can occur when using air inflatable limb splints. Once again, careful monitoring is required to ensure that excess pressures are not generated.

HUMIDIFICATION

At ground level, the air in the respiratory tract is saturated by water vapour and this maintains ciliary function and prevents desiccation of the mucous membranes. At cruising levels of 28 000–42 000 feet the external temperature is between $-40°$ C and $-60°$ C. As a result, fresh air entering the cabin is dry and passengers may complain of dryness of the eyes and nasal mucous membranes, and of problems with contact lenses. A solution would be to increase water vapour levels in the cabin air using a humidifier, but this would incur an unacceptable weight penalty. Nevertheless, humidification is needed by patients when the air conditioning of the upper respiratory tract is bypassed by an endotracheal or tracheotomy tube. The simplest and most appropriate device is a humidifier – the 'Swedish Nose' (Mapleson et al. 1963).

The 'Swedish Nose' is a heat-exchange humidifier which clips onto the end of the endotracheal or tracheotomy tube. It is lightweight and passes fresh gases through a condenser foil on which the water vapour in the expired air condenses, thus humidifying the inspired gases. As an added bonus, there is a degree of heat conservation during the respiratory cycle. The system can maintain a relative humidity of around 50 per cent. A more sophisticated system passes the inspired gases over the surface of a heated water bath with the temperature of the water maintained at $60°$ C which also prevents bacterial growth. The vapour temperature falls to around $40°$ C by the time it reaches the respiratory tract, thus avoiding any possibility of scalding the mucous membranes.

AMBULANCES

The road ambulance, in many countries, is little more than a box on a chassis. The vibrations and poor ride may cause motion sickness not only in the patient but also in the medical team. The speed of the ambulance can subject the occupants to low-frequency vibrations in two ranges (4–10 Hz and 16–28 Hz). When travelling with a police escort at speeds of between 30 and 45 miles per hour (56–72 km h^{-1}), it is almost impossible to carry out nursing care, operate suction equipment or give drugs. However, ambulances with a 'floating stretcher' give an excellent ride as the vibrations are completely damped down, though the cost of this type of stretcher may be prohibitive (Snook and Pacifico 1976). Rotary-wing aircraft may be used in inter-hospital transfers, but there are difficulties involved in operating helicopters. Some major centres have fully equipped helipads, windsocks and high-intensity lighting for night flying, but the vast majority do not have these facilities and use car parks or public parks as landing sites. This requires the presence of police and fire vehicles. A significant problem in helicopter flying can be the weather. The pilot must be informed of the severity of the patient's condition, so that appropriate flight decisions are made for the safety of all concerned (Freilich and Spiegel 1990).

Many ambulance services have access to a police helicopter. Most of these aircraft are small, single-engine machines, offering little space for any sort of treatment to be carried out during the flight. Exceptions to this are twin-engine helicopters. However, the use of a helicopter for somewhat trivial cases has led to the debate whether the saving in time of moving patients by such an expensive means of transport is cost effective. There are two problems. Communication in flight between the members of the medical team and finding one's way around the cabin safely may be difficult. The helicopter cabin can be a large black hole, and a powerful torch is essential to enable checks to be made on the patient's condition. Monitoring, because of vibration, can also be a problem. As far as ventilators are concerned, a small gas-powered ventilator is most suitable. It can be fitted with a valve to deliver 40 per cent oxygen and this will extend the life of the small cylinder. It is advisable to carry a spare cylinder and change over just prior to landing.

THE TRANSFER

So far the problems that may occur during a flight and the measures to deal with the difficulties that may arise have been discussed, and in this way a successful air evacuation can give the impression that such transfers are straightforward and problem free. It is true that most flights fall into this category, but a great deal of thought and planning is required to ensure a seamless operation. In some cases it will be necessary to provide a specialist support team, and it is essential to have a system of priorities, i.e. those who require immediate transfer (urgent), those who require transfer within 24 hours (priority) and those who require transfer within 72 hours (routine). Experience has shown that there are few absolute contraindications to an aeromedical evacuation.

The request to transfer a patient from an overseas location may demand a complex organization, and the success of the transfer will depend upon communications between the overseas hospital and the home base. Time differences, poor local facilities, difficulties in contacting the local medical staff, and, most important, language difficulties, can lead to problems and delay. In the first place, the reason for the transfer must be clear. This may be a move to better facilities, a move to be close to friends and family or even going home to die. When organizing such a flight, it is essential to have the necessary documentation in place with the patient's details (sex, age and home address), appropriate information on the clinical diagnosis and the present condition (very seriously ill, seriously ill or stable), details of the illness or accident and relevant medical history, as well as length of time since admission to hospital. The proposed date of transfer will need discussion, and it is important to find out if relatives wish to accompany the patient.

Details of all investigations (chest radiography and other imaging, biochemistry and haemoglobin) must be made available. Intravenous fluids, catheters, analgesia, antibiotics, plaster casts and respiratory support must be considered together with any specialized equipment, including ventilators and spinal frames. It is also important to establish whether there has been any contact with an infectious disease. Consideration must also be given to the distance from the hospital to the airport with the handling facilities, road conditions, ambulance availability and the likely local weather conditions. This information will provide some indication of timings. Finally, it is always necessary to ensure that adequate funding is ensured.

When all this information has been gathered, it is possible to decide whether the patient is fit for transfer, and the composition of the medical team. In over 90 per cent of transfers there is no need for a doctor. It is also necessary to decide whether a member of the team should be sent out ahead to review the patient's condition, and to ensure that the patient's notes, including translations if necessary, are available along with passports and relevant inoculation certificates. Flight planning will determine the flying times and of these the most important is the turn around time at the airfield. Timing is of the essence when using a charter air ambulance, as flight crew duty times are limited. The nightmare scenario of the patient arriving at the airport with the medical team being advised that the aircrew have exceeded or will exceed their duty hours or that the aircraft is unserviceable must be avoided. It is important to assess the time required to travel from hospital to airport, and the departure from the hospital should commence with confirmation of the arrival time and serviceability of the aircraft.

The needs of the passenger at the arrival airport must be made known to all concerned including loaders, customs, immigration and the police, including whether an escort is required for the road transfer. Helicopter transfer may sometimes be desirable. Prevailing weather conditions can change dramatically at short notice. Potential diversion airports and hospitals must be identified, especially during the autumn and winter months. Should there be a sudden deterioration during the flight, or even death, an administrative as well as a medical problem of some magnitude is present. The make-up of the medical team for the carriage of the seriously ill can vary, but in many cases there has to be at least two nurses with in-flight nursing experience. If a doctor is required, they should be experienced in aviation medicine and not be 'borrowed for the occasion'. In certain cases including major trauma, severe burns and patients requiring in-flight ventilation, a doctor is mandatory. Aeromedical training courses for both doctors and nurses are useful and give a good theoretical background, though it may be difficult to obtain an in-flight nurse with the hands-on experience.

IN-FLIGHT SUPPORT

The flight medical bag should provide the medication needed to cover any general condition that may arise in transit. It is, of course, not possible to anticipate every possible in-flight complication, but a careful pre-flight assessment of the patient and some inspired guesswork can indicate what extra items might be required. It is vital to check, prior to departure, all items against the inventory. Some countries exercise tight control over the carriage of classified drugs, and so it is essential that the documentation is accurate. It is good practice to ensure that the medical adviser to the company operating the flight provides the necessary documentation including details of the flight and authorization to carry drugs. Long delays at customs can be avoided with a detailed declaration.

It has been said that there are only two items which are absolutely essential for resuscitation. These are an adequate supply of oxygen and a reliable suction unit. The same advice can be given for aeromedical flights. Indeed, a suction unit must be available at all times, especially during the descent and approach phase of the flight when unexpected turbulence may induce vomiting. All monitoring and infusion lines should be checked for patency and security, as it is easier to make changes before the transfer than to carry out the task in-flight. It is good practice to change endotracheal and tracheotomy tubes prior to departure from the hospital. Further, a wire cutter should be available for cases with facial or jaw fractures in case the patient should vomit. All limb plasters should be cut before a flight and this is especially important if the fracture is compound, as there may be air in the wound or trapped under the plaster.

It is advisable to delay the carriage of patients with serious burns if the hospital facilities are adequate. A transfer can be more easily arranged when adequate renal and respiratory functions are assured. However, a severely burned patient in an inadequate setting may need an urgent transfer, and this should be arranged with the inclusion, if at all possible, of a specialist in the team. The transfer should not be attempted until the patient's condition is stable. Primary resuscitation can take up to 48 hours. Replacement of blood and fluid loss, adequate urinary output and adequate analgesia are essential, and ventilatory support is likely to be required. At this time a window of opportunity is available to effect the transfer of the patient to a specialized burns unit.

Aeromedical experience in the carriage of certain disorders is useful. Patients with diabetes, if at all possible, should be stabilized before transfer and the insulin regimen planned before departure and given at the same times – all time zone changes ignored. Blood glucose levels should be determined before take-off with an intravenous line *in situ* if there is any risk of hypoglycaemia. A patient with a history of arrhythmia or chest pain can be transferred after 5–7 days as long as a doctor is in the medical team, though if an air ambulance is being used the transfer should be delayed for 10 days. Careful planning is required for the transfer of psychiatric patients. Co-morbidity must be excluded and drug treatment checked. A psychiatric trained nurse may be essential for the flight and the patient must be seated away from all doors, hatches and safety equipment. Penetrating eye injuries and eye surgery with the presence of gas in the posterior chamber is an absolute contraindication to air evacuation at the normal cabin altitude, though it may be possible if the cabin altitude can be maintained at sea level.

As far as subarachnoid haemorrhage is concerned, assuming the necessary investigations have been carried out, it is appropriate to postpone any transfer for 2 weeks. If appropriate investigations are not possible, a difficult decision has to be made. There is always the risk of a further bleed in flight, but transfer is possible with sedation. The patient should be moved carefully under heavy sedation with oxygen supplementation. The risk must be explained to the relatives. As far as cerebral haemorrhage and infarction are concerned, the level of consciousness must be determined, and signs of any improvement noted since the event. Again, a difficult decision has to be made. The balance of risk versus the benefit of a transfer will depend, in part, on the local facilities.

CONCLUSION

Carriage of seriously ill patients requires careful pre-flight appraisal, and the risk of the transfer must be weighed against the benefits. Once a transfer is decided, detailed assessment and planning are essential, taking into account the needs of the individual patient and the features of the cabin environment. Proper preparation will ensure that most patients can be carried safely (Parson and Bobechko 1982).

REFERENCES

Cramer D, Ward S and Geddes D. Assessment of oxygen supplementation during air travel. *Thorax* 1996; **51**: 202–3.

Dolev E. Early evacuation of patients from the battlefield after laparotomy. *Milit Med* 1987; **152**: 57–9.

Freilich DA and Spiegel AD. Aeromedical emergency trauma services and mortality reduction in rural areas. *NY State J Med* 1990; **90**: 358–65.

Kowalzig H. Long distance transportation of the wounded at high altitudes. *Dtsch Militarzt* 1940; **5**: 10–14.

Lam DM. To pop a balloon. Aeromedical evacuation in the 1870 siege of Paris. *Aviat Space Environ Med* 1988; **59**: 989–91.

Loder RE. Use of hyperbaric oxygen in paralytic ileus. *Br Med J* 1977; **1**: 1448–9.

Mapleson WW, Morgan JC and Hilliard EK. Assessment of the condenser humidifier, with special reference to a multiple-gauze model. *Br Med J* 1963; **1**: 300–5.

Parson CJ and Bobechko WP. Aeromedical transport: its hidden problems. *Can Med Assoc J* 1982; **126**: 237–43.

Povey RW. New turning frame. *Br Med J* 1968; **2**: 114.

Rossell J McF. 'Flying doctors' in Australia. *Can Med Assoc J* 1939; **40**: 280–1.

Scholl MD and Geshekter CL. The Zed Expedition: the world's first air ambulance? *J R Soc Med* 1989; **82**: 679–80.

Snook R and Pacifico R. Ambulance ride: fixed or floating stretcher? *Br Med J* 1976; **2**: 405–7.

Stryker H. A device for turning the frame patient. *J Am Med Assoc* 1939; **113**: 1731–2.

Vincent A. Le transport des blessés par avion. *Rev Int Croix Rouge* 1924; **6**: 720–3.

Index

NOTE: page numbers in *italics* refer to tables, page numbers in **bold** refer to figures.